THE VISUAL ENCYCLOPEDIA OF
NATURAL HEALING

THE VISUAL ENCYCLOPEDIA OF
NATURAL HEALING

A STEP-BY-STEP PICTORIAL GUIDE TO SOLVING
100 EVERYDAY HEALTH PROBLEMS

BY THE EDITORS OF
PREVENTION MAGAZINE HEALTH BOOKS
EDITED BY ALICE FEINSTEIN

RODALE PRESS, EMMAUS, PENNSYLVANIA

Cover design by Lynn N. Gano

Library of Congress Cataloging–in–Publication Data

The Visual encyclopedia of natural healing: a step-by-step pictorial guide to solving 100 everyday health problems/ by the editors of *Prevention* Magazine Health Books; edited by Alice Feinstein.
     p.   cm.
  Includes index.
  ISBN 0–87857–928–1 hardcover
  ISBN 0–87596–273–4 paperback
  1. Medicine, Popular—Encyclopedias.
I. Feinstein, Alice.   II. Prevention Magazine Health Books.
RC81.A2V57   1990
610—dc20   90–45937

Distributed in the book trade by St. Martin's Press

        8 10 9   hardcover
2 4 6 8 10 9 7 5 3 1 paperback

———— OUR MISSION ————
We publish books that empower people's lives.
RODALE ✿ BOOKS

NOTICE

This book is intended as a reference volume only, not as a medical guide or manual for self-treatment. If you suspect that you have a medical problem, please seek competent medical care. The information here is designed to help you make informed decisions about your health. It is not intended as a substitute for any treatment prescribed by your doctor.

Contributors to *The Visual Encyclopedia of Natural Healing*

Publisher: Pat Corpora
Editor in Chief: William Gottlieb
Group Vice President, Health: Mark Bricklin
Executive Editor: Carol Keough
Senior Managing Editor: Debora Tkac
Senior Editor: Alice Feinstein
Production Editor: Jane Sherman
Copy Editor: Nancy King-Bennink

Contributing Writers
Claudia Allen
Kim Anderson
Don Barone
Sharon Faelten
Deborah Grandinetti
Brian Kauffman
William LeGro
Judith Lin
Bejou Merry
Russell Wild

Research
Ann Gossy
Anne R. Castaldo
Anna Crawford
Christine Dreisbach
Staci Hadeed
Karen Lombardi
Paris Mihely-Muchanic
Linda Miller
Cynthia W. Nickerson
Sandra Salera-Lloyd

Book Design
Book design by Lynn N. Gano
Layout design by Julie Burris, Lynn N. Gano,
and Lisa Gatti

Contributing Illustrators
Janet Bohn
Mellisa Edmonds
Kathi Ember
Leslie Flis
Margaret Hewitt
Chris Hill
Bradley Keough
John Lane
Mary Laskowski
Scott MacNeill
Susan Rosenberger

Office Staff
Roberta Mulliner
Eve Buchay
Karen Earl-Braymer

CONTENTS

CONTENTS

INTRODUCTION

Ever teach someone how to tie his shoe? Chances are you squatted on the ground, undid your own laces, and broke the whole process down into a series of easy steps. There's a reason why you did that.

Some things are a snap to learn if you can only *see* how to do them. Reading or hearing about how to do a special exercise to ease the pain of arthritis, for example, is not quite the same as seeing someone do it. You want to enjoy the benefits, but you're left with a million questions instead: How high do I raise my arm? What do I do with my legs? How do I hold my head? Am I supposed to lean forward?

Just watch someone actually do the curative movement, and your questions are answered instantly.

We humans are like that. We're very visual. Pictures carry a payload of information that you absorb instantly, effortlessly. When you see something, the information stays with you. You tend to remember what you saw.

So when the editors of Prevention Magazine Health Books got together to plan *The Visual Encyclopedia of Natural Healing*, we had one question in mind: What can best be learned from *pictures?* We sifted through the latest findings of medical science, looking for just the right healing movements, practical curative techniques, and natural practices that prevent and treat health problems.

We found a lot: soothing movements to ease tension, techniques for lifting that protect your back, sleep positions that erase pain, simple exercises that prevent a whole host of painful conditions, body signals that clue you in to disease, massage and acupressure points that bring quick relief, and much, much more.

Of course, no book about natural healing would be complete without sections on food and herbs. That's where the Nutritional Gallery of Healing Foods comes in. These foods have important health-giving properties and belong in your kitchen arsenal for fighting and preventing disease. You probably already have many of the herbs on your spice shelf. The herbs chapter will show you how to use them safely to relieve dozens of conditions.

This book could easily be called a "show-and-tell to natural healing." Picture this: You look at the illustrations. You follow the simple step-by-step directions. And you reap the benefits without having to put in hours of reading.

We hope by using *The Visual Encyclopedia of Natural Healing* you'll "see" your way to better health.

Alice Feinstein
Senior Editor,
Prevention Magazine Health Books

ALLERGIES

Suppose you point out to your neighbor Bruno that his orange pants clash with his bright red shirt. And Bruno reacts by bashing you over the head with a baseball bat. You might say Bruno's response was inappropriate, perhaps exaggerated. You might say it was like an allergy.

An allergy?

You bet. Allergies are "inappropriate or exaggerated reactions of the immune system," according to the American Medical Association.

When you have an allergic reaction, your immune system is acting just like Bruno. It encounters a few harmless specks of pollen or dust and . . . pow! It releases chemicals that give you teary eyes, a runny nose, sneezes, hives, or other symptoms.

The culprits (known as allergens) that switch allergic people's immune systems into overdrive include such things as flowers, grasses, tree pollens, animal dander (little particles of skin and hair), house dust, house-dust mites, various drugs, bee venom, and certain foods, such as milk, eggs, shellfish, dried fruits, nuts, and food colorings. Foods that tend to give adults problems are different from those that trouble children (as you will see illustrated on page 6).

The Mystery of Allergies

Doctors can't say why one person has allergies and another does not, but they do know that the tendency to develop an allergy is inherited. That's not to say that if your father sneezes every time he gets anywhere in the neighborhood of an Old English sheepdog that you will react the same way. What is fairly certain is that if you have allergies, your father or mother probably does, too, although the allergies are not necessarily the same.

Doctors also know that allergies can develop at any age, but new ones very rarely crop up after the age of 40. Food allergies are most likely to appear in children, but outdoor allergies are not usual in children under the age of 3. As the child grows older, however, food allergies tend to disappear, only to be replaced by pollen and other inhalant allergies.

But whether the problem is meals or molds, allergies cause children to miss more days of school than any other illness. Among both children and adults, it is a large problem to a large number of people: Those who suffer include some 40 million in the United States alone.

Walking Away from Your Troubles

What's the best thing to do for your allergies? Simple. Avoid things you're allergic to. This may not sound like very sophisticated medical advice, but you won't find a better tip anywhere. "Avoidance and precaution are the hallmark of allergy management," says Allan Weinstein, M.D., an allergy specialist in private practice in Washington, D.C., a consultant to the allergy section of the National Institutes of

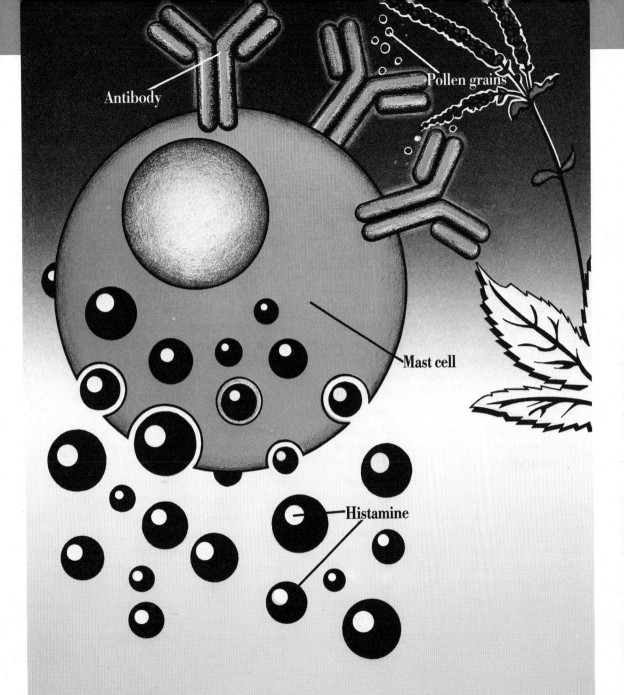

How does a pollen grain produce a sneeze? A mast cell, part of the immune system, encounters the grain of pollen. Between them stands an antibody known as immunoglobulin E. When antibody and pollen clash . . . ker-POW! An explosion is triggered in the mast cell and its arsenal of powerful chemicals, including histamine, rushes out to fight the intruder. Histamine is what causes allergic people more sneezing than a cannon full of pepper.

ALLERGIES

Health, and author of *Asthma: The Complete Guide to Self-Management of Asthma and Allergies for Patients and Their Families.*

Sometimes avoiding allergens is easy. Say you have an allergy to lobster; every time you eat lobster, you break out in hives. The answer to your problem is simple: Stop eating lobster. In the case of allergic reactions to things in the air, avoidance may not be so simple. Just try running from ragweed pollen in Kansas on a windy August afternoon.

Short of escaping to the beach, you might try these other doctor-recommended ways to avoid pollens: Stay indoors on days the pollen count is high; roll up your car windows; shower and shampoo frequently to wash clinging pollen from your body and hair; avoid walks in weedy or damp areas; and take precautions to keep your home as free of allergens as possible.

Naturally, if your chief defense against allergens is to avoid them, it would be extremely helpful to know exactly what you are allergic to. Although you may already have a pretty good idea, an allergy specialist can do a lot to help you zero in on the specific allergies that affect you, says Dr. Weinstein. An allergist will help you to track your good days and bad days, and he will correlate this information with the results of a detailed skin test.

Going beyond Avoidance

Unfortunately, allergens can't always be avoided. So what's your next line of defense?

To some degree, relief for your allergies can be found at the pharmacy. Millions of sufferers turn to a wide array of antihistamines with varying degrees of success. You may have to sample several of the more than 20 different antihistamines on the market to find the one that works best for you. One that works well for your friend may not work well for you.

Be aware that antihistamines often have side effects, such as dry mouth, drowsiness, and blurred vision. If you do feel sluggish, be patient. Experts have found that the longer you take a specific antihistamine, the less it'll make you drowsy. Just don't drive a car or do potentially dangerous work until your alertness is assured.

Antihistamine/decongestant combinations, also available at your pharmacy, have less of a knockout effect. That's because most people find the decongestant to be slightly stimulating, so it cancels any drowsiness from the antihistamine. (Always use antihistamines and decongestants as ingredients in *one* medication—taking two products together could be dangerous.)

It's also important to know that antihistamines ideally should be taken before symptoms develop. Many allergy sufferers don't use these medications correctly. If you're going to be in a situation where you're likely to get a noseful of something you're allergic to, take an antihistamine 30 minutes to an hour ahead of time.

Decongestant nose sprays can also help with allergy stuffiness. Be careful, however, not to overuse these sprays. Use too much for too long and you can have a "rebound effect," irritating your nasal passages and making matters worse. Follow product directions carefully.

Seeking Professional Help

While allergies are not usually life-threatening, they can make your life miserable. So if the nonprescription stuff isn't working too well for you, you may want to consider asking for professional help. An allergist not only can tell you specifically what you are allergic to but also can prescribe medications that may do a better job of preventing or calming your attacks than over-the-counter antihistamines. (There are also prescription antihistamines that don't cause drowsiness.) Or he may advise you to get regular shots.

Allergy shots, says Dr. Weinstein, are usually reserved for individuals who are unable to avoid the offending allergen, who have allergy seasons that are longer than a few weeks, and who have symptoms that cannot be managed with oral medications alone.

Allergy shots are more effective for some allergies than others. Success with allergy shots for hay fever caused by seasonal pollens is as high as 85 percent, says Dr. Weinstein. But the rate of success with dust is only about 70 percent, probably because dust is made up of many components. The success rate for molds is even less satisfactory.

Shots work by actually putting into your bloodstream small amounts of what you are allergic to and gradually increasing this dose. This process reduces your body's sensitivity to the allergen so that when you encounter it in the environment, your body simply says "Oh, it's only you."

The problem with shot therapy is that it takes a long time—usually up to two years—before you feel the effects. And going for biweekly or monthly shots is not most people's idea of a good time. There may also be side effects, such as rashes, itching, and swelling.

Staying out of Touch

Just as with allergies to things in the air, the best defense against contact allergies is avoidance. Substances that frequently trigger allergic reactions when touched include plants such as poison ivy, oak, and sumac (in all three cases, the offending agent is the same—an oily resin called urushiol) and certain chemicals and metals, such as nickel. But some unlucky souls are allergic to all sorts of physical stimuli, even heat, cold, light, and sun rays!

Since poison ivy and its ilk affect so many people—about half the population—we've devoted an entire chapter to the subject (see page 352). As for avoiding the other contact allergens, here are a few suggestions.

If cosmetics designed to improve the look of your skin instead leave it broken out in rashes, switch to cosmetics labeled "hypo-allergenic." If you have questions about which cosmetics are giving you trouble, your allergist can help you figure it out by giving you a patch test, in which a number of substances are applied to your skin and the reactions are carefully monitored.

If you know that nickel is your problem, be aware that almost anything made of metal may contain some nickel. Jewelry, buttons, clasps, and other objects that stay in contact with skin for extended periods of time are the causes of most reactions.

5

ALLERGIES

The best defense against nickel allergy is a simple kit that can easily and safely test any object for the presence of the offending metal—with no damage to the material tested. Ask your doctor where to get such a kit.

Remember that sensitivity to nickel is most acute on hot, sticky days. That's because perspiration allows more of the metal to come into contact with your skin. So if you are only mildly allergic to nickel, you may need to avoid it only during summer heat waves.

The Anti-Allergy Diet

Food allergies are often a tricky business. Sometimes, just as soon as you pop a certain food into your mouth, you get a reaction. It may be stomach pain, diarrhea, vomiting, cramps, hives, swelling around the eyes or lips, or even sneezing and a stuffy nose.

Also, certain foods may provoke a reaction only at certain times. Where troublesome ragweed may always be troublesome, shrimp may bother you only when it is prepared a certain way.

Watch What You Eat

Children's tastes tend to differ from adults', and so do their allergies. Take note—if your five-year-old claims she's allergic to broccoli, she's probably making it up.

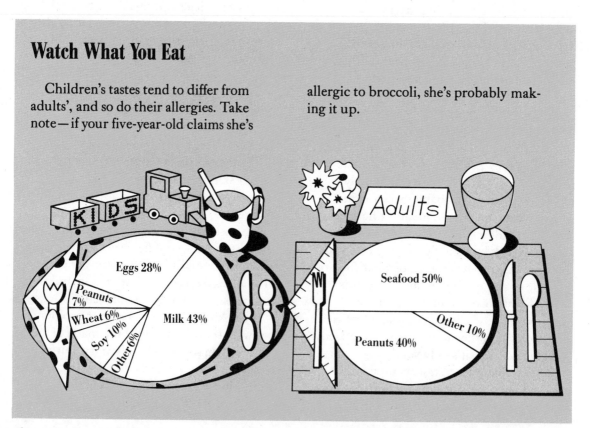

KIDS

Eggs 28%
Peanuts 7%
Wheat 6%
Soy 10%
Other 6%
Milk 43%

Adults

Seafood 50%
Other 10%
Peanuts 40%

Experts say that you can find out just which food is bugging you by experimenting with an "elimination" diet. The elimination diet consists of removing a suspected food from your diet for at least a week, and then adding it back to your diet to see if there is a reaction. If symptoms disappear when you eliminate the food item and return when you start eating it again, you've pinpointed a cause of one of your allergies.

But where do you start to look for foods you may be allergic to? A good place would be the chart on the opposite page, which shows the likeliest culprits.

Russell Wild

Don't Be Rash about What You Touch

Contact allergies are quite common. Listed here are those things that studies show cause problems for the greatest number of people.

Poison ivy, oak, and sumac. In all three cases the offending agent is an oily resin called urushiol.

Paraphenylenediamine. Don't let the name fool you. This chemical is not only found in obscure chemical mixtures, it is also used in hair and fur dye, leather, rubber, and printing.

Nickel compounds. Nickel is found in jewelry, buttons, clasps, and other objects.

Rubber compounds. Chemical additives are the major source of contact allergies to such rubber products as gloves, shoes, aprons—even rubber bands and balloons.

Ethylenediamine. This is a preservative used in cosmetic creams and eye-care products.

What to Avoid to Beat the Sniffles

Inhalant allergies are caused by microscopic particles that find their way up your nostrils to create all kinds of misery on hot summer days. But not everyone reacts to these microscopic terrors. A large government study was conducted to find out what percentage of the population has inhalant allergies. Here's the percentage who reacted to various allergens.

Allergen	People Who Tested Positive (%)
Ryegrass	10.2
Ragweed	10.1
House dust	6.2
Oak	4.7
Bermuda grass	4.4
Alternaria (a mold)	3.6
Cat	2.3
Dog	2.3

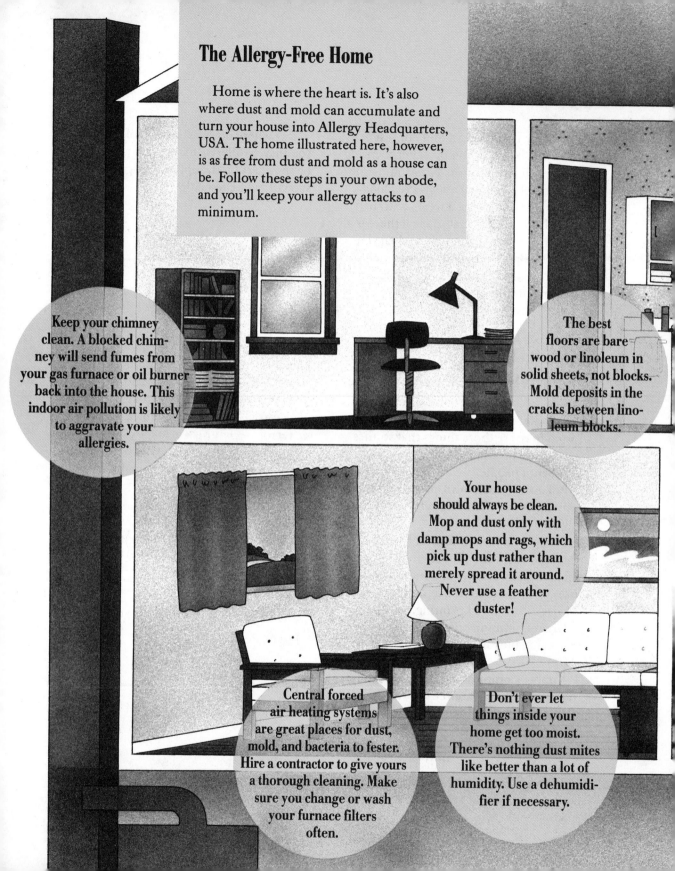

The Allergy-Free Home

Home is where the heart is. It's also where dust and mold can accumulate and turn your house into Allergy Headquarters, USA. The home illustrated here, however, is as free from dust and mold as a house can be. Follow these steps in your own abode, and you'll keep your allergy attacks to a minimum.

Keep your chimney clean. A blocked chimney will send fumes from your gas furnace or oil burner back into the house. This indoor air pollution is likely to aggravate your allergies.

The best floors are bare wood or linoleum in solid sheets, not blocks. Mold deposits in the cracks between linoleum blocks.

Your house should always be clean. Mop and dust only with damp mops and rags, which pick up dust rather than merely spread it around. Never use a feather duster!

Central forced air heating systems are great places for dust, mold, and bacteria to fester. Hire a contractor to give yours a thorough cleaning. Make sure you change or wash your furnace filters often.

Don't ever let things inside your home get too moist. There's nothing dust mites like better than a lot of humidity. Use a dehumidifier if necessary.

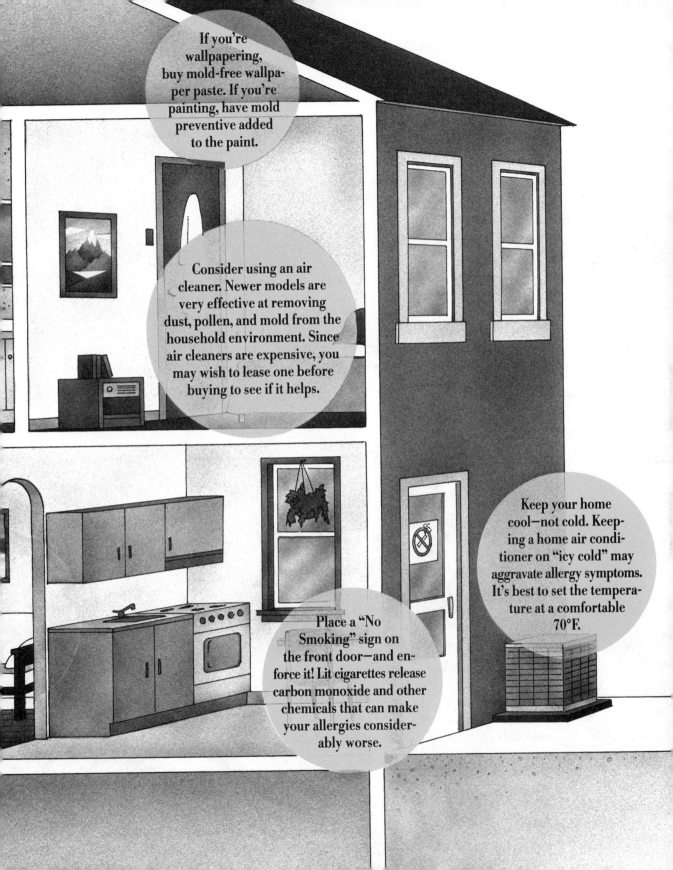

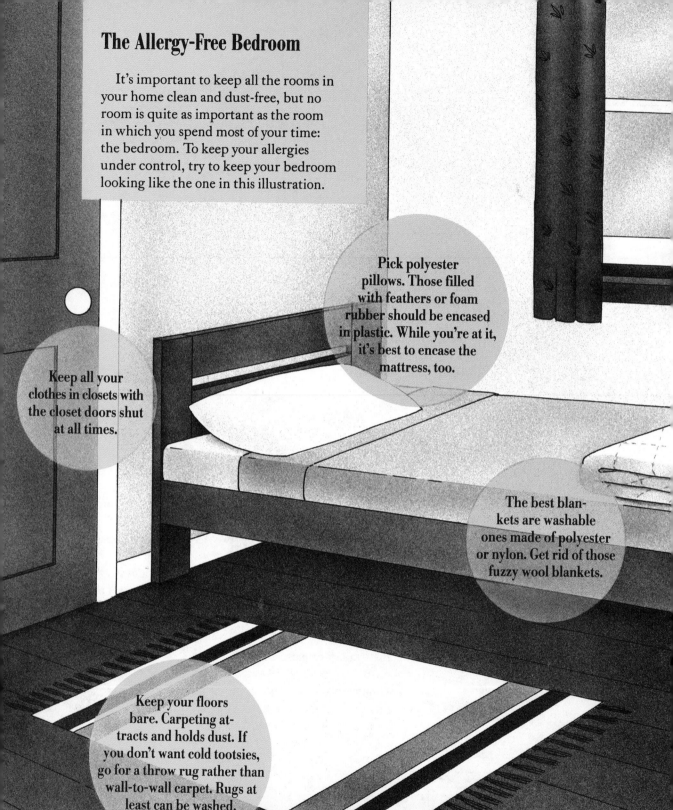

The Allergy-Free Bedroom

It's important to keep all the rooms in your home clean and dust-free, but no room is quite as important as the room in which you spend most of your time: the bedroom. To keep your allergies under control, try to keep your bedroom looking like the one in this illustration.

Pick polyester pillows. Those filled with feathers or foam rubber should be encased in plastic. While you're at it, it's best to encase the mattress, too.

Keep all your clothes in closets with the closet doors shut at all times.

The best blankets are washable ones made of polyester or nylon. Get rid of those fuzzy wool blankets.

Keep your floors bare. Carpeting attracts and holds dust. If you don't want cold tootsies, go for a throw rug rather than wall-to-wall carpet. Rugs at least can be washed.

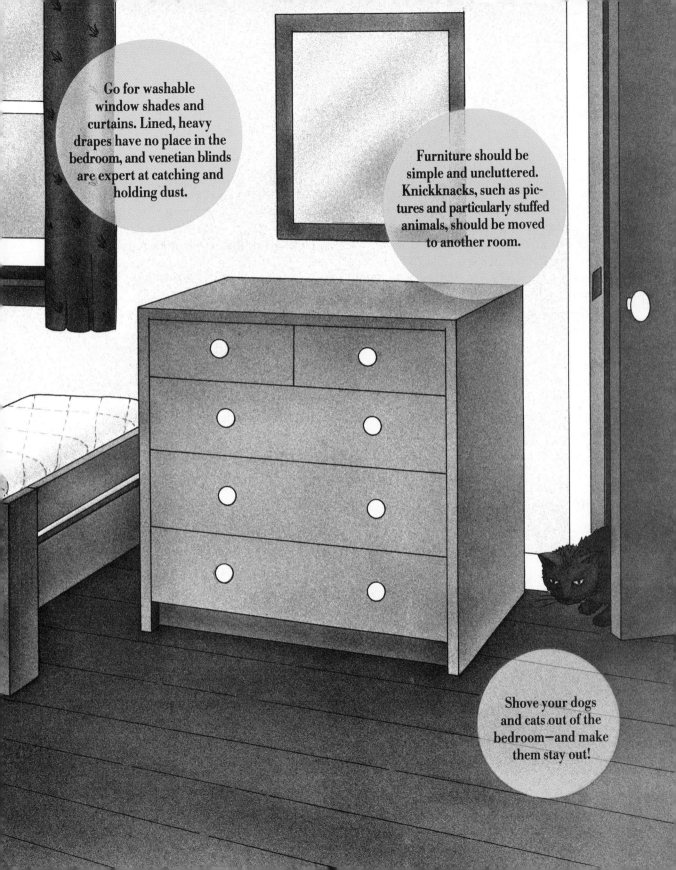

ANGINA

It's hard to say anything nice about coronary heart disease. But it's not impossible. For as mean and ugly and nasty as America's number one killer may be, at least it often gives its victims a warning. No, you don't get an engraved notice in the mail. What you *are* likely to get is a recurrent pressing, squeezing, or burning pain in the chest. Doctors call this warning pain angina pectoris—angina for short.

This pain (which sometimes spreads to the shoulders, arms, neck, jaw, or back) is due to a lack of oxygen in the heart muscle. It is typically triggered by exercise, emotional upset, packing away a large meal, or any circumstance that creates extra demand on the heart. The heart muscle isn't getting enough oxygen because it isn't getting enough blood. It's not getting enough blood because the arteries have been narrowed by fatty deposits clinging to their walls. Doctors call this condition atherosclerosis.

Not all chest pain is brought on by inadequate blood supply to the heart, nor is all inadequate blood supply to the heart due to atherosclerosis. Only if you undergo a few (painless) medical tests can a doctor determine the nature of your problem. If it is true angina you are suffering and the cause is

(continued on page 14)

How to "Block" Nighttime Angina

Tilt the head of your bed 3 or 4 inches, and you may be able to say good-bye to nighttime angina attacks. The reason: Lying flat causes an

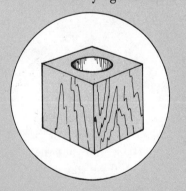

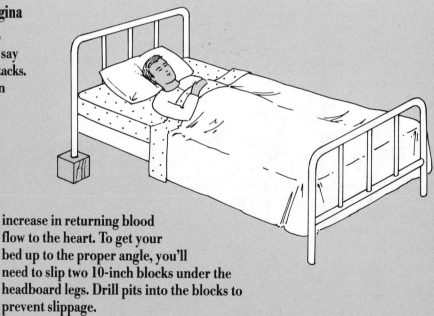

increase in returning blood flow to the heart. To get your bed up to the proper angle, you'll need to slip two 10-inch blocks under the headboard legs. Drill pits into the blocks to prevent slippage.

A Peek inside an Artery

Angina pectoris has been compared to the heart screaming for more oxygen. Because of hardened arteries, the heart doesn't get enough oxygen-carrying blood. And what are hardened arteries? They are arteries that have filled up, or partially filled up, with fatty plaque. The medical term for hardening of the arteries is atherosclerosis. The disease begins with a striped patch on the inside wall of the artery, on which bits of cholesterol and other substances in the blood collect. These substances then harden and thicken, progressively narrowing the space in which the blood can flow. The coronary arteries, those arteries connected to the heart, can be narrowed by as much as 70 to 90 percent and the heart will still have enough blood to meet its needs, at least when it's resting. But when exercise, emotional demands, or a heavy meal make the heart beat faster—requiring more oxygen—the reduced blood flow may no longer be adequate. Doctors call this condition myocardial ischemia, and the symptoms may be shortness of breath or chest pain. That's when we say the heart starts to "scream." That's angina. If the artery becomes completely blocked, an even worse scenario may occur—a heart attack. For this reason, all angina sufferers should be under a doctor's care.

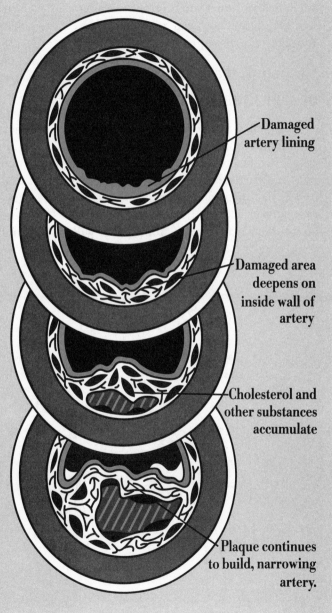

Damaged artery lining

Damaged area deepens on inside wall of artery

Cholesterol and other substances accumulate

Plaque continues to build, narrowing artery.

atherosclerosis, you've just received a serious warning. You should even be grateful for the message, because if you heed the warning and take action now, you might avoid the more serious consequences of heart disease.

Getting to the Heart of Your Problem

Angina is not to be taken lightly. If you have angina, you should be under a doctor's care. He may prescribe medications for you, such as nitroglycerin, which can be slipped under the tongue during or in anticipation of an attack. The medicine will increase the flow of blood to the heart. Your doctor will

undoubtedly suggest many changes in aspects of your lifestyle that might have put your heart in danger in the first place. (See the chapter on heart disease on page 230.)

While you are eating low-fat and low-cholesterol meals, exercising regularly using a program your doctor has prescribed for you, and doing all the things you should be doing to get your heart and blood vessels back in top working order, you can also be taking immediate action to lessen your chances of angina attacks.

Above all, avoid the temptation to cheat on your low-fat diet. Feasting on such things as pork chops, french fries, and ice cream can bring on the pain of angina. This simple

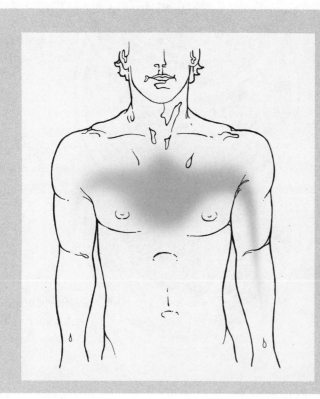

Is it an Angina Attack?

The pain of angina usually follows a particular path. Most often, the attack will first be felt as a dull, heavy, constricting pain in the center of the chest. The pain may radiate into the throat, upper jaw, back, and arms (mostly the left arm). Additional symptoms often include difficult breathing, intense sweating, and nausea.

Arteries in (Double) Trouble

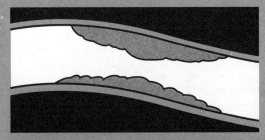

Plaque along the walls of an artery allows less space for blood to flow.

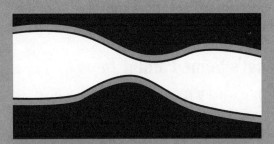

Arteries are subject to spasms, which, like plaque, allow less space for blood flow.

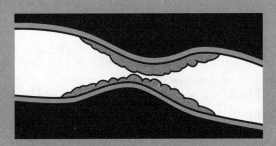

Angina attacks often result from a double whammy of both plaque *and* spasm—narrowing the artery to a greater degree than either would alone.

connection between fat and angina pain was made back in the 1950s in an informal study at the University of Pennsylvania. A doctor there fed glasses of pure cream to 14 angina sufferers and immediately induced chest pains in 6 of them. And subsequent studies have driven home the point again and again: Fat attacks the heart.

How Much Exercise?

Exercise presents a dilemma to angina sufferers. A *lack* of exercise often plays a role in the development of atherosclerosis. But huffing and puffing brings on chest pain. What should you do? Some studies show that exercising just to the point of pain carries no risk. In fact, studies show that regular exercise should improve your tolerance—you will be able to exercise longer before the pain starts. Other studies show that it is uncommon for a heart attack to occur during exertion. So go ahead—if you have your doctor's permission—and exercise. Just make sure you start slowly and don't overdo.

There are a number of other things you can do to turn off those angina attacks. If you smoke, there's no question that you need to kick the habit—fast. Both nicotine and carbon monoxide contribute to the worsening of coronary heart disease—and make angina symptoms more severe.

The good news for angina sufferers is that the clogged arteries that cause such pain can be cleared. With a long-term commitment to following the program of drugs, low-fat diet, and exercise that your doctor outlines for you, you could add many pain-free years to your life.

Russell Wild

15

ARTHRITIS

If this page were handwritten by someone with arthritis, it might look like this.

A nd if you had arthritis, handwriting wouldn't be the only thing you'd find difficult. You might also have a hard time turning doorknobs, climbing stairs, winding your watch, brushing your hair, tying your shoelaces, driving a car, removing a pan from the oven, holding a telephone, or just getting out of bed in the morning.

"Virtually everything you do in life can require special effort when you have arthritis," says Floyd Pennington, Ph.D., group vice president of education at the Arthritis Foundation national headquarters in Atlanta.

Of course, if you have arthritis, you already know how it changes your life. And chances are, if you don't have arthritis yourself, someone close to you does. There are approximately 37 million people with arthritis in the United States alone. That means that one in seven Americans has arthritis, and one in every three families is affected.

Not only that, but six million Americans who have arthritis are not seeing a doctor for the condition, according to a nationwide survey conducted by the Centers for Disease Control in Atlanta. Many people see television ads for painkillers and attempt to treat the condition themselves.

The problem is this: Arthritis can worsen if the only treatment a person is receiving is pain relief.

That's why, if you have arthritis, it's important to know what kind of arthritis it is and to be under a doctor's care.

That's Some Painful Joint

Just what is this thing we call arthritis? Simply stated, arthritis is an "inflammation of the joint." This inflammation can be caused by more than 100 different diseases that attack the joints, the tissue surrounding the joints and the spine, as well as other parts of the body.

What this means is that arthritis is not a single, easy-to-understand disease.

To get a better picture of what arthritis is, it helps to understand the structure of a joint. Simply put, a joint is any place in the body where two bones meet.

The bones are connected to each other by bands of tissue called ligaments. These ligaments hold what's known as the joint capsule in place. The capsule is made of tough, fibrous tissue filled with a lubricating fluid. The ends of the bones, which meet inside the capsule, are lined with a silky covering of cartilage.

When functioning normally, the cartilage and fluid act like a shock absorber, preventing the bones from rubbing against each other. When the joint is inflamed, the result is stiffness and pain.

The Many Forms of Arthritis

The most common form of arthritis is osteoarthritis, also known as degenerative joint disease.

Osteoarthritis is principally a disease of the cartilage. It most often strikes the weight-bearing joints, such as the hips, knees, and spine. This form of arthritis frequently occurs in joints that have suffered previous injury or infection.

Doctors say that everyone who lives long enough will probably get some degree of osteoarthritis.

Rheumatoid arthritis, the next most common form of the disease, can strike anyone, at any age.

Together, rheumatoid arthritis and osteoarthritis account for roughly two-thirds of all cases of arthritis. Scientists aren't certain what causes rheumatoid arthritis, but they have good reason to suspect a virus. Rheumatoid arthritis affects primarily the synovial membrane, the thin layer of tissue that lines the joint capsule.

Rheumatoid arthritis may be serious, mild, or anywhere in between. It generally strikes in the toes, hands, elbows, jaw, hips, neck, and shoulders. Unlike osteoarthritis, which may affect only one or two joints, rheumatoid arthritis often strikes many joints at the same time. Joint pain tends to flare up and subside, only to return again and again.

In addition to these two most common forms of arthritis, there are literally dozens more that can bring on similar pain and inflammation.

Systemic lupus erythematosus, for example, affects about 100,000 Americans. It is what doctors call an autoimmune disease, in that the body's own defense system goes haywire, attacking the lining of joints and other tissues by mistake.

Gout affects 1 in 100 Americans. Juvenile arthritis afflicts 50,000 children throughout the country. Additional thousands of Americans suffer from infectious arthritis, caused by bacteria invading the joints; bursitis and tendinitis, sometimes known as tennis elbow or housemaid's knee; and many less common forms of arthritis, such as scleroderma and ankylosing spondylitis.

When to See Your Doctor

The forms of arthritis are many, but they all share one important feature: Each warrants a visit to the doctor. Knowing which kind of arthritis you have is an important first step in dealing with the illness.

Only your doctor, using a number of tests, can determine exactly what your problem is.

But when do you first know you have arthritis? Look for the most common warning signs:

• Swelling in one or more joints

17

ARTHRITIS

- Early morning stiffness
- Recurring pain or tenderness in any joint
- Inability to move a joint normally
- Obvious redness and warmth in a joint
- Unexplained weight loss, fever, or weakness combined with joint pain

If you have two or more of these symptoms and they persist for more than two weeks, experts at the Arthritis Foundation say it is time to schedule a visit with your doctor for a full diagnosis and proper treatment.

Be forewarned that discovering what kind of arthritis you have may not be an easy task. Some forms of arthritis can be diagnosed only after several visits to the doctor over a period of weeks or even months, during which the pattern of the disease reveals itself. Be a patient patient.

How to Live with Arthritis

Arthritis isn't exactly a modern malady. If fossils are any clue, there were probably a few triceratops who could have used some really big heating pads. And the history of human bones is no less achy.

Hippocrates wrote about arthritis. Socrates said that arthritis was the most common disease in ancient Greece. And in the days of Roman glory, baths were built throughout the empire to treat citizens with painful joints. Emperor Diocletian even exempted those citizens most severely afflicted from having to pay taxes.

As for arthritis treatment, we've come a long way indeed. If you suffered from arthritis back in the days of Julius Caesar, your physician may very well have taken you

to the beach and had you place your feet on the back of an electrically charged fish. And things hadn't improved much by the eighteenth century. At that time your physician would have suggested a little bloodletting to relieve your aching joints.

Today, while we still don't have a cure for arthritis, experts suggest a number of things that can make life easier for you if you have the disease. Although symptoms and treatments vary according to specific forms of arthritis, there are some good general guidelines that can help nearly anyone with the problem.

To begin with, "you need to pace yourself," says Dr. Pennington. Something like cleaning the house can be tough if you have arthritis. If you vacuum one day, put off washing the kitchen floor until the next. By spreading out such tasks over several days, your joints won't suffer as much stress, and you won't suffer as much pain.

Another key to living with arthritis is to use your joints in ways that put the least amount of stress on them. You can do this by using the largest joints possible to perform a given task, says Dr. Pennington. So rather than picking up a coffee mug with two fingers, use both hands to cup the mug. Rather than trying to wrap your fingers around a skinny pencil, wrap the pencil in a sponge hair curler so that you have something fatter to grab. Rather than pushing open a heavy door with your hand and an outstretched arm, open it with the side of your arm and body.

When arthritis flares, you probably feel like curling up in front of the television set and staying there. The last thing in the world you feel like doing is exercising. Many people with arthritis wind up in a self-defeating cycle in which the aches and pains in their joints lead them to live sedentary lifestyles. Becoming inactive, however, is almost guaranteed to make matters worse.

The Need to Stay Fit

Exercise is important for anyone. It's especially important for people with arthritis. Joints that don't see enough action get stiff, and the muscles around them grow weaker and smaller. Sedentary people who have pain in their joints tend to keep those joints in bent positions. But joints that are held bent too long can eventually become locked, resulting in loss of function and possibly even deformity.

Besides helping to keep your joints flexible and your muscles strong, exercise makes life with arthritis easier in a third way: It alleviates pain by activating the release of the body's own natural painkillers.

But what kind of exercise is best? For people with arthritis, vigorous or strenuous exercise is probably out.

Many experts advocate swimming and walking as two of the top exercises for people with arthritis. There is, however, no one activity that will give you all the benefits that exercise can bring. Rather, experts say your best bet is engaging in a variety of exercises designed to build strength. They also recommend exercises that stretch the muscles and increase flexibility in the joints (called range-of-motion exercises).

Stress management also plays a decisive role in dealing with arthritis. At Vanderbilt University in Nashville, researchers have been tracking arthritis patients for more than five years, trying to determine the full nature of the long-suspected connection between stress and rheumatoid arthritis. "There are no good data to show that arthritis can be caused by stress, but once you have the condition, then stress can probably make it worse," says Kenneth Wallston, Ph.D., a health psychologist at Vanderbilt.

Calmness Is the Key

Stress worsens pain by causing people to contract their muscles, says Dr. Pennington. Many arthritis sufferers fall into a cycle whereby the pain of their joints causes stress, which causes muscles to contract, which causes more pain, which causes more stress. You can break the cycle by becoming more active (exercise loosens muscles and relieves stress) and by learning a good stress-management technique like biofeedback, says Dr. Pennington.

Dr. Wallston suggests that a person with arthritis can benefit from sessions with a good stress-management teacher. You can find one through your city or state psychological association, a local hospital, or a community health center. Your physician might also be able to recommend someone.

A good example of a relaxation technique is progressive relaxation. It's simple. Start with a quiet, comfortable environment. Breathe deep. Now, concentrate on tensing and then relaxing various muscle groups throughout the body. Contract the muscles in your feet and lower legs for 5 seconds, then relax—feeling your tension and pain slip away as you do. Repeat the process, moving from one muscle group to another until your whole body feels calm and relaxed.

Does What You Eat Matter?

Now add to these ABCs of arthritis a great big D, which stands for diet. Maintaining your proper body weight is very important in relieving pain from certain types of arthritis. Carrying excess weight puts added stress on weight-carrying joints, such as the hips, knees, and ankles, says Dr. Pennington.

And while you're thinking about dieting, consider not only what you won't be eating but also what you *will.* "Until recently there was no confirmed data that diet in any way helped arthritis, but over the last five years several things have come out that are important," says Carey Dachman, M.D., director of the Division of Rheumatology at Chicago's Edgewater Hospital, a lecturer in medicine at the Chicago Medical School, and director of the Suburban Arthritis and Back Center in Shaumburg, Illinois.

The most promising studies point to the potential power of fish oil and the importance of avoiding foods that might trigger allergic reactions, says Dr. Dachman. (For specifics on what to eat and what to avoid, see "Eat to Beat Arthritis" on page 54.)

When Pain Flares

What can you do when the pain of arthritis flares? Experts at the Arthritis Foundation suggest a number of things: You can use heat, either in the form of a warm bath, an electric blanket, or a hot water bottle wrapped in towels. You also can try applying cold, which you may find particularly soothing on days when your joints are inflamed and hot to the touch. (A bag of frozen peas wrapped in a towel makes a great cold pack.) You might also try alternate hot and cold treatments. That is, dip your hand or foot in warm water, then cold, then warm water again.

When you feel pain, it is also helpful to learn to distract your mind. When walking up a hill becomes painful, name a town or city with each step. When housework brings on pain, mentally rescreen the last several movies you saw.

When pain flares, "tell yourself that the pain will go away, that it is only short-lived," says Dr. Wallston. Another strategy that works for many, he says, is to "look at pain as a challenge as opposed to an obstacle. See your pain almost as a friendly foe that you can enter into a game with . . . a game that you can be sure of winning," he says.

Get the Support You Need

Physical pain is often accompanied by mental anguish. A lot of people with arthritis wind up feeling that "there's no one out there who understands me, no one to whom I can talk, no one to turn to," says Dr. Wallston. "They get the perception that other people just don't know what they're going through." But it is important to remember that you are not alone—you are *far* from alone.

To break out of your feelings of isolation, you may find it extremely helpful to join a support group. In a support group, you can talk with others who are also in pain and learn about their ways of coping with the special set of problems that arthritis creates. Your doctor, the Arthritis Foundation, or your local hospital can help you locate such a group. You might also consider seeing a therapist to help you deal with the mental and emotional aspects of arthritis.

Remember that family and friends can also be of great support, but it is important to clearly communicate your needs to them, says Dr. Wallston. "Be certain to let them know whether you are getting enough support. Be sure to let them know if you're getting *too* much. It's possible that you're being made to feel too dependent. Everyone has a certain need for dignity," he says.

Watch Out for Your Wallet

While you are seeking out people who can offer you emotional support, be aware that there are other people who might offer you a form of "support" you don't need.

There are lots of people out there all too eager to prey upon your physical and emotional needs, people who'd be happy to take your money in exchange for some alleged new cure. The problem is, says Dr. Pennington, "there is no such thing."

Some touted cures, such as copper bracelets or placing sesame seeds in your navel, are harmless enough, he says, "but don't put your faith in them." Other alleged cures may be potentially harmful. Dr. Pennington

includes snake venom therapy and rubdowns with industrial solvents in this dangerous category. (You'll find more on bogus cures in "Beware of the Quacks" on page 56.)

Weeding out the good alternative therapies from the bad is only one of many reasons why a person with arthritis should have a good working relationship with a physician.

Drugs and Surgery

For most types of arthritis, various medications are a vital part of treatment. There are two general groups of medications—those that help with the pain and the discomfort, and those that may help alter the course of the disease.

Where medications, physical therapy, diet, rest, and the proper use of joints aren't enough, a last resort for some people with arthritis is surgery. Operations to "fix" badly damaged joints are very successful, and they continue to improve as doctors learn more about arthritis and sharpen their surgical skills.

Nevertheless, arthritis rarely poses an emergency, so surgery should be carefully considered before resorting to a scalpel.

To find a competent surgeon near you, contact the local office of the Arthritis Foundation. Also ask about the foundation's wealth of literature and programs to help people with arthritis live a full life. Should you have a hard time finding a local branch, the national headquarters is in Atlanta. You can call them at (404) 872-7100, or write P.O. Box 19000, Atlanta, GA 30326.

Russell Wild

21

ARTHRITIS

JOINT-SAVING TIPS

When you have arthritis, even the simplest daily activity, such as opening a drawer, carrying a pot, or lifting yourself from a chair, can become a difficult chore. While you could ask others for help, people willing to lend a hand aren't always available. And besides, you don't always want to ask others for help. You want—and you deserve—your independence.

Remaining independent may be a matter of learning how to do your daily activities in ways that are a bit different from the ways you're used to. You'll need to learn to use your joints in the most efficient manner and, wherever possible, to use the larger joints rather than the smaller.

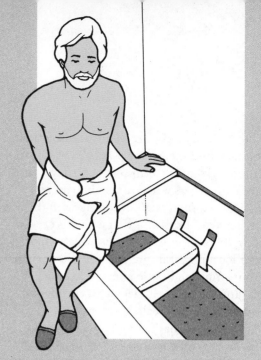

Why struggle getting in and out of the tub? A simple board fixed tightly across the tub should make the going easy. Use a bath seat and rubber mat for safety.

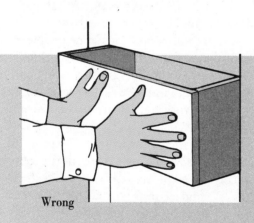

Wrong

Ouch. Shutting a drawer like this—pushing in with your fingertips—creates undue pressure in the joints of the fingers and hands, particularly if the drawer is one that sticks.

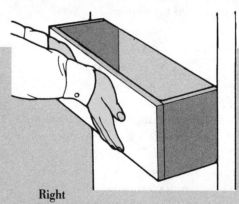

Right

Your hands will applaud you and your joints will cheer you if you shut a drawer like this—with hands and fingers flat. The only joint you'll be using is your wrist.

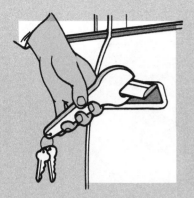

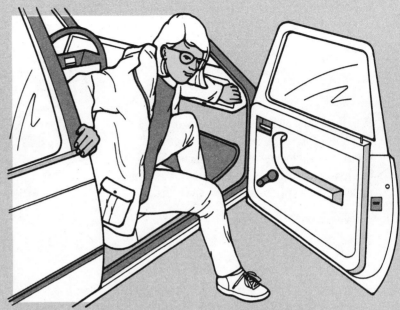

Opening the door to your car becomes hassle-free with this easy-to-make wooden gadget that practically does all the work for you! If you don't know someone who can make one for you, contact the Arthritis Foundation for more information (the address is on page 21).

When your arthritis translates into lower back pain, you know that getting out of a car can sometimes hurt. The key to preventing such pain is to avoid any awkward, twisting movements (as seen here) that put pressure on the spine.

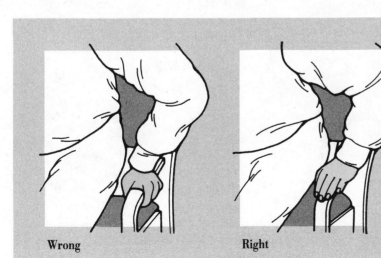

Wrong

Right

Lifting yourself out of a chair like the man on the left is the wrong way to go if you have arthritis. Rather than gripping the chair on your way up, do as the man on the right does—push off with flat hands.

ARTHRITIS

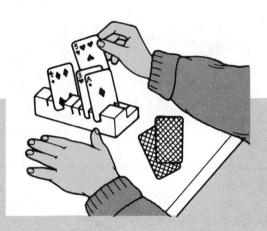

Whether your game is gin rummy or old maid, holding a fan of cards can wipe away the smile and leave you poker-faced. You can avoid all strain on your hands by setting up a simple wooden holder such as this.

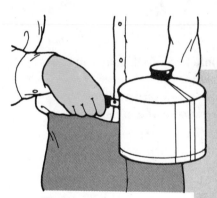

Wrong

Some pots can be quite heavy even when empty, never mind when filled with your favorite dish. Carrying such a heavy load in the traditional manner can be stressful to your arthritic hands.

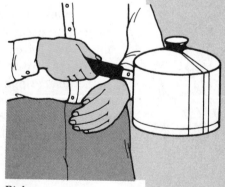

Right

A better way to carry a pot takes all the strain off the joints of your hands. Let all the weight of the pot rest on your *other* arm. If the pot's hot, throw a protective towel over your exposed hand.

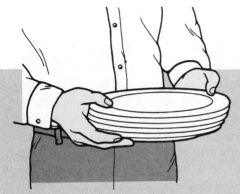

Wrong

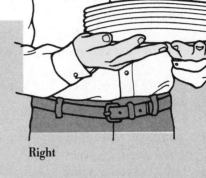

Right

Granted, you don't want to drop your finest china all over the kitchen floor. You don't, however, have to carry the dishes as if you were choking a moose.

A better way of carrying plates is to place your hands flat underneath and carry them as you would a crown for a king's coronation.

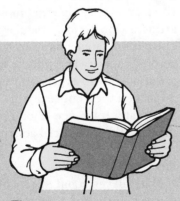

Wrong

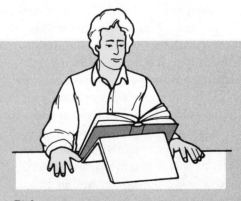

Right

Holding up a heavy book, such as *Webster's Dictionary*, puts a definite strain on the joints in your hands. Give your tender joints a break.

Instead, lay the book down on a table in front of you, resting it on a book rest such as this one. Your hands should feel a considerable amount of relief.

Active Body, Healthy Joints

Sure, you know that exercise is good for you. It's good for your heart. It's good for your lungs. And it's good for your waistline. But did you know that exercise is also good for your joints?

In fact, exercise is *great* for your joints! Especially if you have arthritis.

Just as birds were meant to fly and fish were meant to swim, joints were meant to go back and forth and up and down and twist and turn. And if, by lack of exercise, joints don't get to do what they were meant to do, they start to suffer.

"Without regular movement, the muscles tighten, the tissues become tighter, and eventually there are actual changes in the joint structure," says Kathleen Haralson, a physical therapist who is associate director of the Washington University Regional Arthritis Center in St. Louis, Missouri, and a volunteer with the Arthritis Foundation.

Unfortunately, some people with arthritis use their aches and pains as reasons not to exercise. But this inevitably creates "a vicious cycle," says Haralson. You feel soreness and pain, so you avoid exercise. Because you avoid exercise, your joints get stiffer. Your stiffer joints cause you more soreness and pain, so you avoid exercise. And so on . . .

Ready to break out of this vicious cycle? Then get ready to hop onto an exercycle . . . or into a swimsuit . . . or onto your living room carpet for a few easy movements that will pay off in many ways. You'll find that not only will you be able to move your joints with greater ease, you may also feel less pain and stiffness, and your daily tasks will become easier and easier to do.

One person with arthritis who found out how helpful exercise can be is Billie Jean King. At the age of 18, she was in a car accident that probably contributed to the development of osteoarthritis in both her knees. Instead of letting it stop her, King went on to become one of the most successful players ever in women's tennis.

Today, years later, King promotes exercise as the best therapy for arthritis. "When I don't exercise, I feel worse; it's that simple," said King in an article in the medical journal *Physician and Sportsmedicine.* "When I get the circulation going in the knee joints, it helps a lot."

King is not the only one to have made this discovery. One report from the University of Michigan concluded that most people with arthritis who perform regular aerobic exercise not only make significant gains in aerobic capacity and muscle strength, they are also likely to experience a positive impact on their entire quality of life, including greater tolerance of joint pain, happier moods, and more social activity.

Getting Started

With all you stand to gain by exercising, you may be tempted to overdo it when you first get started. Before you leap into your leotard, there are a few things you should know.

"Before you start exercising, check with a physician," says Arthur I. Grayzel, M.D., senior vice president of medical affairs for the Arthritis Foundation. "Too much exercise can be as harmful as too little. Your doctor, working with a physical or occupational therapist, can help you design a program specifically for your needs."

Particularly if you are over 50, you should have a stress test to make sure your cardiovascular system is okay, says Carey Dachman, M.D., director of the Division of Rheumatology at Chicago's Edgewater Hospital, a lecturer in medicine at the Chicago Medical School, and director of the Suburban Arthritis and Back Center in Shaumburg, Illinois.

If your doctor gives you his blessing, you might want to adopt a new attitude before beginning. Instead of thinking of yourself as a patient trying to overcome a disease, think of yourself as a kind of artist. Just as the ballet dancer performs special exercises to strengthen his thighs and calves, and just as the pianist practices to keep her fingers and arms in shape, you are using exercise to strengthen your joints and keep your muscles in top working order.

Go easy on yourself at the beginning. You may start your exercise program with a mere 5 minutes a day, and that's perfectly all right, says Dr. Dachman. Slowly, you'll want to work your way up to 20 minutes of exercise or more, four to five days a week, he says. One good place to start an exercise program is with the Arthritis Foundation's PACE (People with Arthritis Can Exercise) program. You can get the program's home videotapes, or you can participate in a class taught by trained instructors. Contact your local foundation chapter or the national headquarters in Atlanta (see page 21 for the address). You might also ask them for their free brochures on how to exercise safely.

Your Choice of Activities

What kinds of exercise should you be doing? There are many choices, and the more choices you make, the better. "There are three major types of exercise," says Haralson. There are exercises for endurance, for strength, and for flexibility. Some activities, like weight-lifting, concentrate heavily on only one type of exercise. Others, like swimming and walking, offer components of all three.

That's probably why swimming and walking are tops on the list of activities that experts advise for people with arthritis. Other activities, such as weight-lifting and jogging, which tend to put a great deal of strain on joints, are generally not recommended, although they're not always prohibited.

How Much Should You Push?

Some say, "No pain, no gain." Others say, "Whatever you do—don't strain." Everyone who has ever exercised has had to wonder at some point whether he's putting in enough effort or too much.

Dr. Dachman suggests that you think of a scale going from one to ten, with one representing no effort and no pain, and ten representing obvious pain. Now, with this scale in mind, how far should you push your workouts? "Go to about a five," says Dr. Dachman.

RANGE-OF-MOTION EXERCISES

You might think ultimate fitness means running a marathon, lifting 300 pounds over your head, climbing Mount Everest, or swimming the English channel. But fitness —particularly for the person with arthritis— contains one additional component besides strength and endurance: flexibility, or *range of motion.*

Range of motion refers to the degree to which each joint in the body can be moved in the direction for which it was designed. Range-of-motion exercises, then, are specific therapeutic exercises designed to maintain joint movement, relieve stiffness, and restore flexibility. How important are range-of-motion exercises for people with arthritis? *Very.*

"People with arthritis need a range-of-motion program," says physical therapist Kathleen Haralson, associate director of the Washington University Regional Arthritis Center in St. Louis, Missouri, and a volunteer with the Arthritis Foundation.

"The chief problem with arthritis is joint stiffness and pain. Usually, because of this stiffness and pain, people don't move much, which tends to worsen matters. When people don't move much, the joints grow stiffer," she says, emphasizing that anyone can do range-of-motion exercises.

A good place to start is with the illustrations on the following pages. Before you go too far with your own exercise program, however, you may want to consider having a professional physical therapist set up a complete program for your individualized needs. Your physician can direct you to the appropriate therapist.

How They Are Done

When performing range-of-motion exercises, move the joint slowly and gently until you feel a little discomfort, hold it there for a moment, then move it just a tad farther. "Don't force it and always avoid rapid movements," says Haralson.

Each range-of-motion exercise should be performed from three to ten times, recommends Haralson. Start by allotting just 5 or 10 minutes a day to your program, then try to increase both the number of exercises and repetitions.

The time one should spend doing range-of-motion exercises depends on how many joints are affected—it's really a gray area, says Haralson.

While the order in which you choose to do the exercises is not particularly important, "you should spend the most time on the joints that are the stiffest," she says.

Remember that range-of-motion exercises are not enough to keep you physically fit.

"Range-of-motion exercises are very good to keep your joints lubricated, to keep scar tissue from building up where it shouldn't, and to keep you flexible, but this is where the benefits end," says Carey Dachman, M.D., director of the Division of Rheumatology at Chicago's Edgewater Hospital, a lecturer in medicine at the Chicago Medical School, and director of the Suburban Arthritis and Back Center in Shaumburg, Illinois. In other words, they won't help you ward off heart disease or climb stairs without getting winded.

Hips

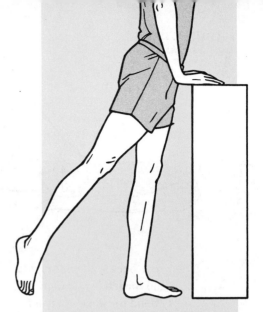

This slow-motion kick should help increase the backward motion of the hip. Standing against a counter, move one leg back, then the other. Keep your knee straight and your hips facing forward.

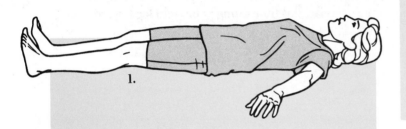

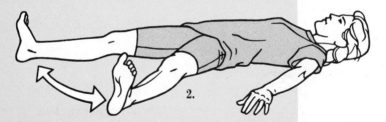

(1) Lie comfortably on your back with your legs straight out, about 6 inches apart. Point your toes straight up to the ceiling. *(2)* Slide one leg all the way out to the side. Return the leg, then do the same with the other. Try to keep your toes pointed up throughout the exercise. Keep your body stable by spreading your arms to the sides.

ARTHRITIS

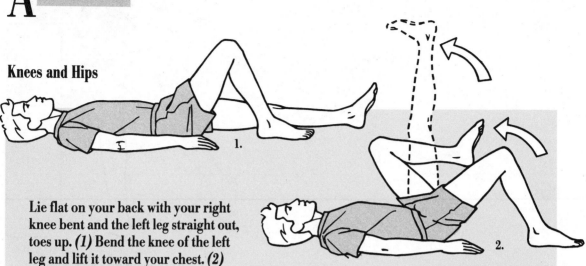

Knees and Hips

Lie flat on your back with your right knee bent and the left leg straight out, toes up. *(1)* Bend the knee of the left leg and lift it toward your chest. *(2)* Now push the left leg into the air, extending it toward the ceiling. Lower the left leg to the floor. Now bend your left leg. Repeat the exercise, this time lifting your right leg toward your chest.

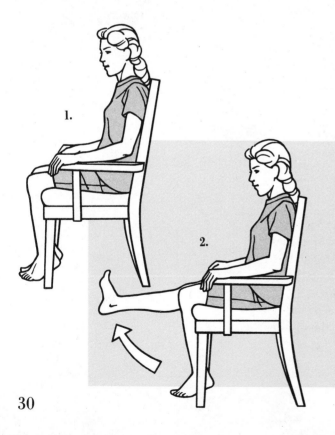

(1) Sit straight in a chair that's high enough off the ground so that you can swing your leg underneath. *(2)* Keep your thighs on the chair and straighten out one leg. Hold it for a few seconds. Let the leg down and continue the movement, bending your knee back as far as it will go. Relax. Repeat with the other leg.

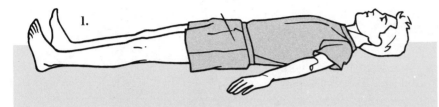

1.

Lie on your back with your legs straight out, about 6 inches apart. Your toes should be pointed up. *(1)* Now roll your hips and knees in and out, while keeping your legs straight. *(2)* To strengthen those knees, try this: Push one knee down against the floor. Tighten the muscle on the front of the thigh. Hold the muscle tight for a count of 5 seconds. Relax. Repeat with the other leg. Keep your body stable by spreading your arms.

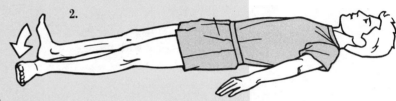

2.

Shoulders

(1) Place both hands behind your head. *(2)* Now move your elbows back as far as they will go. As you move your elbows back, allow your head to roll back as well. Hold a few seconds, then return to your starting position.

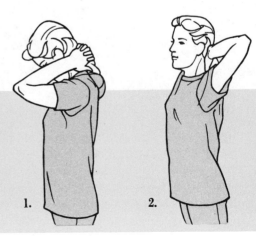

1.   2.

(continued)

ARTHRITIS

Shoulders

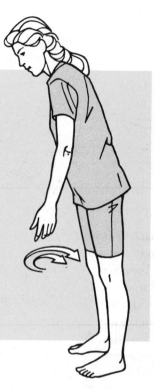

Here's an exercise for stiff or painful shoulders. Standing or sitting, lean forward slightly. Let one arm hang in front of you. Relax. Feel the weight of the arm. Now with the arm straight, like a pendulum, let it swing in small circles that gradually grow larger. Continue until you start to feel discomfort. Repeat with other arm.

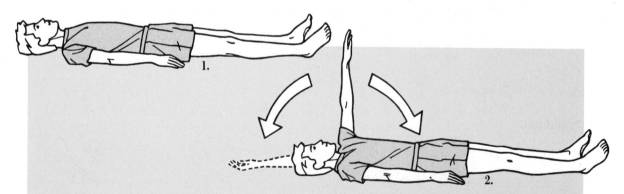

Here is another good range-of-motion exercise for shoulders that have limited motion or suffer from pain. *(1)* Lie flat on your back with both arms at your sides. *(2)* Raise one arm slowly over your head. Your elbow should be straight but relaxed. Keep the arm close to your ear—do not let it swing outward. Return your arm slowly to your side. Repeat with your other arm.

Elbows

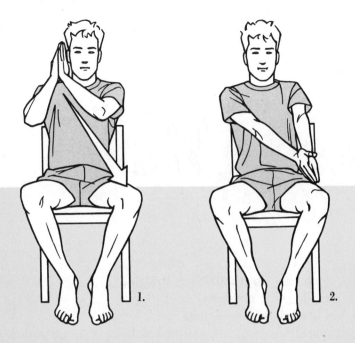

To perform this exercise, picture yourself chopping wood. *(1)* Sitting or standing, place your palms together and bend both elbows until your hands touch your right shoulder. *(2)* Then bring your hands down to touch the left knee. Your elbows should now be straight. Gently push the elbow just a wee bit farther than it wants to go. Repeat on the other side, going from the left shoulder to the right knee.

Ankles

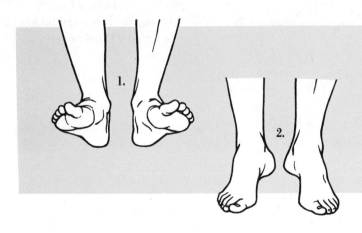

Kick off your shoes and sit down in a chair. *(1)* Keeping your heels on the floor, lift your toes as high as possible. *(2)* Then return your toes to the floor and lift your heels up as high as possible.

ARTHRITIS

Hands

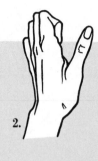

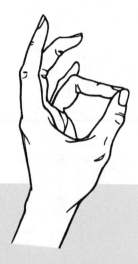

(1) Start with your hand open and fingers straight, as if you were hailing a cab on a busy New York street. (2) Now bend all the finger joints *except* for your biggest knuckles, which you keep straight. Try to touch the top of your palm with your fingertips.

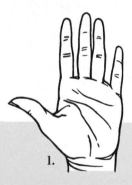

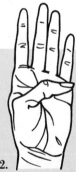

With your fingers spread, one by one touch the tip of your thumb to the tip of each of your other fingers in turn. See if you can form the letter "O" using every finger.

(1) Open your hand with your fingers straight. (2) Reach your thumb across your palm until it touches the base of the little finger. Stretch your thumb out and back. Repeat, using both hands.

Wrists

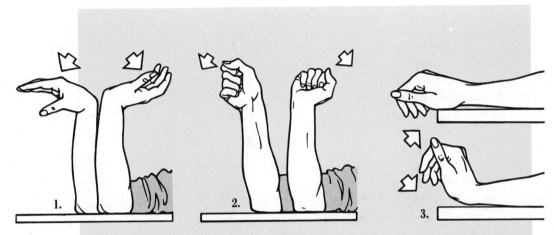

(1) Place your arm on a table. Bend your hand forward (with your palm down), and then bend it back (with your palm up). *(2)* Next, close your fist. With your wrist straight, move your hand forward and back. *(3)* Allow your forearm to relax flat on the table. Now raise your hand with the fingers lightly curled, bending your wrist up as far as it will go. Lower your hand and relax.

Back

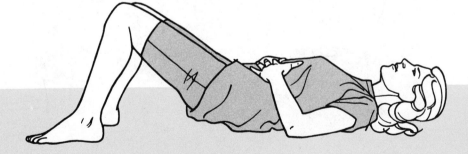

Lie down with your knees bent and your feet flat. Place your hands over your stomach. Now flatten the small of your back against the floor by tightening your buttocks and pulling your stomach in. Think of bringing your pubic bone toward your chin. Repeat.

(continued)

ARTHRITIS

Back

Here's a good exercise for your upper and middle back. *(1)* Sitting on the edge of a chair, straighten your back and bend both of your elbows at approximately a 90-degree angle. The idea is to pinch your shoulder blades together. *(2)* You can do this by moving your elbows back. Gently pull them as far back as they will go without causing pain.

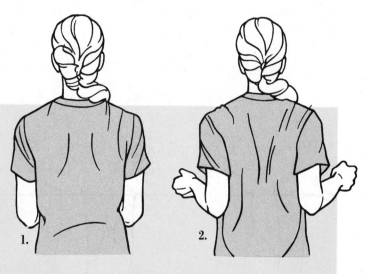

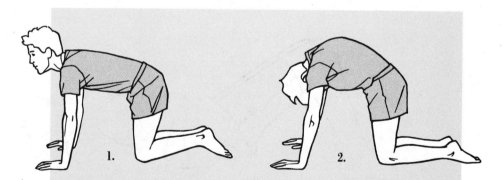

(1) On all fours, make like a cat. Inhale as you raise your back, exhale as you drop your back. *(2)* Lower your head as your back rises and lift your head as your back drops. (Meowing is optional.) This exercise isn't for you, however, if you have problems with your knees, ankles, or hands.

WATER EXERCISES

When the men of *Apollo 11* landed on the moon, they found that the relative lack of gravity there transformed them into supermen —able to leap huge craters in a single bound.

You too can have such powers—and you needn't board a rocket ship! All you need to do is splash into the nearest swimming pool.

"Water can be a great environment to exercise in because there's hardly any stress on the joints," says physical therapist Kathleen Haralson, associate director of the Washington University Regional Arthritis Center in St. Louis, Missouri, and a volunteer with the Arthritis Foundation. "You weigh practically nothing in water. It's easier to move in water, and exercising becomes much less painful."

Water also provides active resistance as the part of your body in motion pushes against the weight of the water. This gentle pushing builds strength, tone, and endurance.

Walk in Water

Just about any exercise you can perform on land can be performed in water. In fact, the selection in water may even be greater. You can do the calisthenic-type exercises as illustrated in this chapter. You can swim. You can even walk.

Walk? If you think walking in water sounds as farfetched as walking *on* water, ask one of the approximately 2,800 people who take regular water walks at the Cleveland County Family YMCA in Norman, Oklahoma. Among the participants, you'll find many who say their arthritis has gotten better since beginning to water walk. "More and more doctors are referring their patients to the program," says John Mikos, aquatics director.

There are many good reasons why anyone— but particularly someone with arthritis—would want to walk in water, says Mikos. To begin with, walking in water offers a great aerobic workout in much less time than a walk on land. One study, says Mikos, shows that one half hour of vigorous water walking can offer the same amount of aerobic activity as a 2-hour hike through the woods.

When you walk in a pool, you run less risk of injury than you do walking among the sticks, stones, and potholes of your average park or city street. As an added benefit, there is no stress on the joints—which, to the arthritis sufferer, means less inflammation and pain. Besides, water walking is fun and keeps you cool, even in the middle of the steamiest summer, says Mikos.

To find a water-walking program near you, check with your local YMCA or YWCA. Not all have water-walking programs, but many do. If you want to try it yourself, you really don't need special instruction, says Mikos. Just find a warm pool, preferably 85° to 86°F. Do your walk with the water at about chest level. Water walking does require more exertion than you might expect, so go easy on yourself.

You needn't limit yourself to walking forward, says Mikos. "There is an infinite
(continued)

Water Exercises—*Continued*

variety of techniques." You can walk backward or sideways, use small, quick steps or long ones, use your arms or just your legs, or try something altogether different—like kicking your legs and touching your toes with every step. "People develop their own techniques as they progress," he says.

Those Y's that don't yet offer water-walking programs usually do offer water-exercise classes, says Mikos. Most chapters offer an excellent program developed jointly by experts at the YMCA and the Arthritis Foundation.

Prepare to Make a Splash

Although water exercises are generally gentle exercises, it is preferable to begin them only with an okay from your doctor. Following are some good beginning water exercises from *The Arthritis Book of Water Exercise* by Judy Jetter and occupational therapist Nancy Kadlec.

The authors advise you to keep your back straight and your stomach flat while performing these exercises. To avoid injury, they say you should never tilt your head backward at a severe angle. Keep your eyes open at all times to help maintain your balance. And don't hold your breath for any reason; none of these exercises requires putting your face in water.

Finally, the authors recommend that you discontinue any exercise that causes pain, unless your doctor specifically has advised you to stay with it.

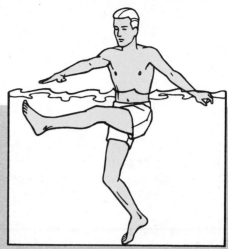

Start your routine with a straight-leg march. With arms stretched out to the side to help you keep your balance, walk forward, lifting each leg as high as you can. Walk briskly for several minutes. Keep your back straight. If you suffer from back pain, skip this exercise.

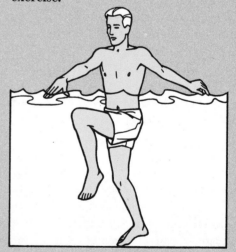

This exercise is like the straight-leg march, above, only now you bend your knee when your foot comes off the floor. The toes of your raised leg should be pointed down. Do not extend your leg forward, just lift it high.

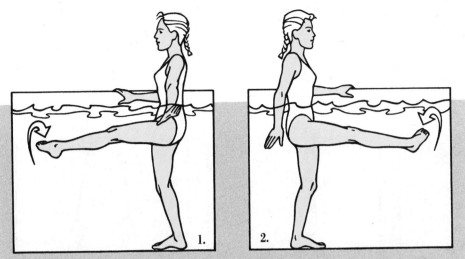

Stand up straight and tall with your head up and hold onto the edge of the pool. *(1)* Raise the outside leg and circle your foot from the ankle. Circle your foot clockwise, then reverse the motion. *(2)* Turn to the other side and repeat the exercise with the other foot. This is a good beginning exercise for sore and stiff ankles.

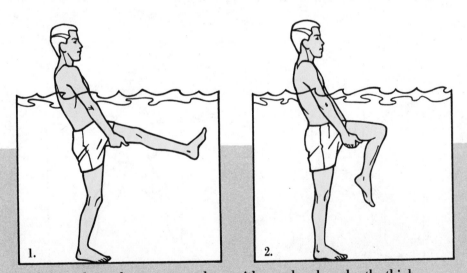

Lift one leg and support your knee with your hands under the thigh. *(1)* Now lift the leg toward the ceiling, pointing your toes up. Try to lift it as high as you can without causing any pain. *(2)* Relax your toes and bend your leg at the knee as far back as it will go. Keep your back straight and your chin level. Feel for the stretch in the back of the lifted leg. Repeat with the other leg.

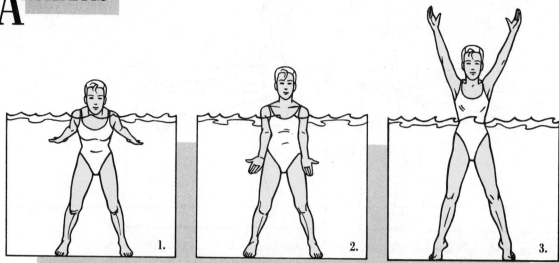

(1) Spread your feet apart about shoulder-width. Breathe in and bend both knees as you lift your arms straight back behind you. *(2)* Now exhale forcefully as you swing your arms forward and up until they're straight up overhead. Allow your knees to straighten as you lift up. *(3)* As your arms swing overhead, lift yourself up by your toes. Swing down to the starting position and repeat. Stop if you start to feel dizzy.

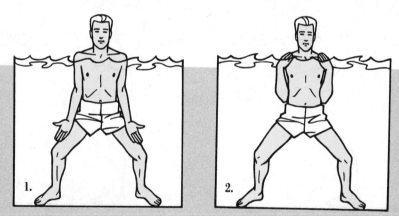

(1) Spread your feet wide apart. Bending at your knees, lower your body until your shoulders are near or in the water. Keep your back straight. Now tuck in your elbows. Turn out your palms with the backs of your hands against your thighs. *(2)* Imagine lifting the water up as you bend your elbows and raise your hands until your fingers touch your shoulders. Lower your arms, making sure that your elbows are still tucked in.

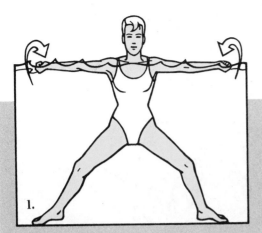 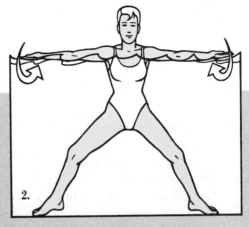

(1) With your feet apart and your knees bent until your shoulders reach the water, stretch your arms straight out to the side at shoulder height, palms up. Now clench your fists. Rotate your fists downward and all the way around, gradually opening your fists until your palms are facing the ceiling once again. *(2)* Return to the starting position and try it again.

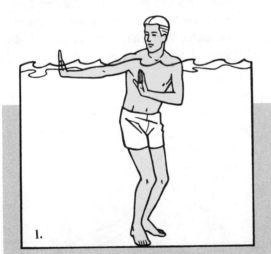 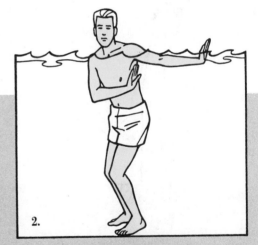

If you've never done the Charleston, it's time to start. *(1)* Stand with your knees slightly bent, toes pointing left, elbows flexed, and fingers pointing upward. Face your palms outward to the right of your body. *(2)* Now pivot on your heels and swing your toes to the right as your arms swing to the left. Pivot on your toes while you swing your heels to the right, swinging your arms back to the right at the same time. You will be moving sideways to the right. Repeat four times, then reverse direction.

ARTHRITIS

AT-HOME WATER EXERCISES

Not everyone has easy access to a pool or beach. If you're landlocked, don't mope. You can still experience the benefits of water exercises. Simply transport your body to a much smaller body of water—the one in your bathroom. From *Bathtub Exercises for Arthritis and Back Pain* by Judy Jetter and Nancy Kadlec, we've selected a dozen easy-to-do exercises that you can perform in either your tub or the shower. Make sure you have a nonslip mat to work on. And ask your doctor about which exercises are best.

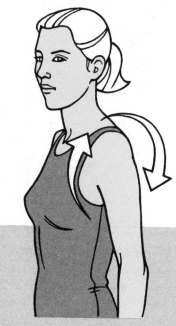

Do this one in the shower. Circle your left shoulder forward. Make the circles as wide as you can without causing pain. Then reverse the direction. Now do the same with your right shoulder. Last, circle both shoulders at the same time, forward, and then back.

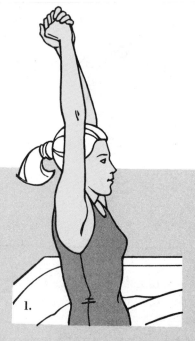

1.

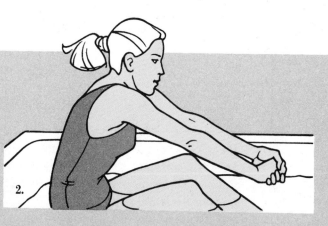

2.

Try this one while you're *sitting* in the tub. *(1)* Imagine you are holding an ax over your head with straight arms. *(2)* Bend forward as you swing your hands downward, as if you were about to split wood. Spread your knees and bring your hands down, all the way to the bottom of the tub.

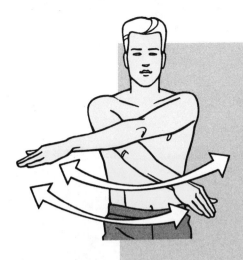

Do this one sitting down if it's more comfortable for you. Stretch both arms out to the side and move them behind your body as far as you can while keeping them straight. Keep your arms as high as possible. Swing your arms past the front of your body, letting them cross until they can go no farther without bending at the elbows. Swing back to the original position. Repeat.

(1) For a good stretch of the torso, clasp your hands behind your neck, or, if this feels uncomfortable, just put one hand on top of the other. *(2)* Straighten your elbows to raise your hands as high as you can with your palms to the ceiling. Hold for a count of three.

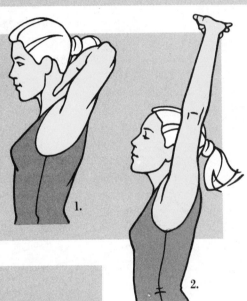

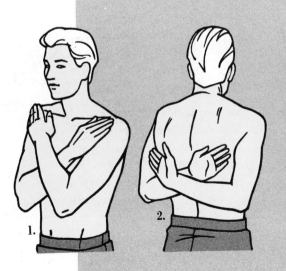

(1) Cross your arms in front, putting your right hand on your left shoulder and your left hand on your right shoulder. *(2)* Now try crossing your wrists behind you in the middle of your back. Repeat, alternating top arm and wrist each time. If you've had surgery, ask your physician if it's okay for you to do this exercise.

ARTHRITIS

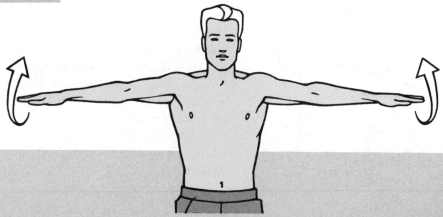

Stretch both arms straight out. Turn your palms down and spread your fingers. (If your tub or shower isn't large enough, just work one at a time.) Inhale and clench your fists as you rotate your hands up to face the ceiling. Exhale as you reverse the rotation and straighten your fingers. Repeat.

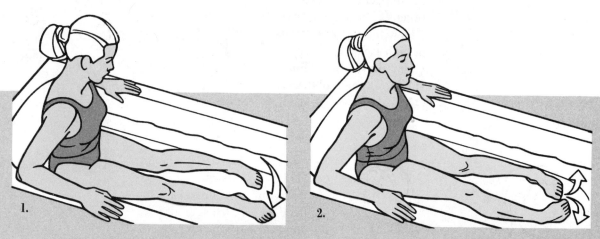

1.

2.

(1) With your back against the tub, extend your legs. Use your hands and your arms to brace yourself solidly. Turn both feet as far as you can to the right so that the outside edge of your right foot and the inside edge of your left foot rest on or near the tub bottom. *(2)* Now rotate both feet in the other direction so that the outside edge of your left foot and inside edge of your right foot rest on or near the bottom. Repeat. Finally, point each foot toward the other and then away as far as possible in opposite directions.

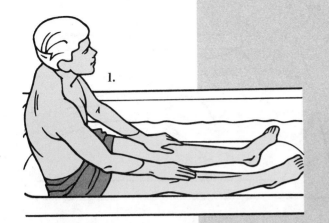

1.

This exercise will flex your torso and back. *(1)* Sit upright and place your hands on your knees. *(2)* Slowly bend forward and touch the tips of your toes. Return to the upright position. Repeat. You may eventually be able to touch the bottom of the tub's front wall. People with pain in the lower back should keep their knees slightly bent during this exercise.

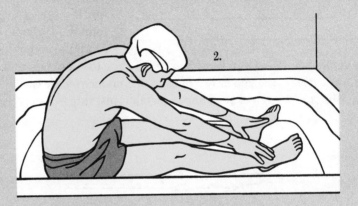

2.

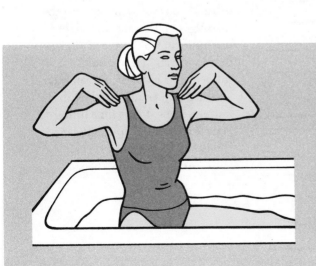

Here's a twister for the waist. With your legs extended, lift your forearms and put your fingertips on the outside of your shoulders (or the front of your shoulders, if space is cramped). Keep your shoulders as far back as you can. Gently twist your torso to the left as far as you can. Reverse direction and twist as far to the right as you can. Repeat. If you have low back pain, be especially careful not to twist too far.

45

ARTHRITIS

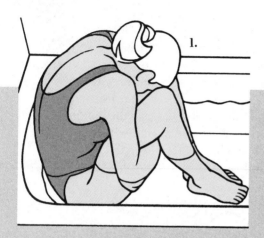

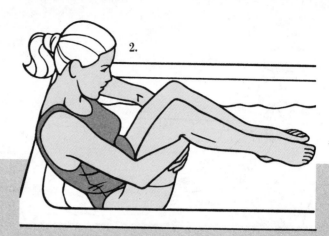

This movement is called the rocking horse. You'll find it's a great strengthening exercise for the tummy. *(1)* Bend your knees to your chest and grasp the underside of each thigh. *(2)* Tighten your abdominal muscle as you keep your knees close to your chest and rock backward onto your buttocks. Make sure you have a nonslip mat under you. Be careful not to rock so far backward that you slip. And if you feel at all uncomfortable, just skip this exercise.

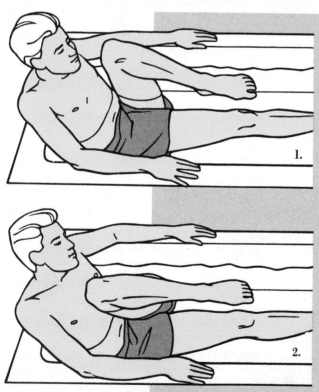

(1) Brace your back against the tub and your forearms against the tub edges and rotate your right hip upward. Hold it there. *(2)* Bend your right knee and lift it toward your chin, then straighten your leg as it returns to the tub bottom. Repeat, this time lifting your knee toward your left ear. Continue. Repeat the exercise with your left hip and knee.

Healing Runs Hot and Cold

Some people like to eat their apple pie hot, others prefer it cold. Some people just love skiing in Vermont in the dead of winter, others beg to be in the balmy Bahamas. Likewise, some people with arthritis swear by heat to relieve pain, and others swear by cold. But which do doctors prefer?

It's basically a matter of half a dozen ice packs on one hand, and six hot compresses on the other, says Robert Karsh, M.D., a rheumatologist at the Overland Medical Center in St. Louis, associate professor of clinical medicine at Washington University Medical School, and a consultant to the Veterans Administration in rheumatology.

Generally, if there's noticeable swelling, you want to apply ice. As the swelling goes down, usually after about 24 hours, then it's time to apply heat, says Dr. Karsh. But aside from this very rough rule of thumb, "whatever makes you feel better is what you should be doing," he says. "I can sound so cavalier since neither heat nor cold can change the course of the disease. If ice makes you feel better—fine. If heat makes you feel better—fine. But you still have to take your medicine."

Heat can be applied in many ways. You can take hot showers and baths, although doctors recommend that you limit your baths to no longer than 20 minutes. You can apply hot compresses. That is, take a towel, soak it in hot water, wring it out, wrap it in a dry towel, and apply the package to the painful area. You also can use a heat lamp to warm aching parts of your body.

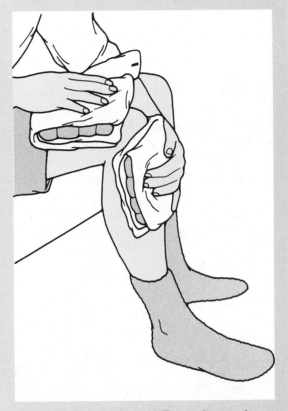

Need help for sore knees? Try cooling and soothing away the pain with one ice pack applied above the knee and another below. Wrap both packs in towels and hold them snugly to the knee for 20 minutes. You'll feel coldness and a burning sensation at first.

To apply cold, you can make a cold compress the same way you do a hot one. Soak a towel in ice water, wring it out, and apply it to the sore area. Covering the wet towel with a dry one, or plastic, will protect your skin from the cold. A cold compress can also be made by wrapping a towel around a plastic bag full of ice cubes or frozen peas.

How to Lay Me Down to Sleep

There is no single best sleep position for all people. For people with arthritis, the best sleep position depends on which joints are involved. According to Kate Lorig, R.N., and James F. Fries, M.D., authors of *The Arthritis Helpbook,* there are certain positions that are best for most people with particular kinds of arthritis. You'll find their suggestions in the surrounding illustrations.

Other than finding the right position, the authors recommend:

- trying a bed with a moderately firm mattress. (Or trying a water bed, which supports the weight of the body evenly and can be kept quite warm.)
- avoiding sedatives and sleeping pills (they rarely help and can be habit-forming).
- going to bed only when you are tired— don't try to force sleep by going to bed too early.

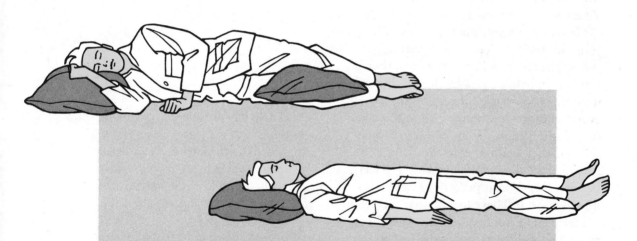

Above left, If you have arthritis but your knees and hips are unaffected, a good sleep position might be on your side with one pillow for your head and another tucked between your knees. *Above right,* If you have hip or knee problems, you want your knees straight and the hips not rotated to the side. The best position for you may be on your back with a small pillow under your ankles.

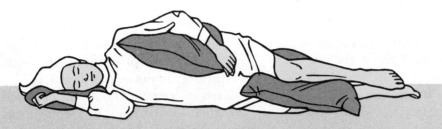

If you have back problems, sleep on your side with your knees bent. Place one pillow between your knees and another under the upper arm to reduce stress on the shoulder joint.

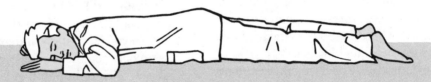

If you have ankylosing spondylitis, a form of arthritis that affects primarily the spine, you may be able to help prevent deformity and loss of mobility by sleeping on your stomach.

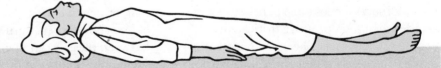

Those with ankylosing spondylitis might also try sleeping on their backs. Try using no pillow at all, except perhaps for a small one between your shoulder blades.

49

ARTHRITIS

PRESS HERE FOR INSTANT RELIEF

It can't be that simple, you say. You mean all I have to do is press right here, and my arthritis pain goes away? Yeah. Sure. And you have a bridge in Brooklyn you're gonna sell me real cheap, right?

While it may be hard to believe, medical science now confirms that the ancient oriental art of acupressure—acupuncture without needles—*can* relieve pain. Millions in China use it, and they have for centuries. In this country you'll find acupressure used in a few major hospitals.

How can pressing a point on the skin alleviate pain? According to ancient Chinese teachings, the acupressure points, or *tsubos*, are places where the body's vital life force, called *chi*, becomes blocked.

Western science offers another explanation: Pressing the points seems to activate the release of endorphins and enkephalins, the body's natural painkillers.

Push Your Own Pain-Relief Buttons

Although acu*puncture* is better known in this country than acu*pressure*, the Chinese actually used their hands long before they used needles, says Michael Reed Gach, the author of several books on acupressure and founder of the Acupressure Institute in Berkeley, California. The use of needles to activate the points is best for dealing with certain problems, but the use of soft, warm fingers is clearly the better choice for dealing with others—such as arthritis pain.

Arthritis pain, says Gach, tends to concentrate around the acupressure points. "Acupressure helps to relieve the joint pain by relaxing the muscles, enabling blood to flow freely . . . with daily practice of acupressure, the arthritic pain can be greatly reduced," says Gach in *Arthritis Relief at Your Fingertips*.

So, where are these points? Finding them really isn't difficult. "Each point can be found in relation to anatomical 'landmarks,' such as the belly button, a specific muscle, or the crease behind the knee," says Gach. The illustrations that follow show you the locations of several important points for arthritis relief.

Getting to the Point

You'll know you have the right point when you feel a slight indentation or depression between the tendons and muscles, says Gach. The right point, generally, will also feel more tender than the surrounding area.

What do you do once you've found the right point? Different acupressure experts suggest slightly varying approaches. Gach suggests you use your middle finger with your index and ring fingers on either side for support, or your thumb. But it's perfectly all right, he adds, to use your knuckles or even round objects such as an avocado pit, golf ball, or pencil eraser.

You should press until you feel "a balance between pleasure and pain," says Gach. Generally, points should be pressed for at least three minutes, as you breathe deeply and relax. The pressure should be applied and released gradually, advises Gach.

If you have trouble reaching a specific point, keep in mind that you can always ask a friend to lend a helping finger.

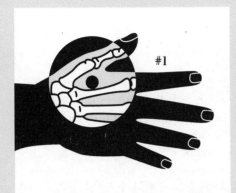

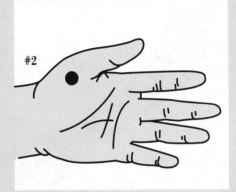

Point #1 can be used for arthritis pain in the hands, wrists, elbows, and shoulders. You'll find it at the highest spot of the muscle where the thumb and the index finger come together. Press in the webbing between the thumb and the index finger, closer to the bone that attaches to the index finger. Angle the pressure toward the index finger bone.

Point #2 is for relief of arthritis pain in the hand. Press on the palm side of the hand in the center of the mound at the base of the thumb. Apply firm pressure into the center of the fleshy pad where the thumb joins the palm of the hand. Not only will this spot relieve you of arthritis pain, but it may also help an upset stomach.

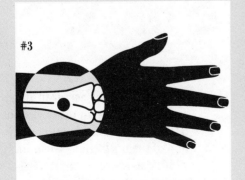

Point #3, helpful for tightness or pain in the shoulders, is found by first flexing your hand backward. The point is on the outside of the forearm, two finger-widths (about 1½ inches) from the wrist crease. Press between the forearm bones. To get firm pressure, wrap your hand around the wrist and use both your fingers and thumb.

(continued)

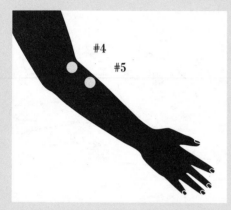

Point #4, good for pain in the hand, wrist, and elbow joints, is found by bending your arm at the elbow and traveling 1 inch toward your hand from the elbow crease. It's where the muscle pops out when you flex your wrist. **Point #5** is located in the elbow joint at the outer end of the crease where your arm bends. It is good for inflammation in the elbow and shoulder.

Point #6 is located between the top of the shoulder bone and the armpit. Good for shoulder and upper back pain, press directly on the muscle. **Point #7,** for relieving shoulder and neck pain, is located 1 inch below the top of the shoulder, between the base of the neck and the tip of the shoulder.

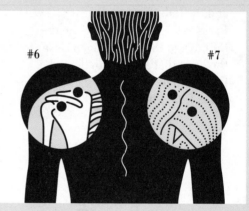

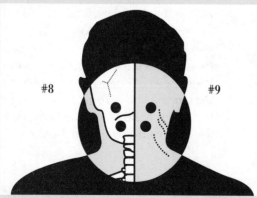

Point #8, for releasing stiffness, rigidity, and pain in the neck and back, is located on the upper portion of the neck about one thumb's-width outside the spine. **Point #9** is located in the hollow below the base of the skull in between two muscles. Good for back pain, stiff neck, and headaches.

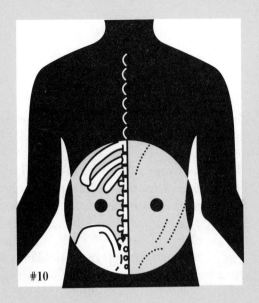

#10

Point #10, for low backaches, is located a few inches out from the spine at waist level. Press the outer edge of the large muscles that run alongside the spine. Use either your thumbs or your fingers, pressing one side at a time or both sides at once. Another way to stimulate these points is to make fists and rub the lower back briskly with your knuckles.

Point #11 is four finger-widths below your kneecap and one finger-width outside of your shinbone. There should be a muscle popping out there when your flex your ankle up and down. Use this point for pain in the knee joint. Use the heel of your opposite foot to stimulate it. Place your right heel on the point on your left leg and rub briskly for 1 minute.

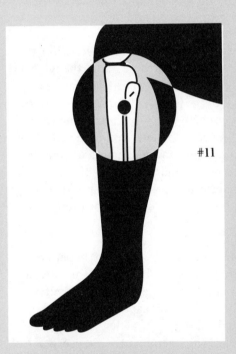

#11

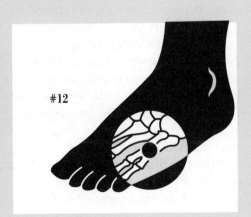

#12

Point #12, located between the fourth and fifth metatarsal bones on the top of the foot, relieves hip and shoulder tension, roving pains, and sideaches. Feel for your bones and place your fingertip between the correct ones, pressing just below the juncture.

ARTHRITIS

Eat to Beat Arthritis

The type of oil that you put in your car has a lot to do with whether it smoothly functions or choppily chugs its way into jalopy heaven. Likewise, research shows that the types of oil you put in your mouth may help to determine whether your joints function smoothly or whether they succumb to the flare-ups of pain and inflammation that arthritis can bring.

The oils you eat don't act exactly like the oils you put in your car. That is, the olive oil in your salad dressing does not ooze its way down into the joints of your fingers and toes and keep them well lubricated. The relationship between dietary oils and your joints is a little more complex than that. Scientists are still reeling in information on which oils help relieve arthritis pain and how they work, but the story seems to be pretty fishy.

Name That Tuna

In one small study of groups of patients with rheumatoid arthritis, half were given fish-oil supplements and the other half placebo (look-alike) capsules. Although the 33 people in the study all had varying degrees of rheumatoid arthritis, every one of them suffered joint stiffness and discomfort.

The study showed that people who took the fish-oil supplements experienced 33 percent less joint tenderness. Furthermore, they were fatigue-free for more than 2½ hours longer each day.

How can this be explained? The theory hinges on substances found in fish oils, called *omega-3 fatty acids*. These acids are thought to inhibit the production of the body

chemicals that are responsible for joint inflammation in people with rheumatoid arthritis.

Luckily, to get all the benefits from fish oil, you don't have to take it by the glassful. Supplements come in capsule form, or—better yet—you can eat delicious fish. You'll be getting plenty of omega-3's if you make fish a regular part of your diet. In particular, you should choose the oil-rich, deep-water types of fish. Good choices are salmon, tuna, halibut, and sardines (packed in water, not in oil).

The Bad and the Not-So-Bad Oils

Of course, most people don't want to limit their oils to the kind that comes from fish. For one thing, fish oil doesn't go well on salads. So what other kinds of oils should you be eating?

As a general rule, vegetable oils constitute a healthy addition to the diet of most people—used instead of butter and lard, they can help lower cholesterol and reduce the risk of heart disease. With a couple exceptions, vegetable oils may not be so good for people with arthritis, however. That's because most vegetable oils are chock-full of the fatty acids called *omega-6's*. Quite unlike their cousins, the omega-3's, the omega-6's *encourage* the body's production of those nasty chemicals that inflame the joints, says George Blackburn, M.D., Ph.D., associate professor of surgery at Harvard Medical School, and chief of the Nutrition/Metabolism Laboratory with the Cancer Research Institute at New England Deaconess Hospital in Boston.

So it's good advice to cut back on most vegetable oils if you have arthritis. That does *not* mean avoiding vegetables, says Dr. Blackburn. Rather, cut back on oil-containing products like salad dressing, fried foods, and margarine. The two vegetable oils that people with arthritis may use are canola oil and olive oil.

Vitamins and Minerals and More

Eating the right kinds of oils isn't the only guideline for a diet that battles the pain and stiffness of arthritis. It's also important to make certain that you eat a well-balanced diet. Nutrients that are especially important for maintaining bone health include calcium (abundant in dairy products, sardines, and collard greens); and vitamins C (citrus fruits, broccoli); D (fish, eggs, most cereals); B$_6$ (avocados, bananas, kidney beans); and beta-carotene (carrots, spinach, sweet potato). Of these nutrients, calcium presents the biggest problem. Many women don't get enough of this mineral, especially if they avoid dairy products. The Recommended Dietary Allowance (RDA) for calcium is 1,200 milligrams for women 11 to 24 years old and 800 milligrams for women 25 and older. You may need a supplement to achieve these totals.

Allergies and Arthritis

For some people with arthritis, there is yet another dietary consideration: food allergies. "A lot of my patients say 'my pain gets worse when I eat tomatoes . . . or orange juice . . . ,'" says Carey Dachman, M.D., director of the

Division of Rheumatology at Chicago's Edgewater Hospital, a lecturer in medicine at the Chicago Medical School, and director of the Suburban Arthritis and Back Center in Shaumburg, Illinois.

Food allergies, unlike inhalant allergies, cannot be determined with a simple scratch test. If you suspect that you are allergic to a certain food and that the food is causing flare-ups of arthritis pain, give that food up for a while and see if the pain goes away. Then, try eating the food again to see if the pain returns.

Theories about the possible connection between arthritis pain and diet abound. For example, Norman F. Childers, Ph.D., a horticulturist who is currently a professor of fruit crops at the University of Florida, gained a following after the publication of his book *Arthritis: Childers' Diet to Stop It!* For 20 years Dr. Childers has claimed that most arthritis is caused by the consumption of certain vegetables belonging to the family Solanaceae, more commonly known as nightshades. Members of the nightshade family include potato, tomato, eggplant, all peppers except black pepper, and tobacco.

Dr. Childers's theory receives little support in the medical community. But while Dr. Dachman does not advocate adherence to Dr. Childers's diet, he does advocate an open mind. "All I know," he says, "is that there are a whole lot of people out there who experience pain when they eat tomatoes. . . . If you find that eating a particular food enhances pain, you should stop eating that food . . . while seeking your doctor's help."

Beware of the Quacks

Pet rocks. Soft drinks for dogs. A lot of things Americans are snookered into spending money on are harmlessly amusing. But some offerings are neither harmless nor amusing. They are simply fraudulent. And there is more health fraud in arthritis than in any other disease, says the Arthritis Foundation—which makes one wonder why people with arthritis are such targets.

The explanation might start with the staggering size of the market. Roughly one in seven people has arthritis; with a market that large and so many dollars available, it's inevitable that quacks will try to hawk their wares, says Robert Karsh, M.D., a rheumatologist at the Overland Medical Center in St. Louis, associate professor of clinical medicine at Washington University Medical School, and a consultant to the Veterans Administration in rheumatology.

There Is No "Cure"

A second reason there's so much quackery in arthritis is that most forms of the disease have no real cure, says Dr. Karsh. "So you have lots of people, many in pain, all looking for a cure that doesn't exist." The fact that there is no cure doesn't stop some people from peddling them and others from eagerly snapping them up.

Third, "there's a widely held myth that doctors can't do anything for arthritis, and that's not true," says Dr. Karsh. This myth causes people to feel helpless and hopeless.

In truth, while your doctor can't cure you of arthritis, there's a whole lot doctors can do to help alleviate your pain and discomfort and help you live a normal life, says Dr. Karsh.

What's Hot on the Market?

You don't want to fall prey to a quack, but how do you recognize one? (It's a known fact that very few carry business cards that say "John Doe, Certified Quack.") First, it might help if you knew what's been hot on the market the past few years.

Here are a few "remedies" from the files of the Arthritis Foundation. These have been categorized by foundation experts as "suspicious." (That is, they are clearly unproven.)

- Anti-arthritis vaccines
- Hormones (male or female)
- Medication "discoveries," such as Gerovital H3
- Sea products (seawater, mussel extracts, seaweed bracelets)
- Vibrators
- Massage products
- Radioactive gadgets
- Magnets
- Copper bracelets
- Sitting in old uranium mines
- Mineral springs
- Homeopathic therapy
- Sesame seeds in the navel

Many of these therapies are not harmful; the big danger is that the person using them is lulled into thinking he's going to be cured and may avoid proper treatment that really can help.

Other occasionally touted therapies, however, can actually do a lot of harm and may even be fatal, says Floyd Pennington, Ph.D., group vice president of education at the Arthritis Foundation national headquarters in Atlanta.

Among these are:

- Snake venom therapy
- Unsupervised fasting
- Steroid drugs
- Very large doses of vitamins
- DMSO (an industrial solvent that some have tried rubbing into their joints)

In addition, the foundation warns against a gadget called Detoxacolon, which is a pressurized enema that could potentially spread infection and perforate the colon wall. They also warn people about visiting Mexican clinics near the U.S. border that offer pills to patients without revealing what they contain.

How to Protect Yourself

Every year Detroit changes its car models, and the fashion industry is forever raising and lowering hemlines. So, too, the marketers of bogus arthritis remedies regularly change their product lines. How can you evaluate a new arthritis product you see advertised to determine whether or not it's likely to help you? Here are a few things to look for.

"Based on a secret formula." Scientists share their discoveries so that other experts can review and question their results. A claim that only its inventor knows about a new discovery signals an unproven remedy, says Cody K. Wasner, M.D., clinical assistant professor of medicine at Oregon Health Sciences University School of Medicine.

"Cures all kinds of arthritis!" There are at least 106 types of arthritis with widely varying causes and treatments. It's highly unlikely that one treatment will ever cure them all, says Dr. Wasner, who teaches medical ethics through the Department of Philosophy at the University of Oregon. "Saying something 'will help all kinds of arthritis' is like saying something 'will fix your car'—that's stupid; you have to know what's wrong with the car."

"Available only through this limited offer!" Treatments for arthritis are available from many different providers of medical care, not just a single person or company. "Sure, it's *possible* that a great breakthrough in arthritis care will come through a post office box somewhere in New Jersey—but you don't want to be the first one to try it anyway," says Dr. Wasner.

"It worked for me! . . . J. P. in Hollywood, Calif." Scientists look for a treatment to show improvement in a large number of people by repeating studies and using statistical tests to show that the results are not due to chance or to wishful thinking. "J.P.," of course, may also be the brother-in-law of the guy who owns the company that placed the advertisement.

ASTHMA

It's easy to take the air we breathe for granted. After all, it's free. But to the asthma sufferer, air is always an extremely precious commodity.

During an asthma "attack," the airways in the lungs narrow. The person having the attack often feels a tightness in the chest, a dry cough, and breathlessness—not to mention fear that sometimes borders on panic. Having one's supply of air gradually squeezed off is anything but a pleasant experience.

Who Gets Asthma?

Asthma is a common disease; more than 10 million Americans have or have had asthma during their lives. The condition often starts in childhood—40 percent of the 10 million people afflicted are under age 16—and tends to disappear or become less serious with age. Boys suffer more frequently than girls.

Asthma attacks are typically triggered by pollens, house dust, animal fur, and other common substances.

Tobacco smoke, air pollution, hair sprays, perfumes, cleaning fluids, and other irritants can all bring on an attack. Stress and anxiety also increase their likelihood. Even exercise, particularly in cold weather, can be a problem.

Whatever triggers it, a bout of asthma can last minutes or it can last days.

Fortunately, learning as much as you can about what brings on problems for *you* and taking certain precautionary measures can lessen the frequency and severity of attacks. And if you *do* have one, knowing how to deal with it can make all the difference.

Step One: Get Tested

If you suspect you have asthma, it's a good idea to see a doctor, says Mark Shampain, M.D., a Pennsylvania allergist and immunologist. The doctor will probably give you a breathing test known as a spirometry. To take this test, you breathe into a tube connected to a machine that measures how much air you can blow out in a given time.

If the test shows that you aren't breathing out as much air as you should, the doctor will have you use an inhaler that contains a medication that opens the air passages in your lungs. If this medication, known as a bronchodilator, actually helps increase your air flow, the doctor will probably diagnose asthma and prescribe an inhaler for you to carry with you. (For some tips, see "How to Use Your Inhaler" on page 61.)

Manage and Prevent Attacks

Making sure you have that inhaler with you at all times is important. Your medication won't do you any good if you feel an attack coming on while you're sitting in a movie theater, and the inhaler is at home in a bureau drawer.

The Strangler Within

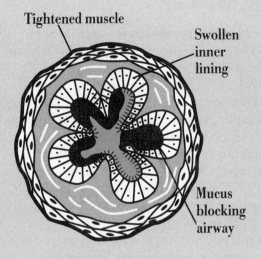

Cross section of normal bronchial tube

Smooth muscle

Inner lining

Cross section of bronchial tube during asthma attack

Tightened muscle

Swollen inner lining

Mucus blocking airway

During an asthma attack, the bronchial tubes—the main tubes through which air passes to the lungs—scrunch up like little fists, leaving hardly any room for air.

What else can you do to deal with those frightening episodes?

It's important to try to relax, says Dr. Shampain. Breathe slowly. If you can make yourself do it, concentrate on relaxing your entire body, right down to your toes, while taking deep, slow breaths. Try pursing your lips as if you were whistling, he says. Breathing through this small opening forces air to stay in your lungs, pushing the breathing tubes open.

You might also find it helpful to drink warm fluids. They help your bronchial tubes relax, says Dr. Shampain. In fact, the best warm beverage may be a cup of coffee. The caffeine in coffee is a natural bronchodilator, he says.

To prevent asthma, avoid whatever it is that triggers your attacks. This advice may not be as easy to take as it is to give. At times, you may be faced with a hard decision, such as whether to give up your beloved kitten or puppy.

To further avoid irritants, wear a face mask when gardening or mowing the lawn. Stay away from damp, weedy areas. Plan your activities for later in the evening and try to stay indoors on hot, windy days. If you have allergies, don't let them get the upper hand.

Allergies can cause the tissue lining in your bronchial tubes to become swollen, which can lead you headlong into a full-blown attack. (See the chapter on allergies on page 2 for other tips on keeping your allergies under control.)

ASTHMA

Exercise Care

Many people who have asthma tend to avoid exercise because they find that it leaves them feeling winded. So they simply don't work out. Actually, it's a good idea to exercise regularly. With time it should make breathing easier. That's the finding of Francois Haas, Ph.D., who directs the pulmonary-function laboratory at New York University Medical Center.

Walking is an ideal exercise. In cold weather, keep a scarf or mask over your mouth and nose to help warm the air before it reaches your lungs. If walking leaves you too winded, try swimming, suggests Dr. Haas. The warm, humid air you breathe while swimming in an indoor pool helps relax the airways in your lungs, explains Dr. Shampain.

Monitor Yourself

Finally, in your quest to prevent asthma attacks, you can easily monitor your breathing by purchasing what's known as a peak flow meter at your local pharmacy for about $20. Some people have a hard time sensing the onset of an asthma attack, and this little device measures the amount of air you are breathing out at any given time.

An early warning will let you reach for that inhaler sooner or take other measures to short-circuit that attack—such as relaxing, leaving a room that might contain suspected allergens, or reaching for a cup of coffee.

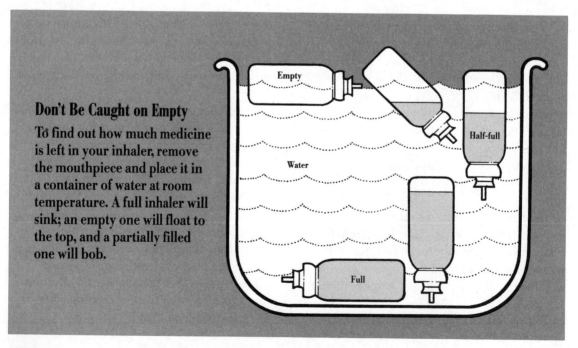

Don't Be Caught on Empty

To find out how much medicine is left in your inhaler, remove the mouthpiece and place it in a container of water at room temperature. A full inhaler will sink; an empty one will float to the top, and a partially filled one will bob.

Empty

Half-full

Water

Full

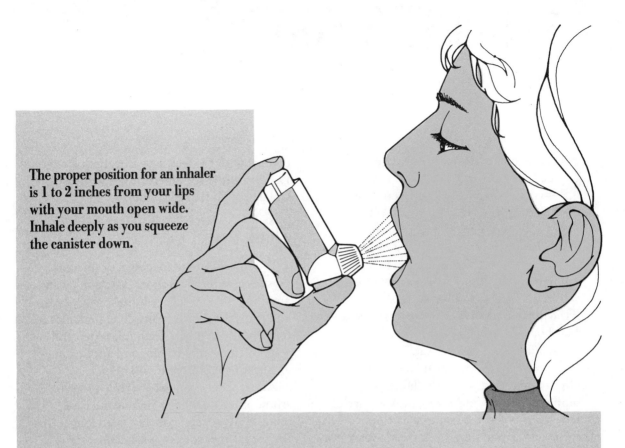

The proper position for an inhaler is 1 to 2 inches from your lips with your mouth open wide. Inhale deeply as you squeeze the canister down.

How to Use Your Inhaler

A tiny canister with a mouthpiece. . . . It looks simple enough, but the medication delivered by this device can literally be a lifesaver for people with asthma.

Actually, the mechanism is deceptively simple. A person whose doctor recommends using an inhaler is likely to have a lot of questions about its proper use.

Inhalers are a first defense against wheezing for nearly everyone with asthma. But the key to getting the most relief from your inhaler is to use it properly. Here are some tips from Thomas Plaut, M.D., author of *Children with Asthma: A Manual For Parents.*

- Put the mouthpiece on the inhaler canister.
- Stand up.

- Shake the inhaler for 2 seconds. (This is extremely important—if you don't shake it, you may get a spray that contains no medication.)
- Hold the inhaler with the mouthpiece on the bottom and the canister above.
- Hold the mouthpiece 1 to 2 inches from your lips and open your mouth wide.
- Exhale naturally, then . . .
- Begin to inhale slowly while you . . .
- Squeeze the canister down on the mouthpiece and . . .
- Inhale deeply for 5 to 6 seconds.
- Hold your breath for up to 10 seconds.
- If your doctor instructs you to take a double dose, repeat this procedure.

SOURCE: Thomas Plaut, M.D., *Children with Asthma: A Manual for Parents* (Amherst, Mass.: Pedipress,Inc., 1988).

61

ATHLETE'S FOOT

Curious name, athlete's foot. There's really nothing athletic about this miserable, itchy fungus, except its persistence. When it takes hold of your toes, it refuses to let go. The moisture produced by the 125,000 sweat glands in each foot offers too hospitable a climate for the fungi to leave willingly. Nasty things like *Trichophyton rubrum* and *Tricophyton mentagrophytes*, two of the many faces of athlete's foot, set up their households. You have to be a little wily yourself if you want to evict it.

Your body will do its share, too. That's why you may find your skin flaking off, taking on a white, oniony look. And that's why you may feel a burning sensation.

One of the best things you can do for a foot so afflicted is to expose it to the light of day. Kick off your shoes and let the sun shine between your toes; enjoy the air circulating freely around them. Applying cool compresses will relieve the inflammation. And a salt-water soak can help soften the skin.

Be sure to protect the rest of you—and your family—from the infected dead skin that's flaking off. Those skin flakes contain living fungi that can reinfect you. So give your shoes at least 24 hours to air out between wearings. Putting them out in the sun for a while helps control the fungus. Remember to protect yourself in public locker rooms and beach houses by wearing thongs or shower sandals.

For your family's or roommate's sake, don't share bath towels, bath mats, or anything moist and porous that comes in contact with the feet, says Elizabeth Roberts, D.P.M., professor emeritus at the New York College of Podiatric Medicine.

Think Dry

When it comes to footwear, don't wear plastic or waterproof shoes. You don't want anything on your feet that makes you sweat and traps the moisture inside. Think clean, too. A daily foot bath with mild soap and water, a thorough drying, and application of an antifungal ointment will help.

Athlete's foot can take a while to heal. Allow at least a month for a severe case. Some really severe cases last even longer. In the meantime, consult your doctor right away if your feet are excessively itchy or if pus or blisters appear. Seeing your doctor is doubly important if you find something strange on a toenail, says Dr. Roberts.

"Athlete's foot is much more difficult to handle once it gets under the nails," she emphasizes. "You may not feel any discomfort, but there may be a discoloration. If you see yellowing or whitening of the nail, or if it starts to separate from the toe, see a doctor."

And don't be a stoic. Don't think you must just suffer through "this little annoyance" until it goes away. Allowed to spread unchecked, athlete's foot can be a foot in the door for a fungal invasion. But with proper care you can give athlete's foot the boot before it creates something more serious than itchy toes.

Deborah Grandinetti

FAST·FREDDY·FOOTSMELL'S
6 EASY STEPS TO BEAT ATHLETE'S FEET!

WEAR THONGS IN THE LOCKER ROOM.

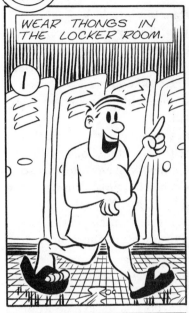

TOWEL DRY YOUR FEET AND BETWEEN YOUR TOES.

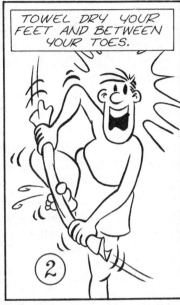

USE A BLOW DRYER ON YOUR FEET AND TOES.

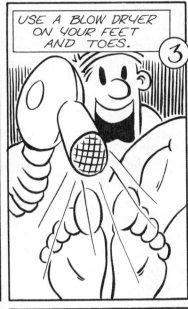

PUT POWDER ON YOUR FEET AND IN YOUR SHOES.

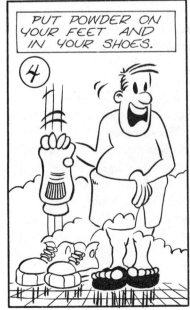

WEAR COTTON SOCKS.

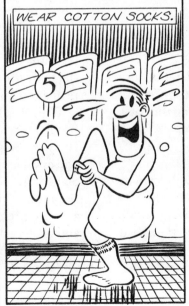

WEAR CANVAS OR WOVEN LEATHER SHOES.

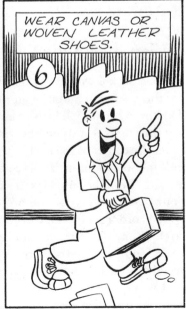

BACK PAIN

Olga Korbut's back sang of suppleness and grace as she arched toward the floor. Peggy Fleming's dazzled as she extended over the ice, her back and leg one continuous line in a breathtaking spin. Baryshnikov's conveys power as he executes a leap.

What a beautifully expressive part of the body the back can be. Yet it's capable of some not-so-beautiful expressions, too. Dull aches. Shooting pains. Prolonged agony.

It's probably back pain that's brought you to these pages, right? Well, you should know that there are ways to short-circuit the pain and prevent its reoccurrence. Once you learn the secrets of the back—how it's built, how you're meant to use it—you can keep yours supple, strong, and pain-free, no matter how many candles are on your birthday cake.

Designed for Action

Your back is worthy of consideration just for the wisdom inherent in its design. Doctors who specialize in treating the back say they marvel at its engineering.

At the center of the back is the spinal column, that continuous line of bone that extends from the base of your skull down to your bottom. This column protects the spinal cord from injury. Curves were built in so this bony structure could keep your head, chest, and pelvis—structures of various weights—balanced over each other.

The 34 bones that comprise the spinal column are called vertebrae. Twenty-four of them are separate but interlocking; the other 10 are fused. In between the vertebrae are the disks—round little cushions of tissue that allow for some movement between the back bones. The disks compress when you lift weight and release like a spring when you remove the load.

Over 140 muscles attach to the spinal column and help support it. The muscles work interdependently; if any one muscle weakens, it can pull the spinal column out of alignment and make it vulnerable to injury. Tendons connect these muscles to the vertebrae, and ligaments connect the bones to each other.

Fanning out from either side of the spine, in the spaces between the vertebrae, are 30 peripheral nerve roots. They extend from the spine to every single part of the body. Think of the spine as the body's central information-relay system. Nerve impulses traveling between the brain and the rest of the body use these nerve pathways as their primary highway.

While the back is beautifully built, it's not problem-free. An estimated eight out of every ten Americans will suffer from at least one episode of back pain in their lives, says Stanley A. Herring, M.D., a Seattle physiatrist and University of Washington clinical assistant professor of rehabilitation medicine and orthopedics. He adds that back pain is the number one cause of disability for people under age 45, and the number three cause for people 45 and older.

And the incidence of back pain is on the

rise. In fact, reports of back pain have increased 14 times faster than the population itself, says David Lehrman, M.D., founder and director of the Lehrman Back Care Center in Miami, Florida, and chief of orthopedic surgery at St. Francis Hospital. He thinks he may know why.

"Our grandparents spent their days exercising and being active—chopping wood, tilling the soil," he says. "These motions work the back, knees, hips, and arms to bring about balance in the body system. Today, as executives and office workers, we're doing more straining than strengthening of muscles. Sedentary lives lead to muscular imbalance."

Why Your Back Hurts

Muscle sprain or spasm is the most common cause of back pain. Remember those 140 associated back muscles? Well, people who use them frequently—day laborers, athletes—sometimes tend to suffer from back pain. But people who make a heavy demand on these muscles every once in a while—weekend athletes and employees whose jobs require occasional lifting—might be in for extra trouble.

Too much demand on a weak muscle can cause it to spasm, which is your body's way of saying, "Cool out. If you push me beyond my limits, I'm going to tighten up so you can't do it again." Sometimes a group of muscles gets into the act, contracting in pain

and immobilizing the injured area.

You experience that contraction as pain. As these contracted muscles tighten, the small blood vessels in them narrow, and that means less oxygen and nutrition from the blood get carried into the muscle cells and more wastes remain. Chronic tension caused by emotion can create the same constricted circulation.

Other times, the problem concerns the relationship of the vertebrae to each other and to the disks. A prolapsed or slipped disk can pinch a peripheral nerve. That pinched nerve may cause problems elsewhere in the body. A disk can become so badly squeezed that part of it is forced out from between the vertebrae. If the disk in question is pressing on the sciatic nerve, a major nerve in the body with branches throughout the lower body and legs, you have sciatica. Sufferers experience this as a burning sensation shooting down the buttocks and thigh.

Sometimes you'll feel back pain even without back injury. Kidney problems, for example, can masquerade as mid- to lower back pain. Other potential sources of back trouble are the pancreas, gallbladder, lungs, heart, and major blood vessels.

Your Mind Can Set You Up

Attention to the way your back works won't exempt you from back misery, however. Modern research suggests you have to take your mind into account, too. The link between emotional stress and muscle tension is well accepted.

In fact, John Sarno, M.D., a physiatrist and professor of clinical rehabilitation medicine at New York University's School of Medicine and the author of *Mind Over Back Pain*, believes that muscle tension resulting from emotional stress causes back pain most of the time. In his view—and it's a provocative one that his fellow physicians aren't quick to embrace—you'll rid yourself of pain if, for example, you confront your inner conflicts.

If you tend toward migraine headaches, stomach ulcers, heartburn, asthma, colitis, or allergies, you could be a victim of what Dr. Sarno calls tension myositis syndrome (TMS). According to his theory, TMS sufferers repress feelings that generate mental conflict. "In the attempt to avoid the unpleasant feelings, the brain creates a painful muscle condition to focus the person's attention on the body rather than on the feelings," says Dr. Sarno. In other words, if you deal with a mental conflict by shutting off your feelings, your back muscles may do the talking for you.

"I think everybody has some of the personality characteristics that make him susceptible to TMS," says Dr. Sarno. "The emotional factors behind the tendency to generate anxiety and anger are virtually universal. Anyone who is concerned about what's going on with his family, his job, is a potential candidate."

Dr. Sarno advises his patients to recognize tension as a source of pain and examine their lives to find the cause of that tension. Face

In Pain? Shift into "Neutral"

Sometimes just changing position will be enough to temporarily halt back pain, says David Lehrman, M.D.

Here are three good postures to try. Start with the one to the right. Experiment—gently—until you find one that eases your pain. The "correct" posture is one that will help support the normal curve in your spine and will place the least pressure on the irritated disk(s) and affected muscles.

"Once you're in 'neutral,' that position where you feel minimal pain, do some basic stretches that don't cause pain," says Dr. Lehrman. "Always start activities in neutral. Progress from neutral."

Find a chair low enough to allow you to lie with your hips on the floor, your feet resting on the chair, and your knees forming a right angle. Place a small, flat pillow beneath your neck. Now relax your jaw, tongue, and forehead. Rest for a few minutes in this position with your eyes closed.

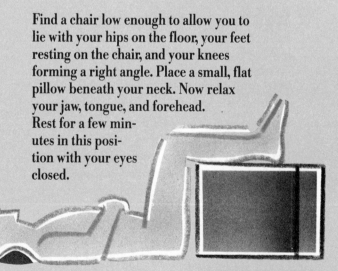

the conflict consciously, and you free the back from its role as mirror of the unresolved conflict, Dr. Sarno says.

Keep Your Back Strong, Supple, and Pain-Free

Your back was built for use. Barring permanent disability, there's no reason not to jitterbug the night away or spend an afternoon digging in your garden. Preventive care can preserve these pleasures for you through the years.

"I think that one of the grossest misconceptions people have about the back is that it is vulnerable, weak, and easily injured," says Dr. Sarno. "That's not true. I always emphasize the strength and power of the back."

To keep yours that way, our experts advise the following: Exercise to keep your back muscles flexible. Learn to lift without injuring yourself. Sit, stand, and walk in ways that use the back as it was designed to be used. Become proficient at releasing tension before it builds up in your back.

Exercise Is Key

Exercise is particularly important. The backs most immune to disabling pain belong to the physically fit.

A University of Copenhagen study of 105 backache sufferers found that long-term regular exercise offered the most improvement by far. Another study of 1,652 Los Angeles firefighters, published in the *Journal*

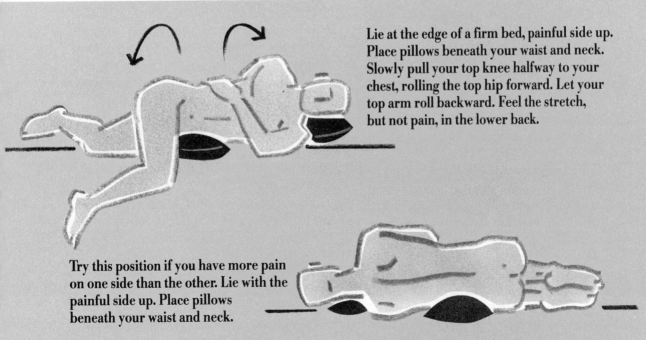

Lie at the edge of a firm bed, painful side up. Place pillows beneath your waist and neck. Slowly pull your top knee halfway to your chest, rolling the top hip forward. Let your top arm roll backward. Feel the stretch, but not pain, in the lower back.

Try this position if you have more pain on one side than the other. Lie with the painful side up. Place pillows beneath your waist and neck.

of Occupational Medicine, found that those who were the most fit were ten times less likely to develop back pain as those with the lowest levels of fitness. Firefighters in the elite, superfit group who suffered back injury did not injure their backs again. Their fitness seemed to offer them a measure of protection against recurrence.

Function Follows Form

Using the back as it was meant to be used is also important. Few people understand the dual nature of the back. If they did, they'd be much less vulnerable to injury from improper lifting.

"The back was designed to be capable of two opposite functions," says David Imrie, M.D., author of *Goodbye Backache* and *The Backpower Program* and director of the Back Care Centre in Toronto. "It can bear weight, and it can move. The foundation of a house can bear weight, too, but it can't move."

Dr. Imrie says the whole secret to having a pain-free back is to separate the moving and the weight-bearing functions. In other words, stabilize the spine before you lift, to eliminate unnecessary movement. But when you're not lifting, move that back tissue plenty to keep it loose.

Correct posture is important even when you're not lifting. If yours is less than ideal, you have your work cut out for you. "Unlearning bad habits takes time," says Dr. Lehrman. "It's a process."

"Most people in their daily routine don't think about back safety," he says. "They're slouched in front of the TV set or reading a book. Slouching and other repetitive low-grade risk postures gradually cause problems."

Dr. Herring agrees. "It's not the one time you bend over to tie your shoes that throws a disk out. That disk was ready to go. It's like the fan belt of a car. You don't know it's bad until it breaks."

Good-Bye Pain

Sometimes when you're in pain and have been for a while, it's hard to imagine you'll ever feel better. But physicians who specialize in back care say that even chronic back pain is treatable.

Dr. Herring says that what surprises his patients most is learning that they'll get better. "A great majority of people, even those with a slipped disk, will get better without surgery," he says.

Take proper care of your injured back, and you're likely to find that time is your ally. Ninety percent of people who suffer an acute episode of back pain feel better within a week, says Dr. Herring.

"With muscular pain, the significant symptoms may resolve in two to three days. Yet you might continue to have some discomfort for 4 to 6 weeks, a mild ache, perhaps, as the tissue heals," he says. "When you tear the fibers of a disk, usually the problems resolve in 3 to 12 weeks."

How can you tell if you have a disk problem? "Usually, you'll have much more difficulty bending forward and sitting down," says Dr. Herring.

If you're in pain right now, here's what you can do, on your own, to get relief.

• If you have muscle soreness, try applying moist or dry heat for 15 to 20 minutes at a time. The warmth will improve circulation to the muscles, helping them flush out wastes. After you apply the heat, try to gently stretch the affected muscles.

- If you've managed to bruise your back, try cold packs for the first day or two. Then switch to heat. Again, be sure to gently stretch the muscles after you apply either cold or heat.
- Get a partner or pro to massage your tense back. (See "Massage to Melt Away Aches" on page 84.) It's always a good idea to see your doctor before allowing deep massage on a troubled back.
- If you suspect stress is contributing to your back pain, try progressive relaxation, visualization, biofeedback, or any relaxation technique that works for you.
- Allow yourself time to heal, but don't overdo the bed rest. Your back—not to mention the rest of you—needs some physical activity.

When You Need to See Your Doctor

There are limits to self-care, however, especially when you're dealing with as vital a part of the body as the spine. Consult your doctor pronto if your back pain is unusually severe and is accompanied by progressive numbness or weakness, loss of bladder or bowel control, or unexplained fever or weight loss.

It's possible the back pain is a signal that something deeper is amiss—a tumor, problems with the kidney, pancreas, or uterus, an infection of the urinary tract or spine, endometriosis, or "any of 100 other things," says Dr. Herring.

Pain-Free Doesn't Mean Fully Healed

You can have the beginnings of muscle strain in your back and not be aware of it until the onset of pain. But even when pain subsides, it doesn't mean the muscles involved are back in perfect shape.

"Absence of symptoms doesn't mean normal function," says Dr. Herring. "The acute injury might heal, but you could be left with functional deficits—poor flexibility, reduced strength—that can cause problems to recur. It's important to assess what changes have occurred in the spine that will set you up for future injuries."

Once you identify the weaknesses, you can gradually begin to strengthen the affected areas or learn how to move in ways that don't add further injury.

A back-care expert can help you tailor a program of exercise and posture correction for your body. You might find a podiatrist helpful, too.

"My bias," says Dr. Herring, "is that there is no one fix for back pain. It's foolish to think you can take a pill or do an exercise or any one thing to correct the problem. Demand a physician who has an understanding of all the causes and is not married to any one solution. I do think there are sound principles that can be followed. It is worth seeking out a physician who understands how to manage your back pain and who can deal with issues of disability."

Deborah Grandinetti

POSTURE: THE BEST BACK INSURANCE

Posture. You hear the word and immediately you think of a set of rules: "Shoulders back, tummy in, backside in, head up." Well, forget the rules. Good posture doesn't come naturally to most of us. Yet there is a posture natural to the body, one that acknowledges its design and recognizes the force of gravity.

Posture is dynamic, too. You need to consider not only the way you stand but also the way you position your body each time you move. The way you cradle the telephone between your shoulder and your ear when you're standing at your sink washing the dishes—that's posture, too. Poor posture.

Your spine was designed to balance your head over your rib cage, and your rib cage over your pelvis, without placing undue stress on itself. The S shape in the spine helps achieve this balance. That's why it's important to maintain the natural curves in your back.

What are the components of good posture? "Your head is over your shoulders. Your shoulders are not thrown back. There is a natural curve in your lower back. Your pelvis is level, not tipped. Your weight is centered over both legs," says Stanley Herring, M.D., a Seattle physiatrist and University of Washington clinical assistant professor of rehabilitation medicine and orthopedics. "You don't want to be too swaybacked or too far bent forward," he adds. "Keeping your lower back in that position allows for proper muscular function and good flexibility of your pelvis, hips, chest, and legs."

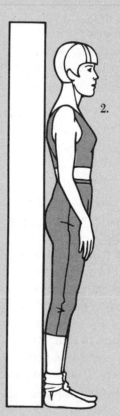

Here's a way to let your body teach you how the correct spinal curve should feel. Stand against the wall. Tuck your chin in and tilt your pelvis forward. This position flattens the spine so the small of your back is closer to the wall. Now stand away from the wall, hold your stomach in, and tuck your tailbone under. Work with this until it feels natural.

To check your posture, stand with your back flat against the wall. Now check the distance between your midback and the wall. There should be enough room for you to slide your fingers between your back and the wall, but not enough room to move your entire hand through the space. If your whole hand fits through, you may need to correct your posture.

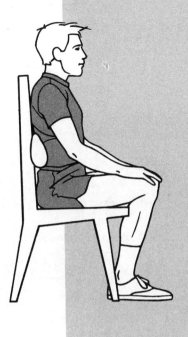

Maintain the natural curve of the spine when you sit by placing a small cylindrical pillow between the chair and your lower back. Make sure the pillow is small enough to allow your upper spine to rest against the chair back. If you can, adjust the chair so your feet rest flat on the floor. A low footrest also can help you keep your back flat. Chairs with arms are good bets because arms allow you to push yourself out of the chair with relative ease.

Adjust the seat in your car so you can reach the pedals and the steering wheel without stretching. Tighten your seat belt so it helps hold the lower spine against the seat back. You might also benefit from placing a cylindrical pillow between the seat and your lower back. Again, be sure to place it so your upper back can rest against the car seat.

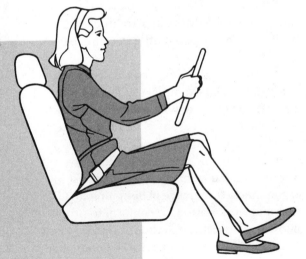

BACK PAIN

WORKDAY STRETCHES TO KEEP YOU LOOSE

So you think your office job is cushier than a construction worker's, huh? Well, your back might not agree.

"Sitting increases the pressure on your disks 300 percent," says David Lehrman, M.D., founder and director of the Lehrman Back Care Center in Miami, Florida, and chief of orthopedic surgery at St. Francis Hospital. "It's a really stressful posture for the lower back. This constant beating on our disks is like overinflating a tire 300 percent. Eventually, the tire will explode."

Give your back a break, Dr. Lehrman advises, by getting up at least every 30 minutes. And really stretch.

"Spend a minute doing neck rotations, working the shoulders, and arching your back. Give every part a little stretch," he says.

If you constantly lean forward over your work station, for example, you'll want to counter the pressure with exercises in which you stretch up and arch back. This will help equalize and normalize the disks.

Standing helps "reset" the back, says Suzanne H. Rodgers, Ph.D., a specialist in ergonomics (the science of designing furniture and work stations to conform to proper body mechanics) and author of *Working with Backache*. "Muscles work with the body skeleton to properly align the body. But they get tired after you've been leaning over a desk for a period. So stand up and reset yourself."

Here are some exercises to get you started. With the right moves, even the standard office chair can become exercise equipment.

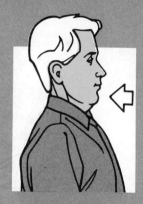

Adjust your neck by sliding your chin back while you keep your ears level. Repeat five to ten times.

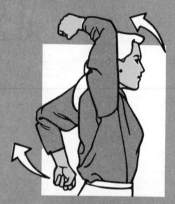

Bend both elbows. Press one above you, the other behind you for a good stretch.

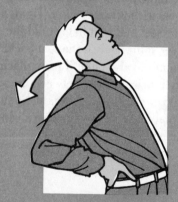

Stand up. Press your palms on your lower back for support. Gently arch up and back; hold for a moment.

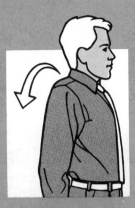

To loosen those shoulders, circle them backward several times, then relax. Now circle them forward.

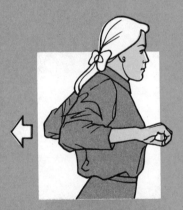

Press your elbows out and back at chest height as far as you can. Hold.

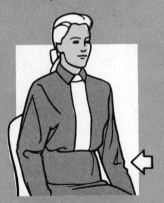

Sit back against a chair. Exhale and tighten your abdominal muscles for a count of ten.

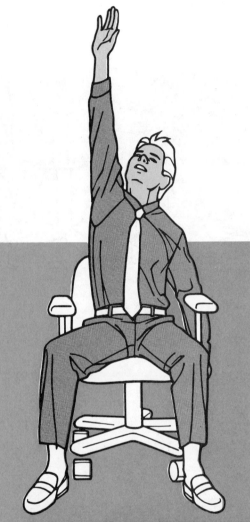

Sit with your back and bottom pressed firmly against a hard, straight-backed chair. Lift your right arm from the shoulder, following the movement with your neck and eyes. Hold for a few seconds and really feel that stretch. Now, lower your arm and relax for a moment before repeating with the left arm. Repeat the entire sequence three more times.

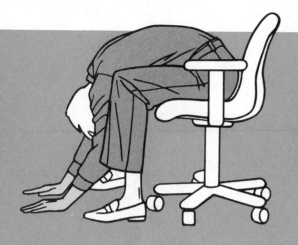

This is a movement sequence. Sit back against a chair. Now reach your arms behind you and grasp the sides of the chair. Arch up and over. Next, lean forward and down, trying to put your hands on the floor and your head between your knees.

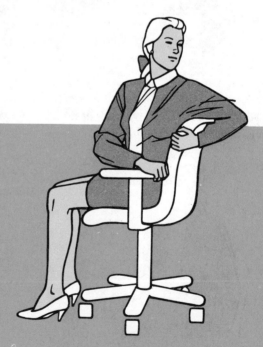

Sit up straight. Place your hands behind your waist, and arch your back. Then grasp the side of a chair on one side and twist at the waist to that side. Repeat on the other side. Then repeat the entire sequence three more times.

LIFT IT RIGHT

Tote that barge. Lift that . . . ouch. Hold it.

Before you hoist that next load you should know that there are specific ways to lift objects so you don't hurt your back. Problem is, most of the time when you lift something you're on automatic pilot. Unless you have back pain to remind you, you simply pick things up without thinking.

Wouldn't it be great if the body could just automatically remember all of the rules of smart lifting?

Well, there is a way to get your body to remember. You'll have to invest some effort initially, but after that, the body responds automatically.

The key is learning how to align your pelvis just so.

If you get your pelvis into proper position, your spine naturally lengthens. In this elongated position, your spine is at its strongest. That makes it capable of absorbing extra weight without straining. Your disks, which act as fulcrums to support the weight being lifted, are more likely to rupture if the spine is strained.

What's the proper position? A "neutral" one, which is midway between a ramrod straight spine (with your stomach muscles pulled tightly in) and swayback (with its overexaggerated curve), according to David Imrie, M.D., author of *Goodbye Backache* and *The Backpower Program* and director of the Back Care Centre in Toronto.

How do you find "neutral"? Here's one way.

Sit in a straight-backed chair. Now scoot out a little bit so you can place your hand in the hollow between your back and the chair. Cross one leg over the other and feel your pelvis push into your hand and the back of the chair. Notice how your abdominal muscles draw in and tighten, making you much more aware of them than you were a moment ago. This is "neutral," the correct posture.

Now uncross your legs and feel how the band of muscle across your abdomen relaxes. This allows your pelvis to tip forward. Your back may begin to arch. You want to avoid this posture.

Cross your legs a second time and again notice the difference. Your pelvis is now balanced in such a way that if someone were to draw a horizontal line across the top of it, that line would parallel the chair seat. Practice this "balanced pelvis" posture until it becomes automatic. You may need to strengthen your back muscles and abdominal muscles before you assume this position naturally without your legs crossed.

How does all this relate to lifting? Well, if you make sure to align your pelvis correctly, the rest of your body will automatically assume a safe lifting position, says Dr. Imrie.

The secret, he says, is to stabilize your spine when you lift. Steady does it. Eliminate all movement of the spine.

Most people aren't strong enough to stop all spinal movement, he adds. Lifting draws on the power in the muscles of our abdomen, back, side, buttocks, and upper legs. If any of these muscles is underdeveloped, you use the muscles unevenly. That can injure the back.

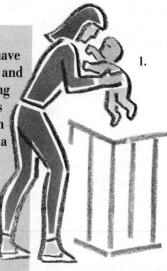

When you have to lean over and lift something up to you, as you do when you pick up a child from a crib, assume a lunge stance first.

1.

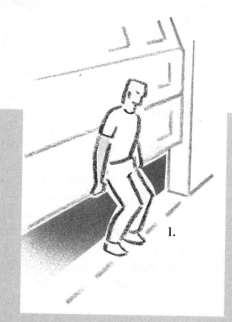

1.

The back-saving way to open your garage door is to turn your back to it, then squat down, and lift it behind you. Opening the door while facing it can strain your back.

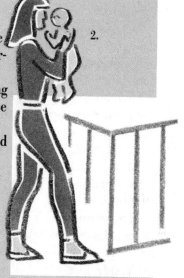

2.

From the lunge stance, bend forward from the hips. Then bring the child in close to your body. Only then should you straighten up. You can use this technique anytime you have to bend down to lift something. Always bring heavy objects in close to your body.

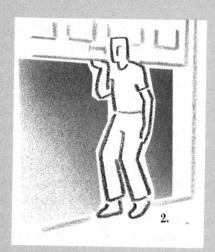

2.

Once you raise the garage door as high as you can, turn to your side. Using one shoulder and arm, continue to lift the door all the way. Let your knees bend.

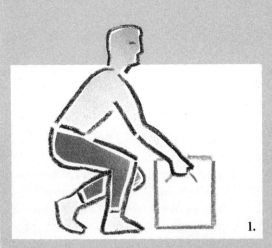

1.

When you're lifting any heavy object, the first part of the body you want to use is your head. That is, *think* first. Make sure you can handle the load. Then bend down at the knees and get as close to the object as you can. Make sure your footing is stable.

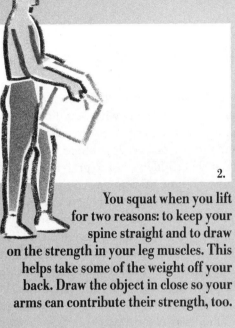

2.

You squat when you lift for two reasons: to keep your spine straight and to draw on the strength in your leg muscles. This helps take some of the weight off your back. Draw the object in close so your arms can contribute their strength, too.

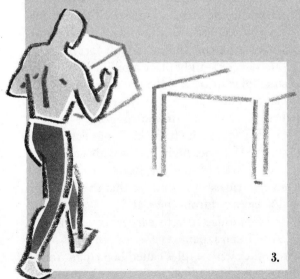

3.

The important thing to remember when you are standing and holding a weight is to avoid twisting your spine. The straighter your spine, the stronger it is, and the more capable of bearing weight. Otherwise, you could cause disk problems.

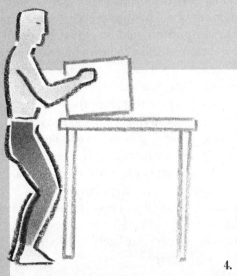

4.

To lower a weight, come in as close to it as possible. Be aware of your spine. Is it straight? Good. Now tighten the abdominal, trunk, and diaphragm muscles. Get a stable grip, then bend your knees as you lower the object.

THE RIGHT MOVES

Back pain can ambush you so suddenly you're left wondering what you did. Was it leaning over the sink to brush your teeth or trying to pry open that jammed window? Was it that sudden twist to grab the phone?

Any of those movements could have been the immediate cause. But chances are, the injury has been building for some time. Think of each improper movement, each step in inappropriate shoes as a drop of water wearing away at stone. Over time, the water will carve right through the stone.

A little knowledge of body mechanics can go a long way toward preventing back pain. Become aware of how your body feels when all the parts are aligned properly, and you'll know intuitively how to move in any activity.

There are good reasons to make the effort. Remember that the back bones house the spinal cord, which transmits the impulses traveling between the brain and the rest of the body. Emerging from the gap between each vertebra are pairs of peripheral nerve roots. These nerves carry messages of vital importance to every part of your body. Damage them, and you may impair muscle function or sensation. Irritate a nerve, and you could trigger your back muscle to clamp tighter and tighter.

Keeping in Shape the Pain-Free Way

If you are vulnerable to back pain, there are three kinds of movement you want to avoid, says Roger Minkow, M.D., founder and director of Backworks in Petaluma, California.

"One is anything that would compress the spine, like over-the-head lifts, such as stacking wood over your head," he says.

"Second is forward or backward bending," says Dr. Minkow. "These movements can increase pressure on the disks if the spine is not kept straight. By bending at the hips instead of the back, pressure can be reduced."

Be wary, too, of activities that require you to twist the torso, like shoveling snow, stacking wood, or freestyle swimming.

Make Your Car a Pain-Free Zone, Too

Your car is another common instigator of back pain, especially on long drives or traffic-jammed roads. Fight back by revamping your car seat. You can buy a metal frame with contouring in it made just for this purpose, or simply place a pillow behind the small of your back. If you're ambitious, you can do a little surgery on the car seat itself. Here's what Dr. Minkow suggests.

"Buy foam 1 inch thick. Cut a rectangle that's 5½ inches high, and as wide across as the backrest of your car. Bevel the edges with an electric carving knife so that the smaller side faces out from the seat."

Then unfasten your car seat covering. "Almost all Japanese car seats are put together with staples called hog rings. You can take these off with pliers and slip a foam cushion inside the seat behind the upholstery. American cars have zippers. Usually, you can reach underneath the back of these seats and unzip them," he says.

Place the foam on the backrest at a height even with your belt line and secure. Then refasten the upholstery. Voilà!

The Morning Swing

Ease out of bed by rolling onto your side. Prop yourself on an elbow. Now swing your legs over the side and use your hands to push up so you're seated.

The Airport Lift

How do you remove luggage from an airport baggage carousel without straining? First, get as close to the suitcase as you can. Then bend at the hips and knees and tense your lower back muscles. Now slowly pull the bag in toward you. Again, that's *in*, not *up*. Easy does it; don't jerk the luggage.

The Backseat Reach

You're in the driver's seat and your briefcase is in the backseat. How can you bring it up front painlessly? First, rotate your body 90 degrees to the right. You can rest your knees on the seat if you want. Then grasp the briefcase and pull it toward you. Don't try to lift it straight up.

Back Pain

The Overhead Juggle

To lift your luggage into a plane's overhead compartment, lift slowly and steadily. Always stand close to the compartment. Tense your back, bring the load in close to your body, and lift in increments. First bring it to your chest, then above your shoulders, then into the compartment. To get your luggage down, reverse the steps. Keep that bag in close.

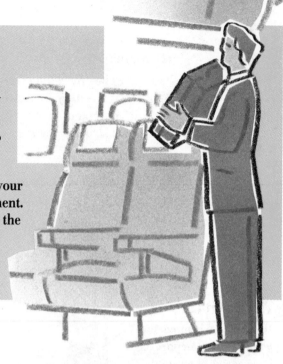

The Shoestring Trick

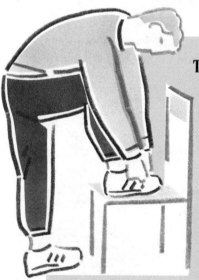

If you want to tie your shoe without aggravating back problems, you have two options. You can get down on one knee or put your foot up on a chair. This way you'll have much less of a reach.

The Gardening Maneuver

Garden to restore your health, not endanger it! Kneeling—on one or both knees—can save your back from the strain of stooping. If you have to, support your weight with one hand on the ground. Short-handled tools and cushioned knee pads can make proper back positioning a cinch. Vive la différence!

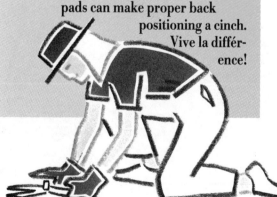

The Bedspread Crawl

The back-saving way to make a bed is to kneel on the bed with one knee. Use the one arm and hand to brace yourself as you smooth the covers with the other.

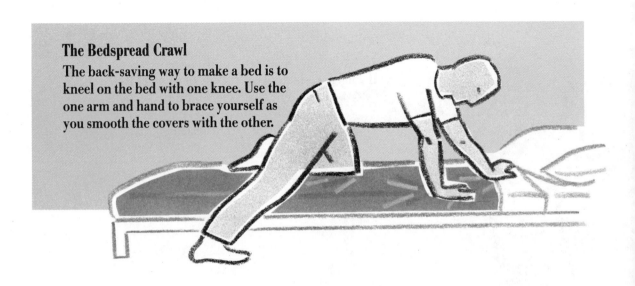

The Car Trunk Caper

To remove something from your car trunk, slide the object close to you. Then bend at the hips and knees, tense your lower back muscles, and hoist the object toward you (not vertically). Keep it in as close to you as you can.

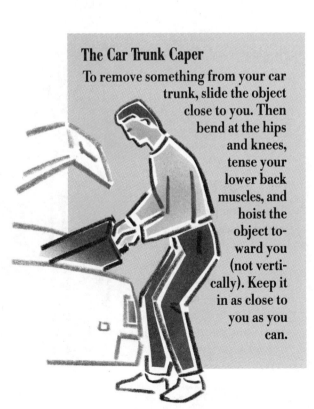

The Beach Chair Shuffle

Lift yourself gracefully out of a low chair by sliding forward toward the chair's edge. Now slide your heels back so that they're even with the edge of the chair. Push off, using your arms.

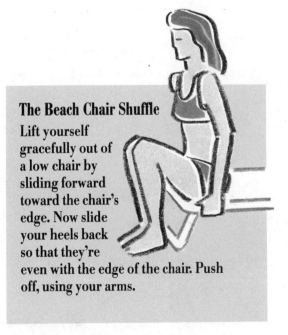

81

BACK PAIN

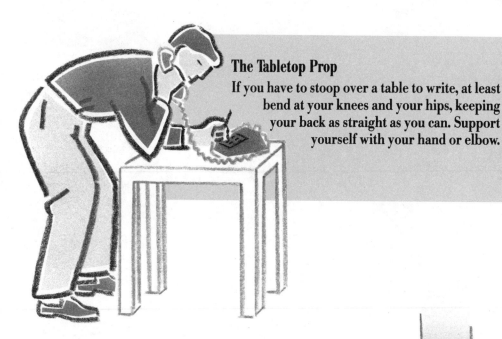

The Tabletop Prop

If you have to stoop over a table to write, at least bend at your knees and your hips, keeping your back as straight as you can. Support yourself with your hand or elbow.

The Lowdown on Scrubbing

Pay attention when you scrub the floor. Don't sit on your heels and bend forward. Instead, get down on all fours. Keep your head in line with your spine. If you place paper towels or old cloth towels under your knees, you can make this position much more comfortable.

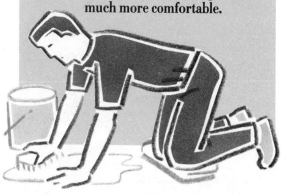

The Painter Principle

How do you paint without inviting back pain? Stand close enough to the wall so you don't have to stretch. Try to move your arms no lower than your waist and no higher than your shoulder. Aids like rollers and paint guns can be real back-savers.

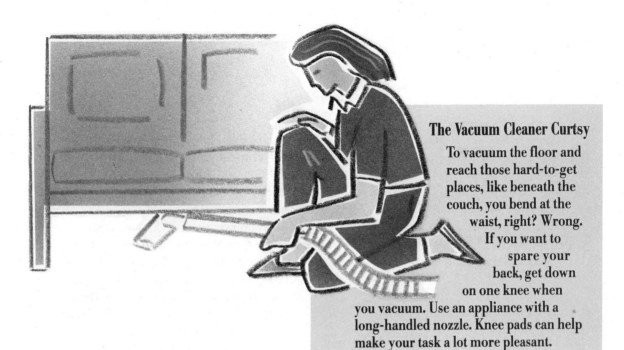

The Vacuum Cleaner Curtsy

To vacuum the floor and reach those hard-to-get places, like beneath the couch, you bend at the waist, right? Wrong. If you want to spare your back, get down on one knee when you vacuum. Use an appliance with a long-handled nozzle. Knee pads can help make your task a lot more pleasant.

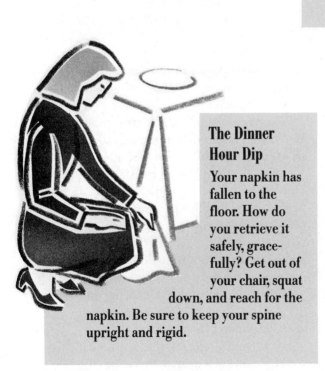

The Dinner Hour Dip

Your napkin has fallen to the floor. How do you retrieve it safely, gracefully? Get out of your chair, squat down, and reach for the napkin. Be sure to keep your spine upright and rigid.

The No-Backache Bow

If you have to get into something that sits low to the ground, such as a filing cabinet, the oven broiler, or the dishwasher's lower shelf, bend one knee or squat down. Don't bend at the waist.

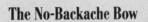

83

BACK PAIN

MASSAGE TO MELT AWAY ACHES

"Oo-oo-oo-oo-oh, yes. Right there."

It feels so good you could just melt. What a difference between now and how you felt 5 minutes ago, pain burning through your lower back, your neck and shoulder muscles soldered together in one sorry, aching clump.

This is the magic of massage. Under your partner's soothing hands, muscles start to unfurl, so new blood can bathe the tissues. The blood carries fresh oxygen and vital nutrients and carries away pain-producing metabolic wastes.

As the massage continues, that marvelous sensation of healing touch triggers your nervous system to release endorphins, the body's natural painkiller. Soon your stepped-up circulation carries this elixir of bodily bliss throughout your system. As the massage ends, you feel so great, you may be half-inclined to rush right out and do all those jobs the back pain kept you from.

Do yourself a favor. Don't. Safeguard your comfort. Give your muscles time to remember how good it feels to relax. And if that means resting in a quiet room and ignoring the jangle of the phone, do it. Better yet, head straight for the bathroom. Fill the tub with warm, scented water and ease into it for a good soak.

Sound tempting?

If you decide on a professional massage, find someone who can give you what's known as an "active" massage, says Gene Arbetter, information director of the American Massage Therapy Association (AMTA), located in Chicago.

"You want something that moves the legs,

lifting and stretching them. The therapist will do some softening of the tissue, but there should also be an active component—stretches where the client resists or uses muscles as directed by the therapist."

Realize, however, that massage is no substitute for proper medical care. If you suspect the problem is a displaced disk or an injured nerve, consult your doctor. A good massage therapist will want to know the diagnosis so he can respond appropriately.

"If you have a disk problem that's not properly diagnosed, you wouldn't want deep tissue work in muscles surrounding the spine," says Arbetter.

And if your pain is caused by muscle strain due to poor posture or movement habits, know that massage can only bring you short-term relief.

"Massage is usually a safe treatment plan. But there's no proof that massage alone shortens the disability," says Stanley A. Herring, M.D., a Seattle physiatrist and University of Washington clinical assistant professor of rehabilitation medicine and orthopedics. "In my practice, I use some types of massage to get soft tissue relaxation and flexibility. But rarely do I prescribe massage as the only form of treatment."

With those cautions aside, bring on the massage oil. Your best bet is a pro who knows just what to do.

If you need a referral, the AMTA can give you the name of a nearby therapist who has had at least 500 in-class hours of training in an AMTA-approved school or the equivalent experience.

Basic Massage Strokes

Begin with *effleurage,* a French word for a light, gentle stroke. This warm-up stroke acquaints your partner with your touch. Begin by gliding your hands along the torso, from the neck to the base of the spine; from the shoulder to the fingertips. You can use the palms of one or both hands, your knuckles, fingertips, or the ball of your thumb.

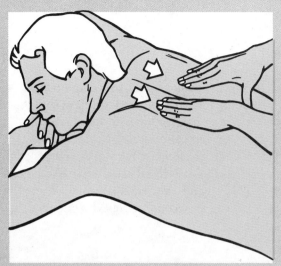

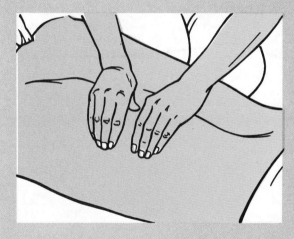

With one or two hands, or with your thumb and fingers, carefully "pick up" muscles and lift them away from the bones. Then roll, wring, and squeeze. This move is called *petrissage.* Direct pressure with your thumbs may be helpful on people who have thick, well-developed muscle. Massage experts say *petrissage* increases circulation, which helps speed the removal of toxins like lactic acid.

Now use thumb and fingertips to trace deep circles near the joints and other bony areas such as the sides of the spine. Also circle the central part of large muscles. This "friction" stroke breaks down knots that result when muscle fibers bind together, giving new flexibility to joints, tendons, and muscles. Follow immediately with *effleurage.*

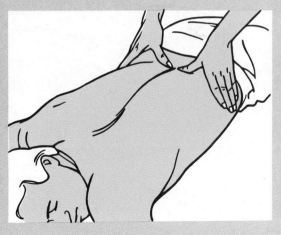

(continued)

The short chopping stroke called *tapotement* can be done many ways. You can chop with the edge of your hand or tap with your fingertips. Clap with your palms or the flat surface of your hands and fingers. You can even beat with the edge of a closed fist. Use *tapotement* for a few seconds to stimulate the muscles or for 10 or more seconds to relieve a cramped muscle.

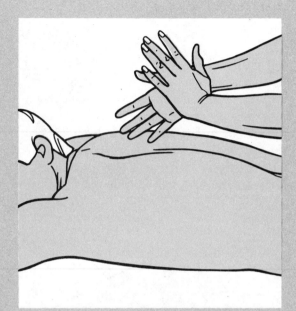

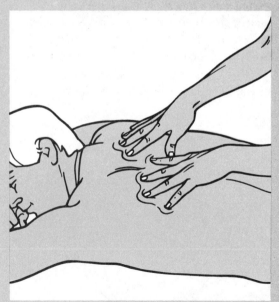

To stimulate the nervous system, increase the activity of the glands, and boost circulation, use a massage stroke known as vibration. Spread your hands or fingers out on your partner's skin, press down firmly, and rapidly shake for a few seconds with a trembling sort of motion. This stroke can help increase the power of the muscles to contract.

To begin the massage, warm a small amount of oil in your palms before applying it to your partner's back. Now you're ready to try *effleurage*, the long gliding stroke. Be sure to lean into the stroke to minimize the strain on your own back. Begin at the neck, slide down the back and up again. Repeat the movement several times.

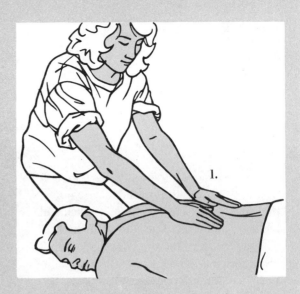

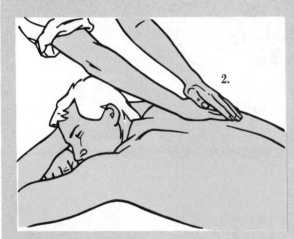

Now that you've acquainted your partner with your touch and helped to warm up the muscles, it's time to work deeper. Place one of your hands on top of the other, press into it, and stroke one side of the back at a time. Repeat several times. Once you get the hang of this movement, feel free to be creative. Have your partner give you feedback on how the movements feel.

Continue the long, soothing, gliding strokes of *effleurage*, alternating light and deep strokes according to your partner's preference. Try using your forearms as well as your hands and fingers. Be careful not to put too much weight on your partner's back.

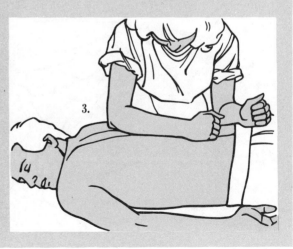

(continued)

You can now move into deeper *petrissage* strokes. With your thumb and forefinger, "pick up" the muscles all along the back and shoulders and gently knead them. Be extra thorough working the shoulder blades, an area where tension seems to collect. If you're not sure how much pressure to use, ask. Take your time with this portion of the massage; rushing ruins the effect.

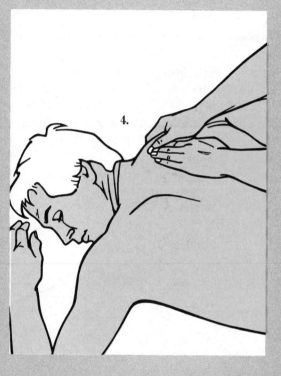

4.

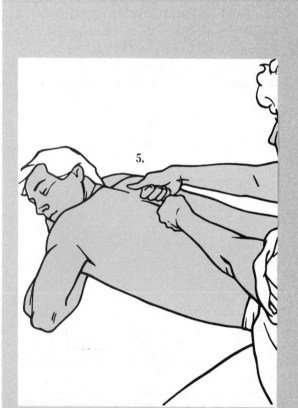

5.

Next, roll your knuckles down the muscles along the spine. Be careful not to apply massage strokes on the spine itself. Go slowly and steadily. Let your partner feel each vertebra. You may want to repeat this stroke a few times and try a variation in which you use a rocking motion of the fingertips in the grooves on either side of the spine.

Petrissage in the lower back can help ease stiffness and pain. You can make it easy on yourself by sitting beside your partner with your legs straight in front of you. Lean away slightly while kneading the muscles just below the waist. Think of yourself as kneading out the knots in the muscle fibers. Have your partner tell you how vigorous you should be.

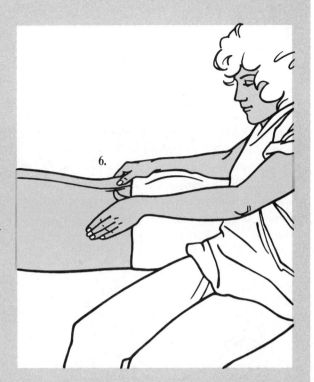

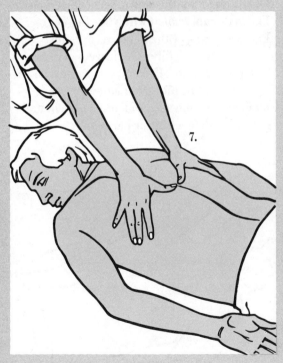

Now that you've thoroughly warmed the back, apply friction by inserting your thumbs in the indentations along the vertebrae and then pressing them out away from the spine. Keep up a nice rhythm. Speaking of rhythms, is your breathing slow and relaxed? Or tense and uncertain? Remember that your own feelings while doing the massage can influence the feelings your partner receives from it.

(continued)

Continue to stimulate the muscles and increase circulation by applying *tapotement*. Cup your hands into a "C" shape and let the sides of your hands make contact with your partner's back. Strike the muscles up and down the back with a chopping motion for several seconds. Keep a steady rhythm. Be vigorous, but make sure you don't hurt your partner.

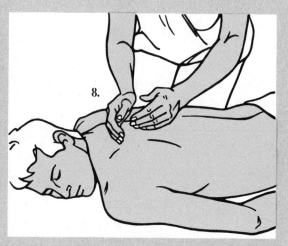

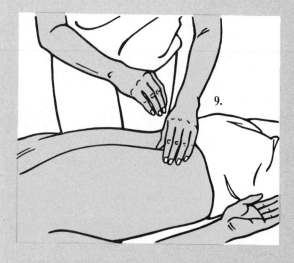

Once you've got this down, see what it feels like to do *tapotement* with your fingers, knuckles, fists, or the flat of your hands. Experiment with different degrees of pressure, different rhythms. Pretend you're a percussion player. The more you enjoy the movement and the more confident you are in it, the better it will feel to your partner.

Vibration is next. Place your fingers at the sides of your partner's spine and press down. Then vibrate them rapidly for several seconds. Move up and down the back. You can also try this with your palms. You can keep the palms separate when you vibrate the back, or make it more intense by placing one palm on top of the other. Remember to breathe calmly as you develop a rhythm.

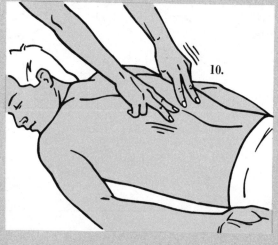

LENGTHENING
AND STRENGTHENING

Maybe you don't need the mighty strength of a Hercules all the time, but you'd sure like to be able to count on your back power when you need it. On those wintry afternoons when you haul in the firewood or when you haul out the trash after a seasonal housecleaning. Or on those days when you lug your bulging suitcase clear across the airport to reach your gate.

What exactly does flexibility have to do with lifting a bundle of firewood? Well, a long muscle is a strong muscle. A muscle has the most strength when it's stretched to 1.2 times its relaxed length, says Suzanne H. Rodgers, Ph.D., a specialist in ergonomics (the science of designing furniture and work stations to conform to proper body mechanics) and author of *Working with Backache.*

So your first step on the road to a stronger back is to help all the tight muscles in your back ease back to their optimum resting length.

"We tend over the years to lose movement by a natural process of sedentary activity," says David Lehrman, M.D., founder and director of the Lehrman Back Care Center in Miami, Florida, and chief of orthopedic surgery at St. Francis Hospital. "Because most people don't exercise beyond a comfortable range, they tend to lose their range of motion, their flexibility."

The muscle groups you need to be concerned about for back strength are the back extensor muscles (the ones along either side of the spine); the abdominal muscles, and the muscles that encase your hip bones, buttocks, and upper legs.

Let's understand why each of these muscle groups is important.

The back extensor muscles help keep the spine in place, and together with the hip muscles, keep you from falling flat on your face when you reach down to lift that firewood. The hamstrings (along the back of your legs) and gluteus muscles (in your buttocks) also help support the spine and allow for movement in the hips.

The stomach muscles (two bands of muscle that reach from the rib cage to the pelvis) keep the spine in place when you turn and twist. When properly toned, they exert a pressure that helps support the front of the spine.

You'll have the greatest range of motion, of course, when your muscles are relaxed and ready to stretch. The trouble is, most of us spend a lot of time flexing our muscles in one direction.

"When you sit or bend forward, you're flexing," says Dr. Lehrman. Flexing a muscle in one direction for long periods of time can shorten and weaken it.

Here is one of his favorite floor exercises to counter the constant forward flexing of your body. This exercise works the hamstrings. Lie on your back on the floor. Bend your right knee, leaving your right foot flat on the floor. Now slowly and gently bring the left leg straight up, foot toward the ceiling. Hold this stretch 20 to 30 seconds. Repeat the exercise, bending the left knee and raising the right leg.

The exercises on pages 92 to 94 will help you gain strength and flexibility.

BACK PAIN

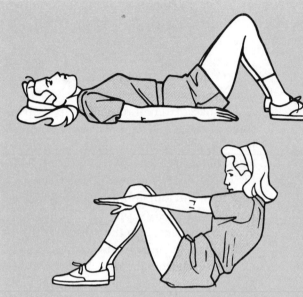

(1) Be sure to warm up before you try this exercise to strengthen your abdominal muscles and help you correctly position your pelvis. Lie down with your arms at your sides, your feet flat on the floor, and your knees bent at a 45-degree angle.

(2) As you exhale, gradually curl your head, shoulders, and upper back off the floor. Keep your chin tucked. Hold for a count of five, focusing on keeping your pelvis in position. Then release slowly. Repeat four more times.

Lie on your left side with your left arm supporting your head and your right arm balancing the body. Position your pelvis as shown at right. Raise the upper leg slowly about 12 inches, then slowly lower. Repeat nine more times on each side.

Once you've warmed up, you're ready to tone the muscles that help stabilize the spinal column. Lie on the floor with your legs straight and your arms at your sides. Lift your right leg as high as possible. Hold for 5 seconds. Repeat five times, then reverse legs.

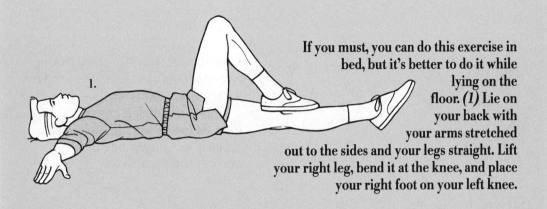

1.

If you must, you can do this exercise in bed, but it's better to do it while lying on the floor. *(1)* Lie on your back with your arms stretched out to the sides and your legs straight. Lift your right leg, bend it at the knee, and place your right foot on your left knee.

(2) Keeping your arms extended and your right foot on your left knee, slowly drop the knee toward your right side. Go only as far as you can; don't strain. Remember to keep breathing steadily.

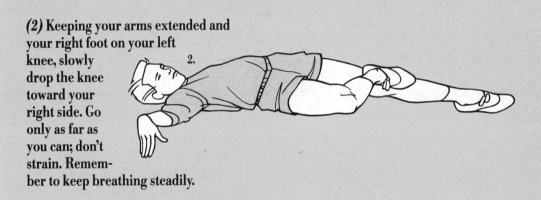

2.

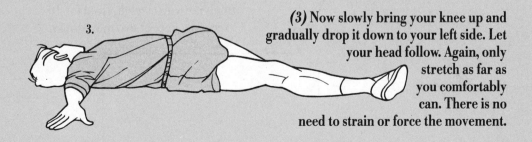

3.

(3) Now slowly bring your knee up and gradually drop it down to your left side. Let your head follow. Again, only stretch as far as you comfortably can. There is no need to strain or force the movement.

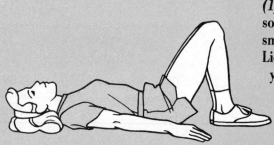

(1) You can use this exercise as a warm-up, so take extra care to make the movements smooth. Do them slowly without jerking. Lie on your back, bend your knees, and rest your feet flat on the floor. Raise your hips from the floor. It is important not to strain too far with this movement. It's okay to come up only slightly if that feels comfortable for you. Hold.

(2) Now slowly return to the original position. Slowly. Try feeling each vertebra as you ease yourself down. Rest a moment. Feel the tension ease. Repeat ten times with a rest between repetitions. Be sure to coordinate your movement with your breath. Exhale when you exert yourself; inhale during the easier movement.

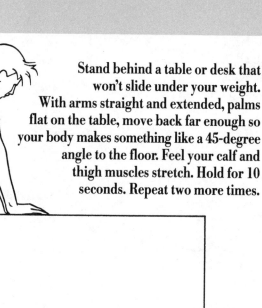

Stand behind a table or desk that won't slide under your weight. With arms straight and extended, palms flat on the table, move back far enough so your body makes something like a 45-degree angle to the floor. Feel your calf and thigh muscles stretch. Hold for 10 seconds. Repeat two more times.

SLEEPING OFF BACK PAIN

For the sufferer of back pain, sleep can offer a blessed refuge.

Even just easing into bed can make a world of difference. How welcome the softness of it, the familiarity, on a day when your back feels so alien.

There are ways you can make going to bed even more soothing. If you're going to be sitting up in bed to read or watch TV, make sure to put a small pillow behind the small of your back, says David Lehrman, M.D., founder and director of the Lehrman Back Care Center in Miami, Florida, and chief of orthopedic surgery at St. Francis Hospital.

And when you're lying down, be sure to choose a position that allows you to keep your spine straight, rather than flexed, says Roger Minkow, M.D., founder and director of Backworks in Petaluma, California.

In other words, don't curl forward into a ball, or you may find yourself waking up with a sore back.

On the next page, we show you how to use pillows to help you keep the spine straight and ease the pressure on it. Placing a pillow beneath the legs, when you lie on your side, is just one way to be extra considerate of your back.

Make sure, too, that your mattress isn't sabotaging your back pain prevention efforts. If yours is about as firm as pudding, chances are your back muscles are under strain every hour you sleep because your spine is bending, causing pressure to build in your muscles, ligaments, and disks. A piece of plywood placed under the mattress and box spring can help you get more mileage out of a mattress that bows in the middle.

Dr. Minkow also advises people with back pain to buy an egg-crate mattress topper made of high resiliency foam, specifically 2.8-pound foam with 30 ILD, a compression measure your mattress salesman will understand. Make sure the foam has some body to it. Place the foam right on top of the mattress. "It will add softness if the plywood makes your mattress feel too hard," he says.

If you have trouble falling asleep, "an ice pack is comforting to use," says Dr. Lehrman. Sometimes switching position will be enough to temporarily ease the pain. If that doesn't work, try changing the mattress. Yours could be too old. A mattress that's too old and soft may also keep you locked in one position all night. That's not good either. Your body is meant to move even while you sleep.

Above all, don't let your backache cheat you out of intimacy. You and your spouse may need to be a little more innovative about positioning yourselves, but there's nothing like good loving to dissolve tension and saturate your system with the body's natural pain relievers.

"Sex is the best relief you can get," says Dr. Minkow. "There are a few points here that are important. It is not uncommon for people with back problems to suffer problems with interpersonal relationships, simply because the partner is listening to a whole bunch of complaining all the time."

Making time for sex can help, says Dr. Minkow. "Don't be afraid of it. You need to relax and experiment to find a position that's comfortable."

Back Pain

Lying flat on your back creates unnecessary strain. See if you can get comfortable lying on your side. If you must lie on your back, minimize the strain by putting a small pillow under your neck and two good-sized pillows under your knees. These pillows will help reduce the curve in your lower back.

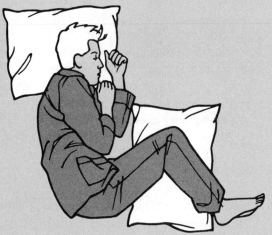

Sleeping on your side with two pillows may be cozier and easier on your back. Place one semifirm pillow beneath your head and a second one between your legs. That cushioning reduces the pull your legs exert on your lower back.

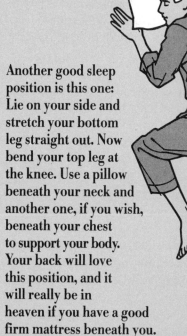

Another good sleep position is this one: Lie on your side and stretch your bottom leg straight out. Now bend your top leg at the knee. Use a pillow beneath your neck and another one, if you wish, beneath your chest to support your body. Your back will love this position, and it will really be in heaven if you have a good firm mattress beneath you.

BITES AND STINGS

It's a perfect day for an outing; the sun at work, the wind at play. So you hike in the woods, explore a marsh, or picnic at stream's edge.

Go ahead and enjoy yourself, but beware. The great outdoors swarms with tiny creatures hoping to feast on you. Other creatures have no interest in you as a source of nourishment, but they may attack to defend their turf.

That painful bite or sting could come from a bumblebee, mosquito, or tick, a snake, dragonfly, or scorpion, a wild animal, or even your neighbor's ill-mannered dog.

A little knowledge is a good repellent. Here's what you need to know to defend yourself and respond appropriately.

Back Off from Bees, Wasps, and Hornets

Common sense and awareness can help you avoid most bee and wasp stings. Let the seasons be your guide. In the spring, keep away from wasps. Some varieties are especially irritable when nest-building. In the summer, watch out for the nests of bees and yellow hornets. Be sure to check that open can of soda for bees before you bring it to your mouth. And don't go barefoot on the lawn.

In late summer through fall, watch out for yellow jackets, particularly in woodpiles. Before you lower your unprotected hands to move logs, check a woodpile to see if it harbors yellow jackets. If you see even one, back off. There are likely to be more.

If you are stung by a honeybee, the only insect that actually leaves its stinger behind, remove the stinger (we show you how on page 98). For any type of sting, apply ice to the area to slow absorption of the venom. Ask your doctor about taking an antihistamine, which may help ease painful swelling. Aspirin also can help.

If you know you're sensitive to bee stings, be sure to keep epinephrine on hand when you're outdoors. It comes in a convenient, easy-to-administer form, very much like a fountain pen. If you have had severe allergic reactions to stings in the past, get medical attention immediately.

Sidestep Spiders

There are two kinds of spiders you need to watch out for: the black widow and the brown recluse. If you are bitten by either one, get medical attention immediately. Both spiders are easy to identify. Black widows have a red hourglass design on their tummies, and brown recluses have a fiddlelike design on their backs.

Treating Animal Bites

Respond to any animal bites by flushing the wound well with soap and water. Consult your doctor about the need for a tetanus shot. If the animal is a pet dog or cat that has

97

not been vaccinated against rabies, quarantine it for ten days.

If you've been bitten by a wild animal and you can capture it, contact your local health department. They can test the animal for rabies and determine whether or not you require treatment. If the animal has escaped, consult your local health department and your doctor for treatment.

Treating Jellyfish Stings

Jellyfish might look like soft, harmless blobs, but these sea creatures can inject venom-coated threads into your skin with a pressure equivalent to 2 to 5 pounds per square inch. These tiny, dormant stinging capsules lodge just under the skin. Don't flush the areas with water, or you'll stimulate the release of irritants. Rather, soak the area with vinegar or meat tenderizer. If you have access to baking soda, make a baking soda-and-water paste. If you're at the beach, rub wet sand into the area—it will work as a counterirritant. But use sand only if you've been able to neutralize the toxins from the sting.

If pain does not subside in a few hours, see a doctor. If you experience nausea, muscle pains, and/or signs of shock, see a doctor immediately.

Get Help for Snakebites

If you are bitten by a snake, there is really not much you can do by way of self-treatment. "The less you do, the better," says Nancy Mellor, a registered pharmacist and poison information specialist with the Arizona Poison Control Center. "Stay calm and, if practical, elevate the bitten area to heart level. But don't take a lot of time with it." The best thing to do is go straight to the emergency room.

And don't use ice, warns Mellor. Snake venom is damaging enough to skin, and an ice pack can give you frostbite on top of that, she says.

How do you avoid snakes? "Just keep your eyes and ears open and look where you're putting your feet," she says.

Deborah Grandinetti

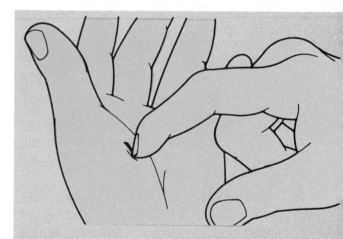

The Right Way to Remove a Stinger

There's a right way to remove a honeybee's stinger and a wrong way. Don't reach for the tweezers or squeeze the stinger because that will only inject more venom into the wound. Instead, use your fingernail, a nail file, or a knife blade to flick it out. Then apply a cold compress to reduce pain and swelling.

Dodge Dogs Before They Bite

You've never seen this strange dog before, and its owner isn't around to vouch for it. How do you judge whether the dog merely wants to give you a "hello" sniff or if it is ready to attack?

In the illustrations to the right and below, we show you how to read dog body language.

If a dog seems threatening, don't look directly into its eyes or it may perceive you as an aggressor. Instead, lower your head and keep your hands down. Speak in a soothing voice, turn slowly to the side, and lean slightly away from the dog.

Here are five more important don'ts.

- Don't trespass on the dog's turf.
- Don't make any loud noises or abrupt movements.
- Don't bother a dog if it's eating or sleeping.
- Don't get between a mother dog and her puppies.
- Don't approach a dog that is injured.

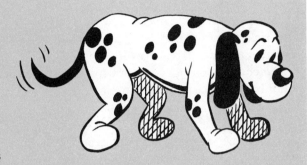

You've heard the phrase "hang-dog look." Well, that's how a friendly dog looks. Its ears are flat, its tail is tucked down, and its body is low. The dog may even expose its throat or grin. Most likely, it won't look directly at you unless it wants your attention. Be aware, however, that even "friendly" dogs can bite if they're provoked.

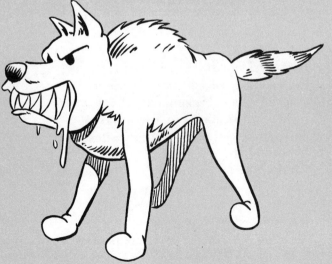

The dog you need to watch out for is the one that tenses its ears and holds them forward, bares its teeth in a snarl, and raises the hair across its shoulders and rump. If the dog stares intently at you, it may be sizing you up for confrontation. Be extra careful if you see the dog stiffen its legs or slowly wag a high, arched tail.

99

Tiny Ticks Can Cause Big Trouble

What you can't see *can* hurt you. Consider the tick, that tiny relative of the scorpion, mite, and spider. If you are bitten by an infected tick, you can come down with any number of unpleasant diseases, including Lyme disease, which can lead to a crippling form of arthritis if untreated.

There are various kinds of ticks and various kinds of medical treatment that are specific to the bite of each. But the best way to protect yourself is to prevent yourself from getting bitten in the first place.

Common sense dictates that you avoid tick-infected areas. Local health officials can help you identify them. If you're unsure, suspect woodlands, marshes, grassy areas—and anywhere deer run free. You can check for tick infestation by dragging a stick with a white cloth attached to it through the underbrush in the area you intend to explore.

When you hike, keep your body covered. Wear a long-sleeved shirt that buttons at the wrist, long pants, and socks. Tuck the pants into the socks to prevent the ticks from crawling up your leg.

It's a good idea to wear white or light-colored clothing because ticks are easier to spot against a light background. After your hike, be sure to examine your skin and your clothing thoroughly. And make sure that ticks don't hitch a ride home on your pet.

Ticks are fairly small until after they bite. Then, engorged with blood, they resemble a blackened blood blister with legs.

If you do get bitten, the tick will hold on for dear life. The sooner you can remove the tick, the better. (We show you how on the next page.) Don't be squeamish about pulling out a little skin with it. The sacrifice is worth it, as fast action may prevent infection.

If you don't find any ticks when you and your partner check each other out, don't assume you're safe. The tick that causes Lyme disease is so tiny you may have a hard time spotting it, and a tick bite isn't likely to be painful enough to attract your attention. Pay attention to your body for the next four weeks; if you find any rashes or red spots that

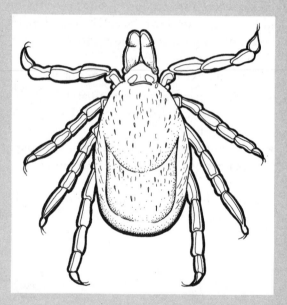

Look closely or you might miss that tick. Tick larvae are about the size of pinheads. Nymphs, the name for a tick in its second season, are about twice that size, while a fully mature tick is about ¼ inch long. The tick has small legs jutting out from its sides and, at its mouth, a sharp probe with backward-pointing barbs on it. The probe is what enters you, draws blood, and injects bacteria.

you can't account for, have your doctor check them out. It's especially important to see your doctor if the rash is accompanied by flulike symptoms.

Depending upon the region and the type of tick, these troublesome little bugs can transmit a whole host of diseases with exotic-sounding names, including Lyme disease, Rocky Mountain spotted fever, Colorado tick fever, tularemia, and babesiosis.

Lyme disease is most common of all. The tick that causes it is so tiny most people don't even know they've been bitten until a rash resembling a bull's-eye shows up.

Rocky Mountain fever will give you a rash two to three days after the onset. Most likely it will break out on your wrists and ankles first, then spread to your trunk, palms, and soles of your feet. Colorado tick fever sets in three to five days after the bite. Expect recurring fever, chills, a headache, and perhaps nausea and vomiting as well.

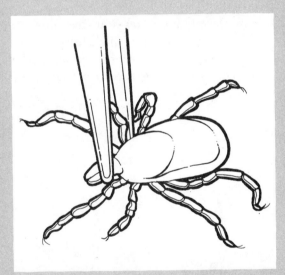

Remove a tick quickly, before it can inject disease-causing bacteria into you. Use tweezers or—even better—thin, curved forceps your druggist can sell you. Grasp the tick as close as possible to the part sticking into the skin. Now pull steadily up without jerking until the tick comes loose. Then disinfect the wound with rubbing alcohol or antiseptic. It's a good idea to keep the tick. Your doctor may want to see it or have you take it to the local health department.

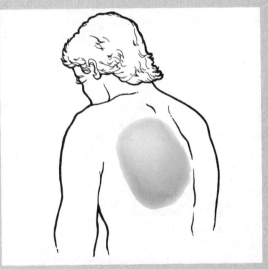

Lyme disease can bring on a characteristic skin rash. Frequently, you'll find a red area that looks somewhat like a bull's-eye at the place where you were bitten. There may be a small welt in the center and a red ringlike rash encircling it. The rash usually appears two to five days or up to four weeks after the tick draws blood from its victim. Left untreated, the rash may reappear at another site on the body. Often the rashes go unnoticed, but they should not be ignored.

BLEMISHES

Amazing, isn't it? We can fly astronauts to the moon and transmit broadcast signals around the world, but we still can't find a cure for that common scourge, acne vulgaris.

Could it be that acne serves some sort of useful purpose—a marker at the crossroads of childhood and adolescence? A mystery of the body/mind continuum that the afflicted adult needs to decode?

The answer may be hidden in the riddle of why a certain small percentage of the population never gets pimples. And why every other mammal in the world is free from acne, even though their hides contain the same trouble-making components.

When you have acne, it means that your body is screwing up two jobs necessary for the maintenance of healthy skin. Your hair follicles aren't getting rid of dead cells fast enough. And the sebaceous glands at the base of the hair follicles pump out too much sebum, the oil that makes your face shine. Dead cells stick to a hair follicle full of sebum and provide perfect conditions for the growth of *Propionibacterium acnes*, the type of

The Oil Crisis

(1) Below each pore, near the base of the hair follicle, are sebaceous glands. They secrete sebum, an oily substance that helps lubricate the skin. Healthy skin excretes sebum and sloughs off dead cells. *(2)* But if dead cells stick to the follicle and the glands secrete too much sebum, the waxy buildup can clog the pores. *(3)* This blockage invites bacterial growth, and pus forms. A plug exposed to air creates a blackhead. (A plug that ruptures the follicle wall becomes a pimple.)

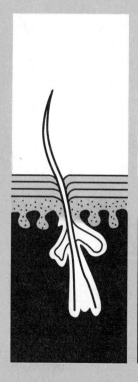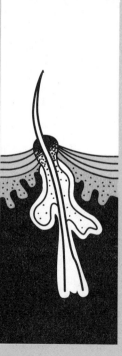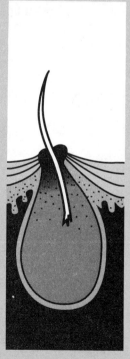

bacteria responsible for the skin eruptions. And that's where the trouble starts. (See "The Oil Crisis" on the opposite page.)

You can help control acne with regular preventive maintenance of your skin. Your first order of business is to loosen oil plugs and rid yourself of acne-causing bacteria. Maintenance requires careful cleaning and the application of an over-the-counter acne medication. Cleaning doesn't mean scrubbing the bejabbers out of your skin, however. In fact, overenthusiastic scrubbing can weaken the follicle walls and make your skin more likely to become irritated by your topical acne cream. Most dermatologists recommend washing your face with a mild soap.

Once you clean your skin, apply a topical preparation to reduce the acne bacteria. Clinical trials have shown benzoyl peroxide products help by reducing the acne bacteria and inflammation, enhancing blood flow to the skin and speeding the rate at which the body excretes sebum.

Try a 2.5 percent solution of benzoyl peroxide before you try any of the stronger solutions. Doctors maintain that for most people, the percentage of benzoyl peroxide in a product doesn't make any difference in terms of its effectiveness.

In addition to caring for your outer covering, also take a look at the inner you. The problem with acne, you should pardon the expression, may be more than skin deep.

Anxiety and anger were found to be significant contributors to severe cases of acne in one University of Southern Florida

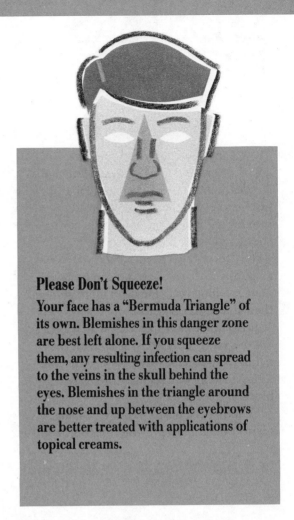

Please Don't Squeeze!
Your face has a "Bermuda Triangle" of its own. Blemishes in this danger zone are best left alone. If you squeeze them, any resulting infection can spread to the veins in the skull behind the eyes. Blemishes in the triangle around the nose and up between the eyebrows are better treated with applications of topical creams.

study. Another study, published in the *Journal of Laboratory and Clinical Medicine*, showed that acne sufferers had an increase in pustules days after the study team induced anger during an interview. These same researchers found that suppressing anger helped make acne worse. If anger and anxiety are your constant companions, you might consider seeing a professional counselor to help you deal better with stress—for more reasons than just clearing up your complexion.

Deborah Grandinetti

103

BLISTERS

Maybe you've gripped your pruning shears too tightly and too long, or absentmindedly reached for a burning pot handle. Maybe you've jammed your feet into hiking boots that don't respect the contours of your feet.

Whatever the irritant, when your skin responds with a blister, you can be sure your body is telling you, "Hey, I'm more vulnerable than you think. Careful!"

Blisters are most likely to form where skin doesn't yield easily, like the skin on the palms of your hands and the soles of your feet. Movable skin seems more resistant to blisters.

Whether the blister is large or small, your main concern is to prevent infection while it heals. For a small blister, the wisest thing you can do is protect it, perhaps with a moleskin if it's on your foot, and then let nature take its course. The fluid will gradually be reabsorbed and the top skin will peel off as layers of new skin push up from beneath it, says Andrew Lazar, M.D., clinical instructor of dermatology at Northwestern University Medical School, Evansville, Illinois.

But if the blister is likely to pop, go ahead and drain it. (We show you how below.)

"Don't unroof the blister," warns Dr. Lazar. "The roof acts as a barrier to infection. If you remove it, you're down to the floor and that area isn't protected. Remember, we all have bacteria on our hands and feet."

Deborah Grandinetti

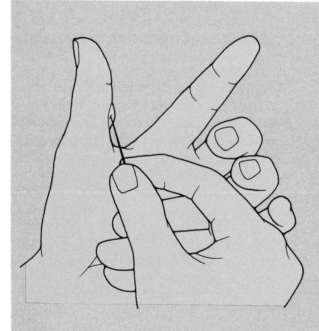

Home "Surgery" for About-to-Break Blisters

To lance a large blister that is likely to break, assemble soap, a needle, gauze, 70 percent isopropyl alcohol, and an antiseptic. First, wash the area with soap and water and swab with antiseptic. Disinfect the needle with alcohol, then use it to lightly puncture the roof of the blister in just a few places. Press the blister gently to drain, but be careful to leave the roof of the blister intact. This protective covering will help prevent infection. After you've drained the blister, apply an antiseptic and cover with sterile gauze.

Boils

Colloquial expressions aren't always precise. For instance, everyone knows that blood doesn't literally boil when you get mad. But the skin *can* boil, especially in places where it gets rubbed the wrong way a lot. Exhausted, the top layer of skin lets down its guard. Before you know it, a noxious gang of bacteria slips through and picks a fight.

The body responds with a vengeance, and the resulting immune system warfare causes inflammation, swelling, and an unsightly accumulation of pus.

Such battle sites—known as boils—are common on the arm, groin, back, buttocks, inner thighs, and "anyplace where skin gets rubbed," says Andrew Lazar, M.D., clinical instructor of dermatology at Northwestern University Medical School, Evansville, Illinois.

If you see a boil developing, apply warm compresses several times a day to help bring it to a head. Continue the compresses for a few days after the boil opens to help drain the pus.

You might also want to take showers instead of baths to minimize the likelihood of the infection spreading to another area. And be sure to wash your hands well before you touch food. The germs that cause the boil can multiply in warm food and produce toxins that cause food poisoning.

If the boil fails to open or if you have recurring boils, consult your doctor.

You should also consult your doctor if the boil is particularly tender or under thick skin like that on the back.

Deborah Grandinetti

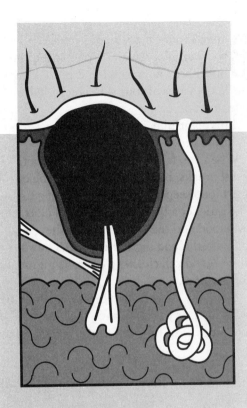

When Your Skin's Aboil

To you a boil may seem like no more than a tender, red bump. On the microscopic level, however, it's a battlefield. A boil is your body's response to staph bacteria that have managed to sneak past the protective barrier of your skin. Surveillance cells from your immune system detect the intruders and dispatch white blood cells to wipe out the invaders. Pus forms as these blood cells, bacteria, and dead skin cells collect.

BRUISES

anged yourself again, did you? Maybe you weren't even aware of it at the time, but there's no mistaking it now. All of a sudden, an area of your skin fancies itself a kaleidoscope.

This colorful parade reflects what's going on inside you.

When you fall or suffer a blow, a blood vessel breaks, blood escapes, and some of that blood seeps into the surrounding tissue. The quicker a broken blood vessel clots, the less blood and the smaller the bruise. As spilled red blood is gnashed to bits by your white blood cell clean-up crew, its pigmentation changes.

A healthy body heals a bruise in about 10 to 14 days. As the body ages, healing may take longer. Aging is not the only factor that needs to be considered in healing, however.

Certain medications interfere with the body's clotting mechanisms. When you take aspirin or ibuprofen (Advil or Motrin, for example), you bleed more easily because it affects the function and number of platelets in the body. That means your bruises may take longer to heal.

There's not much you can do to make the bruise go away faster, says Recia Kott-Blumenkranz, M.D., a Michigan dermatologist.

If you sustain an injury that you expect will cause a bruise, apply a cold compress. This will help to control the swelling and relieve the pain. If the bruise or pain persists for more than 14 days, see your physician.

Deborah Grandinetti

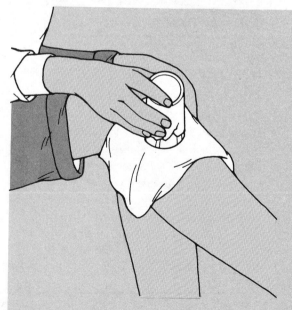

Keep Relief in Your Freezer

Ka-thwa-akk! Expecting a bruise? Soothe it with ice. Fill paper cups with water and put them in the freezer, so you'll have them when you need them. The Mayo Clinic recommends this method of treating a bruise: Elevate the injured part above the level of the heart. Then peel away the top of an ice cup. Place a cloth on the bruised area and circle the area with the ice. Continue the ice massage for no more than 30 minutes. Repeat two to four times a day.

BRUXISM

Did our cave-dwelling ancestors instinctively grind their teeth to razorlike sharpness so they could better chew their pterodactyl teriaki? We may never know. But some New Zealand researchers suggest that a primitive tooth-sharpening instinct may explain why as many as 80 percent of all adults grit and grind their teeth at night.

To be sure, only about 20 percent of us meet the criteria for a serious form of bruxism: unconscious nighttime chomping so hard and loud that it can actually break our teeth, strain our jaw muscles, give us headaches, and—because of the grinding noise—sometimes even endanger our marriages.

It's no wonder that the practice does such damage: During a typical grinding session, 200 pounds of mouth pressure per bite is exerted—fairly intense teeth gnashing for a tired roommate to endure. "When you have that much force coming together, something's got to give," says Noshir Mehta, D.M.D., of the Gelb TMJ Center at Tufts University in Boston. He says he's seen patients who have reduced their molars to "stubs," only to do the same to their new dental work.

The caveman theory—which suggests that like most rodents, ancient man instinctively ground his teeth sharp—isn't exactly gospel in the medical community. In fact, most doctors aren't sure what causes bruxism. Because of the higher-than-normal incidence of it among victims of Down's syndrome,

some experts suspect that genetics may be at the root of the problem.

Other experts think stress plays a significant role, says Elliot Gale, Ph.D., director of the Oral, Facial, and TMD (temporomandibular disorder) Disorder Clinic at the State University of New York at Buffalo. Anticipatory stress (such as the kind experienced the night before you ask for a big raise) probably sets the choppers chomping more often than events that have already transpired (such as the boss saying no), Dr. Gale says.

To avoid tooth damage in severe bruxism cases, doctors often prescribe dental appliances, usually small plastic mouth guards that prevent teeth from striking against each other. Dr. Gale also advises patients to make sure their teeth touch only when they're chewing or swallowing—the rest of the time the jaw should be relaxed with the teeth slightly apart.

But in at least some cases, reducing stress has apparently been successful in halting bruxism. Researchers at the University of Western Ontario were able to completely eliminate bruxism and jaw pain in a 20-year-old woman in just four weeks, using relaxation techniques.

Warm compresses will help soothe the jaws of nighttime gnashers if they are painful. And avoiding foods that are hard to chew may prevent them from becoming sore, says Calvin J. Pierce, Ph.D., assistant professor of behavorial science at the University of Pittsburgh.

Brian Kauffman

BRUXISM

GIVE THOSE WEARY JAWS A BREAK

It's bad enough that bruxism damages teeth, dental work, and sometimes (because of the noise) even marriages. But if you have it, you probably know how relentless it can be.

Although there's no known cure, stretching may help soothe away some of the tension that contributes to the problem. Exercises for the neck, shoulders, and face can also help reduce stress. Unwinding while you're awake just may keep you from tooth grinding while you're asleep.

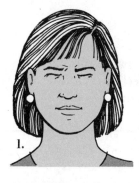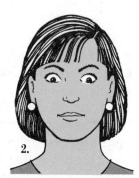

Concentrating on paperwork or a computer screen can short-circuit your facial muscles. *(1)* Close both eyes tightly. Tighten all your facial muscles for a full 10 seconds. *(2)* Then open your eyes wide and relax all the muscles. Repeat.

Ease Facial Tension

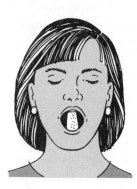

Stretching your jaw muscles helps relieve soreness. Place a cork upright between your top and bottom front teeth for 3 to 4 minutes. Make sure the cork is ¼ inch smaller than your mouth at its widest.

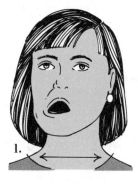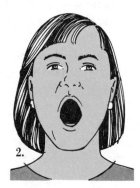

Avoid the mirror when trying this one: You might scare yourself. First, relax your facial muscles. Next, open your mouth and eyes wide and stick out your tongue. Hold and repeat.

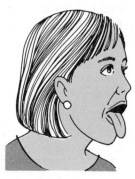

Here's a movement that will help stretch your jaw muscles. *Above left,* Open your mouth, then carefully shift your jaw from left to right. Repeat several times. *Above right,* Another face relaxer: Open your mouth as wide as possible while dropping your lower jaw. Repeat.

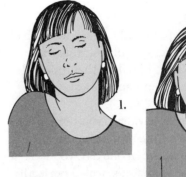

Tension lives and breeds in the neck and shoulders. Slowly rolling your head clockwise and then counterclockwise will help relax and soothe those muscles.

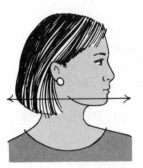

It sounds simple—but sometimes the best advice is. Holding your your head straight, slowly look over your right shoulder, then your left. Carefully repeat ten times slowly, and then ten times at a faster pace.

Relax Your Neck and Shoulders

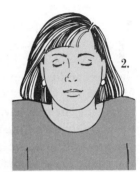

Shoulder shrugs strengthen the neck and shoulder area and help work out the kinks associated with stress. Shrug each shoulder, hold for 2 seconds, and repeat on the other side. Then shrug both shoulders. Repeat several times.

Massage, Don't Grind

Massage alone is no cure for bruxism. For someone who's spent most of the night clenching his jaw and grinding his teeth, a gentle rub along the side of the neck and head should provide soothing relief. Using the acupressure points along the jaw also can ease the pain of toothache caused by bruxism. While you're at it, don't forget the shoulders and upper back. People with bruxism tend to hold a lot of tension in those areas.

To stimulate the acupressure point that relieves aching teeth, place a single finger on the jaw just below the ear and press firmly. Repeat until you obtain relief.

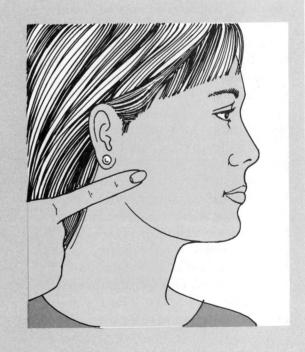

BURNS

You grab the pot handle, feel a hot stab of pain, and quickly pull your fingers away. Too late. The flesh that touched the hot handle reddens and stings. A blister forms.

During the next few days, you remember the accident each time something brushes against your burn. Then one day, you look at your hand and find that it's healed perfectly. There's no more redness. No more blister. No more pain.

How did your body do that?

Modern science wishes it had a better answer for you. The best brains in the business have yet to figure out just how your body can react with such aplomb to an insult like a burn and go about the business of rebuilding with nary a conscious directive from you.

Researchers do know that a burn has the best chance of healing completely if at least one layer of the outermost portion of skin remains intact. This outer skin is called the epidermis, and it includes the skin you can see and the layers immediately underneath it. Burns that go deeper are likely to leave scars.

Healing begins instantaneously, as soon as you remove the cause of the burn. The cells of the damaged tissues produce chemicals that initiate a whole flurry of activity. Doctors call this the inflammatory response. One type of chemical directs the blood vessels to dilate. (That's what turns your skin red.) Dilation allows extra blood, with its extra nutrients, to flow to the damaged zone, speeding the proliferation of new cells.

Other chemicals direct specialized cells to produce the various materials needed for repair. Still other chemicals see to it that the specialized white blood cells clean up dead tissue and prevent infection.

"It all happens in a very sophisticated, very complex way," says Karl Kramer, M.D., clinical professor of dermatology at the University of Miami School of Medicine. "Only some of it do we understand at this point. I think the next phase of research will focus on figuring out how to make more of the growth stimulators so we can help heal wounds faster."

The Threat to Your Immune System

The deeper the burn, the graver the problems for your immune system. Healthy skin serves as a protective envelope for the body. It keeps out bacteria, helps regulate body temperature, and maintains the body's water content. Nerve endings in the dermis, the skin layer underlying the epidermis, monitor changes in the external environment.

Burn yourself, and you may burn much more than your skin. The sebaceous glands, which lubricate your skin, plus nerve endings, and blood and lymph vessels are also at stake.

Sustain a second-degree burn, which sears off deeper layers of skin, and your lymph fluid begins to seep through to the surface.

Bacteria thrive in this nutrient-rich medium. And you have little immediate protection from infection if the burn has sealed off the adjacent blood and lymph vessels.

A third-degree burn poses even more of a challenge to your body's disease-fighting powers. Some burns reach clear to the muscle. Such a severe burn usually leads to a heavy loss of body fluids, depriving your circulatory system of the volume it requires to send white blood cells and antibodies where they're needed. The loss of fluids also means a reduction in the salts, vitamins, and proteins your immune system looks to for basic building materials.

Meanwhile, the deep hole in the skin is extremely vulnerable to infection. It's not uncommon for a physician to order a tetanus shot for someone with a bad burn, or to prescribe antibiotics.

On-the-Scene Care

Taking the proper measures immediately after burning yourself can limit damage and improve your chances for full recovery.

On these pages you'll find step-by-step directions for treating first-, second-, and third-degree burns, and those caused by chemicals. Familiarize yourself with these procedures now, so you can quickly recall what needs to be done when the time comes. Because it is often difficult, even for doctors, to categorize a burn, it's a good idea to see your doctor for any serious burn.

The very first thing you need to do is remove the source of the heat. If clothing or hair is on fire, extinguish the flames with a flame-retardant blanket or cool water. If the source is chemical, flush the area with lots and lots of water. Remove all hot or contaminated clothing that is not stuck to the skin, even if you have to cut it away.

If the source is electrical, turn off the current. If you are helping another, insulate yourself by standing on nonmetallic material, such as a pile of dry newspapers. Then use rope, a rubber car mat, or dry board to push or pull the victim away from the source. Make sure these items are bone dry before you use them.

Then assess the burn. (See "The One, Two, Three of Burns" on page 113.) If you have reason to suspect a small third-degree burn in the middle of a milder surface burn, treat the entire area as you would a third-degree burn.

After you treat the burn, cover it with a clean dressing, if you can easily do so. Don't use cotton or any fluffy material that could stick to the wound. If you are on your way to the emergency room, make sure the covering can be removed without doing further damage to the skin.

Make a Burn First-Aid Kit

You can prepare ahead for such emergencies by preparing a simple burn kit. Then you'll know you have everything you need in one place. The kit should contain:

Burns

- a pair of scissors, to help remove hot or contaminated clothing and to cut bandages.
- clean or sterile cloths in several sizes. You'll want a long piece of cloth to tie off a bandage.
- a record of when you and family members last received tetanus shots.
- emergency telephone numbers.

If you create a second kit for your car, you'll also want to include a clean pail, a jug of fresh water, and a clean blanket.

How to Prevent Shock

You don't have to worry about the burn victim going into shock when the burns are superficial. But if he is losing lots of fluid through the skin, the potential for shock is there. When the body loses too much fluid, blood pressure drops, disrupting normal circulation. Once circulation to the brain is disrupted, a person looks sweaty and pale and can become dizzy, confused, and eventually lose consciousness.

To guard against shock, lay the person face-up. Loosen any tight clothing. Make sure the legs are raised about a foot off the ground, unless you suspect a head or neck injury. This position will help blood flow from the legs to the upper body. If the victim is unconscious, place him in the recovery position. (See the chapter on heat exhaustion and heatstroke on page 238 for instructions.) You can help prevent heat loss by wrapping the person in a coat or blanket.

Shock is a serious condition that requires urgent medical attention. Once blood pressure drops below a certain point, the body cannot recover on its own.

Follow-Up Care for Burns

If the burn is mild enough to care for at home, you should give it 24 hours to heal on its own before applying any kind of ointment or antibiotic preparation. Cover with clean, dry gauze.

What's good to use on a burn? Try:

- fresh aloe vera from the aloe plant or an aloe cream. Some studies suggest that aloe vera can speed healing, stop burn damage from progressing, and control the growth of bacteria in the wound. Aloe vera is particularly soothing on sunburns.
- an over-the-counter povidone-iodine cream or solution like Betadine. You can also try Sugardyne, a new over-the-counter product that combines granulated sugar with povidone-iodine ointment and solution. Richard A. Knutson, M.D., a Mississippi orthopedic surgeon, tested this remedy on more than 1,000 burn patients and found that it soothes pain and promotes normal, unscarred regrowth of tissue, while guarding against bacteria and fungus.
- an ointment containing chlorophyllin copper complex, available over the counter as Prophyllin.

What about vitamin E? Some people have found it helpful. Dr. Kramer suspects that it isn't the vitamin E itself but the act of rubbing it on the wound that helps.

"There is evidence that pressure on wounds will help them heal with less scarring. In fact, with severe burns, after they have healed, special pressure dressings seem to decrease the amount of scarring."

Deborah Grandinetti

112

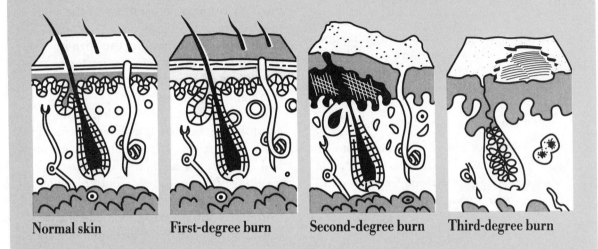

Normal skin   **First-degree burn**   **Second-degree burn**   **Third-degree burn**

The One, Two, Three of Burns

If you have a burn, the very first thing you need to do is assess how bad it is. Treatment strategies differ for first-, second-, and third-degree burns.

Here's how to tell the difference.

First-degree burns. Your skin reddens, but it doesn't break or blister. It feels hot and tender to the touch. Most likely it hurts.

You've damaged just the outermost layer of your skin. If you have pain, you've also irritated the nerve endings.

First-degree burns are often the result of staying out in the sun too long or minor household accidents like grabbing the hot handle of a pot on the stove or getting your fingers too near the base of the iron.

Second-degree burns. This type not only burns the outermost layer of your skin but also layers of skin below. This deeper

damage releases body fluids, causing the skin to be moist and blister. Your skin may redden or turn a mottled red and white. And the burn is likely to hurt intensely.

What causes second-degree burns? Severe sunburn, scalding with a hot liquid or steam, and flash burns from flammable liquids such as gasoline.

Third-degree burns. This type burns all the way through, damaging all the layers of the skin, the sweat glands, and hair follicles in the area. Hair in the burn area falls out easily.

You may not feel any pain because the nerve damage is so extensive. In fact, you may require a skin graft for it to heal.

The skin will look dry and leathery. Discoloration will be evident too. Your skin could be pearly white or brown-black.

113

First Aid for First- and Second-Degree Burns

The way you respond to a burn in the first few minutes can make an enormous difference in the way you heal. The right approach can limit the damage, ease pain, and prevent infection.

Seek medical care immediately if:

- a second-degree burn covers more than 10 percent of the total body area. (To help you calculate, figure that your hand accounts for 1 percent of your body area.)
- the face, neck, hands, feet, or genital area sustains second-degree burns.
- there is smoke inhalation. A doctor must check for damage to the respiratory system.

If you are treating a minor burn yourself, begin by running cool water over the injured area.

Flushing or submerging the burn is important because it removes heat, cleans the wound (decreasing the chance of infection), and helps relieve pain.

During the first 24 hours, don't put anything on the burn but water. Antibiotic ointments are best applied after the burn has had 24 hours to heal on its own. And speaking of don'ts—grease, butter, and ice *never* belong anywhere near a burn.

You may still need to seek medical attention after you've applied first aid if blisters form over the wound.

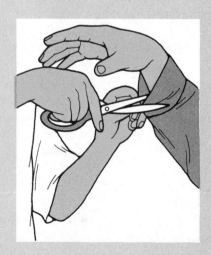

1. If a burn causes the skin to swell, jewelry or constricting clothing near the burn could become even tighter. It's best to remove it now. But don't touch any clothing that has adhered to the skin. Leave that for a doctor.

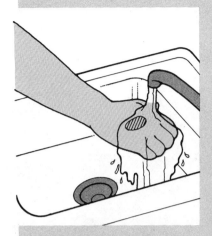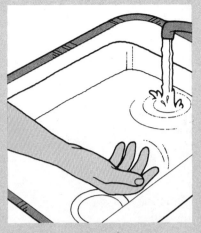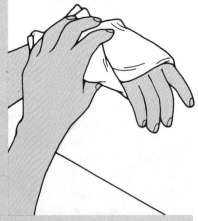

2. Immediately cool the area by placing the burn under cool running water. You don't want the faucet on full force, however, or it could break blisters and really hurt.

3. The other way to cool the tissue is to immerse the burn in cold water. Don't add ice to the sink. Do let the cold water run over the burn as the sink is filling up, so cooling is immediate.

4. If the burn is on the face, or you're outdoors and you don't have access to a tap or a sink, apply a cold wet compress. Be sure to use a clean cloth so that you don't infect the wound.

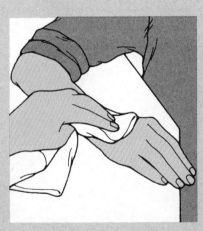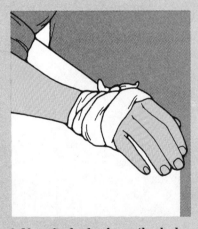

5. Continue cooling the burn for at least 5 minutes or until pain subsides. Then, use a sterile cloth to pat the area dry. If you don't have a sterile cloth, try to use something freshly laundered.

6. Now, find a fresh sterile cloth (or a clean one) and loosely cover the burn. Secure in place by tying another piece of cloth around it. Don't use an adhesive to fasten it.

How to Treat Third-Degree Burns

The right response to a third-degree burn depends on its size. If the burn is larger than a silver dollar, all you can do while you're awaiting medical care is to remove constricting clothing and jewelry. Applying cold water to a large third-degree burn increases the likelihood that the burn victim will go into shock. If the injury is smaller than a silver dollar, administer first-aid care as illustrated.

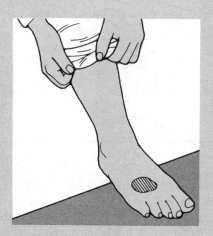

1. Remove clothing or jewelry from the area of the burn. Let a doctor remove any clothing stuck to the wound. Trying to remove anything stuck to a burn yourself may promote scarring.

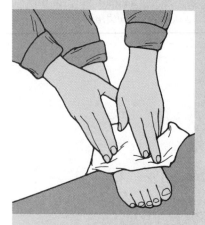

2. If the burn is smaller than a silver dollar, you can help prevent the damage from spreading by cooling the tissue with cold water. A cold wet compress is one method.

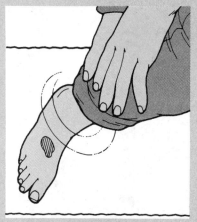

3. Immersing the burned area in a sink of cold water helps cool the injury quickly. Don't treat burns larger than 2 inches across with cold water. Larger third-degree burns require medical attention.

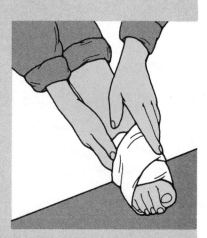

4. Pat dry. Cover with a clean, nonfluffy cloth. Cover the cloth with a dressing and fasten loosely with another piece of cloth.

How to Treat Chemical Burns

Caustic chemicals continue to burn as long as they remain on the skin. The only way to put out the "flames" is to remove contaminated clothing and flush with water—fast. Flush for 15 to 30 minutes.

If you're alone, you'll want to do this even before you call a doctor or emergency medical technician.

But do call the doctor. Chemical burns *always* require a doctor's attention.

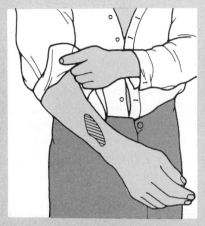

1. Immediately remove any clothing, including shoes and socks, that has become soaked with the offending chemical. Leave any bits of cloth that remain stuck to the wound.

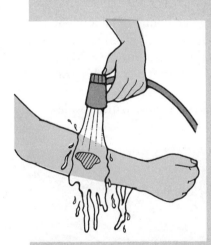

2. Flush the burned area immediately with large quantities of cool water from a shower, faucet, pail, or hose set on comfortable pressure. Flush for 15 to 30 minutes.

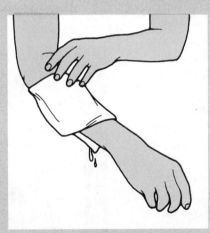

3. After you've thoroughly flushed the wound and the burning has stopped, you can help relieve the pain by applying cool wet compresses until medical care is at hand. Use a sterile cloth.

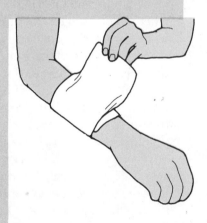

4. Use a nonfluffy, clean cloth and make a dry, loose dressing for the wound. Cover it. Do not open blisters or remove dead skin.

BURSITIS

First of all, relax: You probably don't have bursitis. Most people who think they have it actually have tendinitis. The same activities cause both conditions: swinging at tennis balls, kneeling in the garden, lifting heavy weights, bumping into things, using a jackhammer, carrying those plastic shopping bags with handles.

If your pain comes on suddenly, sharply, and intensely, though, bursitis is a possibility. It occurs when the bursa become inflamed. These little sacs of fluid are located throughout the body, primarily in the joints. They serve to cushion points where muscles or tendons rub against bones or ligaments. They're especially important in the shoulders, elbows, hips, and knee joints. And that's where you most often get bursitis.

The actual cause of bursitis is usually overuse or injury of the joint. And the usual treatment is rest combined with medication, like ibuprofen or aspirin. This is followed by ice and moist heat. The "rest" part of the treatment is easy: You can't move your shoulder anyway.

Whatever it is you've been doing to aggravate your bursa, stop doing it for at least ten days. Rest does not mean total immobilization, however. Doctors caution that complete nonuse of a joint can cause it to "freeze up," a condition that can result in permanent impairment. Even though it may hurt a little, doctors advise gently extending and flexing the affected area once or twice a day to maintain range of motion.

Take ibuprofen or aspirin to reduce inflammation. Inflammation of the bursa can be so intense that the skin surrounding the joint is hot to the touch. This is the time to use an ice pack or gel pack, which also reduces inflammation. Protect your skin with a towel or washcloth between the pack and the skin. Leave the pack on for 10 minutes, remove it for 10 minutes, then replace it for 10 more minutes, until the heat is gone.

A moist heating pad comes in handy when the pain isn't too severe and the joint itself isn't hot. If that's the case, alternate cold and heat treatments—10 minutes of cold, 10 of heat, and so on.

After a few days the intense pain subsides.

William LeGro

The Cushions between Muscle and Bone

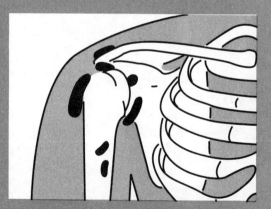

A bursa, a soft sac that contains a lubricating liquid, is tucked between tendons and bones or other tissues in your shoulder.

CALLUSES

You get calluses because you need them. You're walking barefoot on asphalt on a hot summer afternoon. Your high-fashion shoes are rubbing your toes and heels the wrong way. Your hands are gripping an ax. Your body says, "If I don't thicken my skin, my bones are going to poke through." And voilà! A callus is born.

A callus is the skin's armor plating, a symptom of pressure, imbalance, or injury. Dead, thickened skin builds up at the pressure points where bones underneath don't have enough of a cushion of fat or tissue. Or a callus can form around a splinter, a wart, or a scar. In most cases the callus is no problem, but sometimes it can become very painful, such as when it puts pressure on a nerve or cracks open on your heel. Not to mention the fact that its yellowish, dead-looking color is not a pretty sight. Then you want to get rid of it.

Start with the right shoes. You pay for the high-heeled look with thick yellow calluses on the balls of your feet; for long, narrow, pointy-toed shoes with calluses on your toes; for loose-fitting shoes with calluses on your heels. Get shoes that fit properly. Special shoe inserts may also help.

If your feet have already grown a crop of unsightly, uncomfortable calluses, don't despair. Twice a day soften calluses by soaking your feet for 15 minutes in warm water. Follow up with a moisturizing lotion. When your calluses have softened, rub them gently with a pumice stone or callus file to smooth and soften them still more.

A number of callus pads are available to reduce friction, like Dr. Scholl's Callus Cushions or moleskin. Other pads are medicated with salicylic acid, which can eat away the callus, but may attack normal skin as well. If you use these medicated pads, make sure they come in contact only with the callus.

You can make your own salicylic solution: Crush six aspirins into powder, mix with a tablespoon of lemon juice and a tablespoon of water, and stick the paste onto your calluses—but be sure to treat *only* the yellowish areas. Then put your callused foot into a plastic bag and wrap it in a warm towel for 10 minutes. After unwrapping, rub the calluses away with a pumice stone.

William LeGro

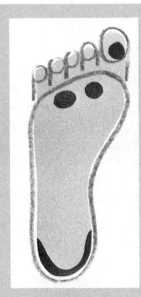

Saving Your Sole

If walking irritates certain areas of your foot, calluses may form to protect the sore spots. Calluses are most likely to form on the big toe, on the ball of the foot underneath the bones leading to the toes, or on the heel, depending on your stride.

119

CANCER PREVENTION

ancer. Even the word is scary to most people. Part of what makes this disease so frightening is the belief that it is beyond our control. Many believe that cancer strikes like lightning—that if it's going to hit, there's not much you can do to get out of its way. The problem is that this belief is *wrong*. There's a lot—a whole lot—you can do to prevent being hit by cancer.

If we know anything about this disease that makes cells grow wild, it's that it is often related to the way we live. In fact, "studies show that a full 75 to 80 percent of all cancers may be connected to lifestyle," says Ernst Wynder, M.D., president of the American Health Foundation.

What does that mean to you? It means that by making a few changes in your lifestyle, you can *drastically* reduce the chances of ever getting cancer.

Follow the Anti-Cancer Diet

A good place to start an anti-cancer lifestyle is at the dinner table. "Changing your diet is not a guarantee against cancer, but there's a lot of evidence to show that the two are linked," says Paul F. Engstrom, M.D., vice president for population science of the Fox Chase Cancer Center in Philadelphia.

The American Cancer Society tops its list of diet recommendations with these seven tips:

- Avoid obesity.
- Cut down on fat.
- Eat more fiber.
- Include foods rich in vitamins A, C, and E in your diet.
- Eat cruciferous vegetables.
- Limit your consumption of cured, smoked, and nitrite-cured foods.
- Drink alcohol in moderation, if at all.

Let's take a closer look at each of these recommendations:

Keep your weight down. When the American Cancer Society did a major study of obesity over a 12-year period, it found an increased incidence of uterine, gallbladder, kidney, stomach, colon, and breast cancers among people who are overweight. Among people 40 percent or more overweight, women showed a 55 percent greater risk and men a 33 percent greater risk of cancer. The key to controlling weight is decreasing your calorie intake while increasing your physical activity. (See the chapter on overweight on page 327 for many specific tips on how to get your weight under control.)

Forgo the fat. People who eat too much fat, whether saturated or unsaturated, plant or animal, may be at a greater risk of developing cancers of the breast, colon, and prostate. Most Americans consume between 30 and 40 percent of their total calories as fat. A much more prudent diet, says Dr. Engstrom, would have only 15 to 20 percent fat. To follow this ideal anti-cancer diet, avoid things like high-fat dairy products, oils, and pastries. Instead, reach for vegetables, fruits, and whole grains. Select lean meats, poultry without skin, and fish.

Favor the fiber. Vegetables, fruits, and grains provide more than low-fat calories; they also provide fiber. And many doctors believe that a high-fiber diet helps ward off certain cancers, particularly colon cancer. Studies of various populations provide the evidence in countries where people eat high-fiber, low-fat diets: The incidence of cancer there is lower than in countries such as the United States, where people eat lots of processed, high-fat, fiber-deficient foods. The average American could stand to triple his daily intake of fiber, says Dr. Engstrom. Foods particularly high in fiber (and also low in fat) include whole-wheat bread, popcorn, raisins, peaches, apples, spinach, and kidney beans. For extra fiber insurance, include a few teaspoons of bran with every meal, says Dr. Engstrom.

Be a vitamin ACE. Although science is still pondering whether certain nutrients have cancer-fighting abilities, doctors are confident that there are a few vitamins that should be included in an anti-cancer diet. These four-star cancer fighters include the ACE vitamins—that is, vitamins A, C, and E. Vitamin A is abundant in carrots and other orange or yellow vegetables, as well as dark green, leafy vegetables like kale. Foods rich in vitamin C include citrus fruits, broccoli, cantaloupe, and strawberries. Vitamin E is found in many foods, particularly in grains and vegetable oils.

According to the National Cancer Institute, well over 500 nutrients have shown some promise of fighting cancer in either laboratory or population studies. Among those receiving lots of attention are the minerals calcium and selenium and the fatty acids found in fish oil. Calcium, abundant in dairy products, spinach, and collard greens, has shown some protective power over intestinal cancer. Selenium, plentiful in seafoods, organ meats, and some grains, may offer a degree of protection against breast, lung, and colon cancer. And the oils from your fish dinner may possibly slow the growth of cancerous tumors. To get enough of all the nutrients you need, eat a diet with lots of variety and consider taking a daily multivitamin supplement, says Dr. Engstrom. He warns, however, that high-dosage supplements of certain nutrients (like vitamin A and selenium) can be dangerous. Don't take supplements of single nutrients without the supervision of your physician.

Eat cruciferous vegetables. Vegetables in the cabbage family may be among the most potent anti-cancer foods you can sink your teeth into. Some studies of large groups of people have suggested that eating these vegetables may reduce the risk of cancer of the gastrointestinal and respiratory tracts. Cruciferous vegetables include broccoli, brussels sprouts, cabbage, and cauliflower.

Hold the bacon. Having a lettuce and tomato sandwich without any bacon may not be your idea of a yum-yum lunch, but be aware that too much bacon and other cured and pickled foods may increase your risk of stomach and other cancers. In countries like China and Japan, where cured and pickled foods are common, so are stomach and esophageal cancers. So don't overindulge in foods that are salt-cured, pickled, smoked, or that contain nitrites. Examples of such foods are pickles, bacon, ham, sausage, and smoked cheeses.

Drink in moderation. For most of us, an occasional cocktail probably does no harm. But heavy drinkers, especially those who also smoke, have a high risk of developing cancer of the mouth, larynx, and esophagus. Women should be especially cautious about drinking, particularly those who are overweight or have a history of breast cancer in the family. If you are one of these people, you might consider the value of a sober lifestyle.

Go Organic

There's been a lot of talk about pesticide residues in our food. A report by the National Research Council concluded that pesticide residues clearly warrant concern.

What can you do about it? Buy organic, when possible. Choose domestic over foreign-grown produce. Discard the outer leaves of lettuce and cabbage. And peel your carrots, cucumbers, and turnips. Produce that can't be husked or peeled should at least be washed well before eating.

Steer Clear of Tobacco Road

First Man: Hey buddy, got a match?
Second Man: Yeah, cigarette smoking and cancer.

Regardless of what you think of "Second

Man's" sense of humor, he certainly knows what he's talking about.

"It's been estimated that about 30 percent of all cancers are related to tobacco," says Dr. Engstrom. For certain cancers the figure is much higher. Lung cancer is the leading cause of cancer deaths in the United States, and perhaps 80 to 90 percent of all cases are linked to tobacco, he says. "The surest way to decrease your risk of cancer is to quit smoking, or, if you've never smoked, don't start."

But smokers aren't the only ones who should be concerned about tobacco. Smoke from the cigarettes of *others* also puts you at higher risk of certain cancers, says Dr. Engstrom. Studies in this country and Japan show that if you live with a smoker, your risk of developing lung cancer is three to five times greater than if you lived in a smoke-free home.

And don't think that chewing tobacco or sniffing it (as snuff) is any safer than smoking the stuff. Simply read the government's warnings on the side of any package of so-called smokeless tobacco: *Warning: This product may cause mouth cancer. Warning: This product is not a safe alternative to cigarettes.*

Prevention: Made in the Shade

After watching your diet and avoiding tobacco, perhaps the next most important thing you can do to protect yourself against cancer is to limit your exposure to the sun, says Dr. Engstrom. The sun's ultraviolet rays have been linked to skin cancer, melanoma, and cataracts. Unfortunately, this link may become stronger over time. Most scientists agree that the earth's ozone layer, which protects us from ultraviolet rays, is being eaten up by man-made pollutants.

What can you do? Aside from writing your congressman to urge pollution control, limit the time you spend in the sun, particularly in the middle of the day. Use a sunscreen with an SPF (sun protection factor) of at least 15 that will block out 98 percent of the sun's damaging rays. Wear protective clothing, including a hat. And wear sunglasses designed to filter out ultraviolet radiation (check the label).

Although anyone can get skin cancer, you are most susceptible and should take the most precautions, if you are fair-skinned. Similarly, people with blue eyes are more susceptible to eye cancer (a rare disease compared to most cancers), the theory being that the protective pigment in blue eyes is distributed unevenly.

Walk Away from Cancer

Nobody knows for sure whether being physically fit can help prevent certain types

Spotting the Suspicious Mole

Certain kinds of moles are signs of melanoma, a particularly dangerous form of cancer. Because melanoma is so deadly, and because there's almost a 100 percent chance of curing it if detected in its earliest phase, doctors recommend that you check your body monthly for any moles that look suspicious.

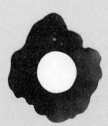

A mole of many colors, perhaps shades of brown, black, and red

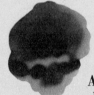

An asymmetrical mole—one half doesn't match the other

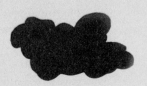

A mole with edges that are irregular, ragged, or blurred

A mole that's bigger in diameter than a pencil eraser or is growing

123

of cancer, but the latest studies seem to indicate that may be the case.

Colon cancer is the one cancer on which physical activity may have an impact. Sedentary people are about 60 percent more likely to develop colon cancer than more active people, says Mary Catherine Schumacher, M.D., a research assistant professor in the Department of Internal Medicine at the University of Utah School of Medicine. Exercising does not compare to giving up smoking as a tool for preventing cancer, she says, but it is nonetheless something to take seriously. The American Cancer Society agrees.

More research will be needed before anyone can recommend an exercise program specifically designed for preventing cancer. In the meantime, any exercise is surely better than none, especially if it helps keep off extra pounds. The American Cancer Society heartily recommends frequent brisk walks.

Come Home to a Safe House

Lifestyle is only part of the cancer picture, however. "If we could control the behavior of all individuals relative to smoking and diet, there would still be cancers," says Dr. Engstrom. Part of the reason is that we are exposed to things in the environment that can trigger cancer. We can protect ourselves from the sun's ultraviolet rays, but what of other environmental hazards?

One environmental hazard you can do something about is radon—the odorless, colorless, radioactive gas that seeps into buildings from underground rocks. Radon is

believed to be the leading cause of lung cancer among nonsmokers. Its effect on smokers is even greater. Their risk from radon is ten times that of nonsmokers. The Environmental Protection Agency estimates that 8 to 12 percent of the nation's homes have dangerous radon levels.

You should test your home for radon gas with commercially available monitoring devices. Kits can cost less than $25 and are simple to use. If your home's radon level registers high, retest at least once more to be sure the reading is accurate.

There is a lot you can do yourself to eliminate the danger from radon. Opening basement windows should help. So can sealing cracks and openings in basement floors and walls. If radon levels are still high after taking these measures, consult a radon-control company.

Fight Pollution

Other pollutants in the air you breathe come not from under your house but from outside it. Studies have shown that lung cancer rates are higher in heavily industrialized areas. City people get certain kinds of cancer more frequently than country folk.

Drinking water is also something to think about. Proven cancer-causing chemicals have been found in drinking water, and several studies have reported a link between chemical contamination of water supplies and cancer rates.

"There is evidence that industrial pollutants in our air and water contribute significantly to cancer risks. In light of this, if you have a choice about where to live and bring up your family, the quality of the environment should be one of the considerations. At the same time, it's very important that all citizens press for protective regulation by getting in touch with their representatives at the local, state, and federal levels," says Frederica P. Perera, D.P.H., an associate professor at the Columbia University School of Public Health.

You also should test your home drinking water for contaminants or ask your municipal water authority for the results of their routine tests. Determine whether there are any hazardous waste sites in your community —the toxins from those sites can leach into your underground water supply or run off into rivers and streams. If you feel you are in danger of toxic contamination, have the Environmental Protection Agency test your home for toxic pollutants.

If needed, you can install a good (if expensive) water purifier in your home.

Say No to Needless X-Rays

It has been known for years that radiation can cause cancer. The risk of developing cancer following exposure to even low levels of radiation may be three to four times higher than previously estimated, according to the National Research Council.

Medical X-rays are a common source of radiation. X-rays are sometimes necessary, but not always. Many times, they are given as a matter of routine. Sometimes doctors give an X-ray only because they think that patients expect to get one as part of a checkup.

Russell Wild

How to Do a Testicular Examination

You'll be happy to know that cancer of the testis is rare. It is also completely curable—if diagnosed early. Doctors recommend that a man perform a self-exam once a month. It's not difficult to do, and it will only take about 3 minutes of your time.

The best time to check yourself is after a warm shower or bath, when the skin around the scrotum is most relaxed, so that it's easier to feel what's underneath. What you're looking for is any hard lump.

Using both hands, gently roll each testis between your fingers and thumbs. One at a time, roll it backward, forward, and sideways.

You should know the location of the epididymis, a sausage-shaped organ that runs up and down the back of the testicle. It feels like a bump when you touch it, but rest assured it's no cause for worry. If you're in doubt, however, you should by all means ask your doctor.

If you feel any hard lump that is clearly not your epididymis, see your doctor without delay. Testicular cancer can spread through the body and prove fatal. If you catch it quickly, it is almost always treatable by surgery.

125

CANCER PREVENTION

How to Do a Breast Examination

Just being born female puts you at risk for breast cancer. There's nothing you can do about that. But you can give yourself a monthly self-examination. Breast cancer is one of the most controllable cancers there is.

Ideally, a woman should begin examining herself regularly in her late teens or early twenties. Cancer isn't likely at that age—it's quite unlikely. That's why it's the perfect time to learn the unique consistency of one's own breasts without anxiety over cancer.

As years go on, so does the chance of developing breast cancer. Those most susceptible include women over 50 years old, those with histories of breast cancer in the family, and those who have had breast cancer already.

But—remember—any woman can get it. So it's important to know the signs: (1) a lump or thickening in the breast; (2) a change in breast shape; or (3) discharge from the nipple. The steps to a thorough self-exam are illustrated here. The best time to do a breast exam is two or three days after your period.

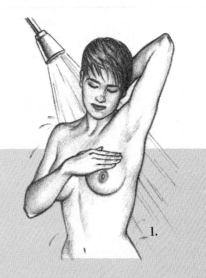

Start your breast examination in the shower or bath, when your skin is wet and you can glide your hands over it easily. With your fingers flat, move over every part of each breast. You want to check for any hard lump or thickening.

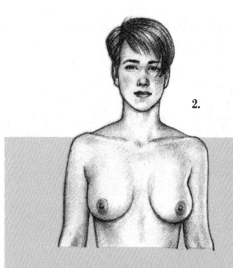

After your shower, stand or sit before a mirror in a well-lit room with arms down by your sides. Are there any changes from the last time you examined yourself? Are there any dimplings of the skin or a pulling in of the nipple?

126

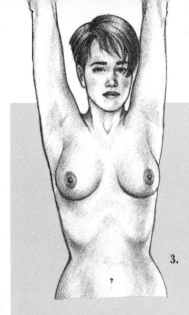

Lift your arms high over your head. Look for any changes in the contour, or any signs of swelling in either breast. Look for dimples or changes in the nipple, such as a crustiness or scaling. Also note any discharge.

3.

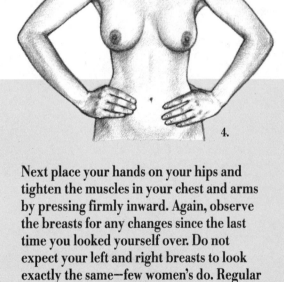

4.

Next place your hands on your hips and tighten the muscles in your chest and arms by pressing firmly inward. Again, observe the breasts for any changes since the last time you looked yourself over. Do not expect your left and right breasts to look exactly the same—few women's do. Regular self-examinations will give you a notion of what is normal for you.

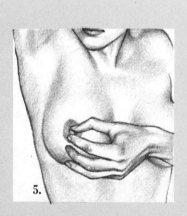

5.

Squeeze the nipple of each breast gently between your thumb and index finger. Note any discharge, whether clear or bloody. It should be reported to your physician. Milky-looking discharges, however, are not uncommon and are caused by harmless changes in the breast.

127

CANCER PREVENTION

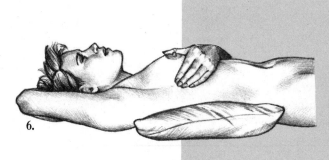

6.

For the next few steps in your self-exam, lie flat on your back with a small pillow or folded towel under your right shoulder. Raise your right arm overhead. With the left hand slightly cupped and fingers together, reach across to your right breast. Using the flat of the fingers, not the tips, feel for any unusual lumps or change in the texture of the breast skin.

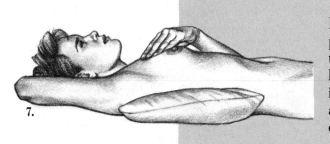

7.

Begin either at the outer edge of the breast, proceeding in a circular direction toward the inner areas of the breast, or examine half of the breast at a time. Avoid compressing the breast tissue between the thumb and fingers as that may give the impression of a lump that is not actually there.

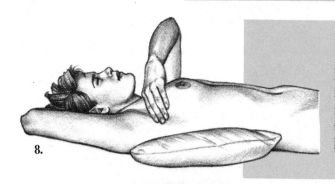

8.

Pay special attention to the outer area between the nipple and the armpit, including the armpit itself. It's here that a majority of breast cancers occur. A ridge of firm tissue in the lower curve of each breast, however, is normal.

Transfer the towel or pillow to the left shoulder and repeat the process, using the right hand to feel the left breast. Usually, any lump the size of a pea or larger can be felt. If you discover a lump, or anything that you think is a lump—see your physician.

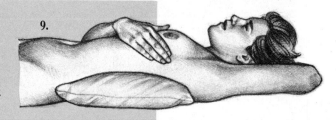

9.

CARPAL TUNNEL SYNDROME

Bill Mondschein couldn't figure out why he was experiencing a tingling sensation in his wrists and thumbs—or why his hands were always falling asleep.

That was two years ago. The 40-year-old shop foreman from eastern Pennsylvania had never heard of carpal tunnel syndrome (CTS), an ailment that experts estimate one in ten Americans will develop.

CTS occurs when tendons, bones, or ligaments press against a major nerve running through the wrist, causing a sort of short-circuit. Ordinarily, the bones and ligaments form a protective "tunnel" around the nerve and tendons, but something happens with CTS that pinches or presses on this tunnel.

Although no one knows exactly what causes it, "there's tremendous evidence that CTS is work-related," says Peter C. Amadio, M.D., of the Mayo Clinic in Rochester, Minnesota. "How else could you explain the fact that the people who debone meat in one particular meat-packing plant have a 20 percent surgery rate for CTS, while only 5 percent of their co-workers in nonboning activities require surgery?"

Mondschein has never worked deboning anything, but, he says, "I've worked all my life with my hands—writing, drawing, cutting patterns, or doing mechanical work." This is almost assuredly what caused his condition, says his doctor. Of all CTS sufferers, many hold jobs that require repetitious motions. That means that certain people may be at higher risk—meat cutters,

data processors, cashiers, assembly-line workers, truck drivers (who keep their hands on the wheel for long stretches), and certain musicians.

A second common cause of CTS is sleep-related, says John E. Castaldo, M.D., a Pennsylvania neurologist. Many people with CTS have developed it by sleeping on their stomachs with their arms and wrists bent and flexed under them. If you sleep in any position that puts continuous pressure on your wrists, you risk damaging the carpal tunnel.

The first signs of CTS are typically numbness, pain, weakness, and a tingling or pins-and-needles sensation in the thumb, index finger, and middle finger. If untreated, the pain can radiate to the elbow, upper arm, and shoulder. Eventually, the nerve impulses in the wrist may be short-circuited, causing nerves in the thumb, index, and middle fingers to "starve" and the thumb muscles to progressively waste away. Some people lose the use of their entire hands.

That's why it's important to recognize and treat CTS symptoms early, before any lasting damage occurs.

Once you've been diagnosed as having CTS, you may be referred to a physical therapy program. In mild to moderate cases of CTS, physical therapy is an effective, inexpensive treatment. "Our focus is on teaching people how to use their hands in a safer, easier, more comfortable way," says Glenda Key, a physical therapy consultant in Minneapolis.

129

CARPAL TUNNEL SYNDROME

Protecting the Tunnel

One approach to battling CTS is to immobilize the wrist with a forearm splint, allowing the fingers to wiggle freely while giving the wrist a chance to heal. Some people wear the splint at night, when they are likely to sleep in positions that bring on or worsen CTS symptoms, says Dr. Castaldo. Others just learn better sleep positions that don't strain their wrists. Dr. Castaldo recommends learning to sleep on your back with your hands resting on your thighs.

To reduce pain and inflammation, you can try a nonsteroidal anti-inflammatory drug like aspirin or ibuprofen. Don't take acetaminophen, though. While it reduces pain, it doesn't do anything for inflammation.

Cold packs can also help to bring down swelling. Heat packs might feel good, but avoid the temptation—heat tends to increase swelling.

In recent years, therapy using large amounts of vitamin B_6 has been widely publicized as a treatment for CTS. The jury is still out on vitamin B_6 therapy, however, so talk to your own doctor before trying it yourself.

Russell Wild

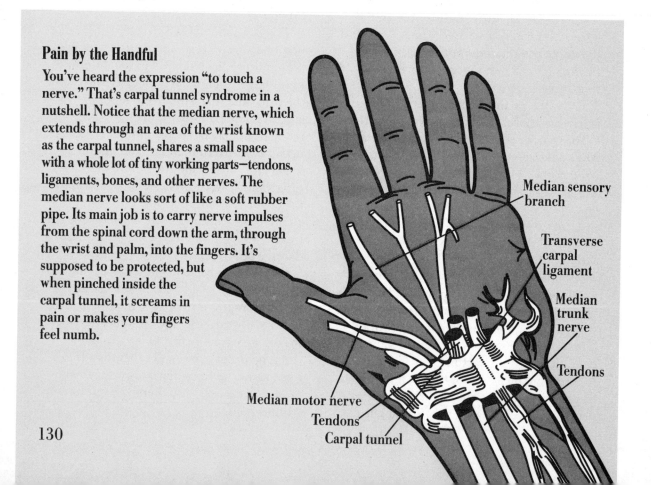

Pain by the Handful

You've heard the expression "to touch a nerve." That's carpal tunnel syndrome in a nutshell. Notice that the median nerve, which extends through an area of the wrist known as the carpal tunnel, shares a small space with a whole lot of tiny working parts—tendons, ligaments, bones, and other nerves. The median nerve looks sort of like a soft rubber pipe. Its main job is to carry nerve impulses from the spinal cord down the arm, through the wrist and palm, into the fingers. It's supposed to be protected, but when pinched inside the carpal tunnel, it screams in pain or makes your fingers feel numb.

Median sensory branch

Transverse carpal ligament

Median trunk nerve

Tendons

Median motor nerve

Tendons

Carpal tunnel

Exercises for Relief

The primary symptom of carpal tunnel syndrome is a hand that feels numb, tingles, or has fallen asleep. What's the best way to wake a sleeping hand? An alarm clock won't help, but a few simple hand exercises might do the trick. The three exercises shown here are suggested by Susan Isernhagen, a physical therapist in Duluth, Minnesota, and consultant to hospitals and industries to help reduce work injuries and rehabilitate injured workers. It's important to regularly exercise all the muscles that are giving you problems, says Isernhagen. These exercises should be practiced at least four times a day.

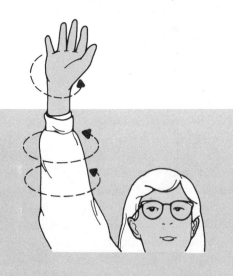

Lift your arm above your head and rotate your arm and your wrist at the same time. This gives your shoulders, neck, and upper back a break and relieves stress and tension.

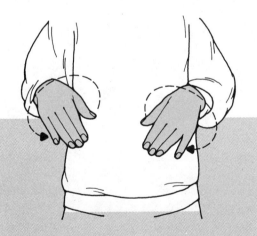

Circle your hands gently at the wrist for about 2 minutes. This exercises all the muscles of the wrist, restores circulation, and gets your wrist out of the position that brings on the symptoms of carpal tunnel syndrome.

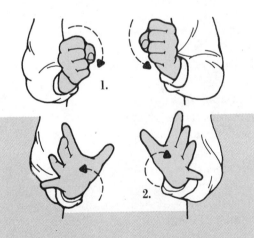

Gentle squeezing motions of the fingers should help to relieve that tingling feeling. Curl your fingers and press them lightly into your palm, then stretch them way back and hold. Repeat several times.

CARPAL TUNNEL SYNDROME

Do You Have CTS?

Your doctor should have a number of tests to determine whether or not you have carpal tunnel syndrome. You can try two of them yourself—the Phalen's wrist flexor and the median nerve percussion. The wrist flexor test brings on symptoms in a good percentage of people who have carpal tunnel syndrome (and about 20 percent of people who *don't* have it). The percussion test brings on symptoms in about 44 percent of people with the syndrome (and about 6 percent of people who *don't* have it).

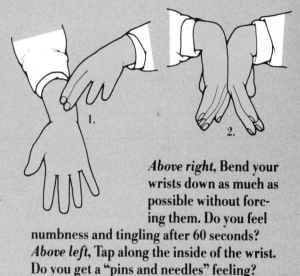

Above right, Bend your wrists down as much as possible without forcing them. Do you feel numbness and tingling after 60 seconds? *Above left,* Tap along the inside of the wrist. Do you get a "pins and needles" feeling?

Preventing Carpal Tunnel Syndrome

Among those susceptible to carpal tunnel syndrome are meat cutters, data processors, cashiers, assembly-line workers, jackhammer workers, and truck drivers—people who spend long stretches of time with their wrists bent. If your job forces you to make repetitive motions with your wrists, try to rotate tasks with your co-workers to give the wrist an occasional break.

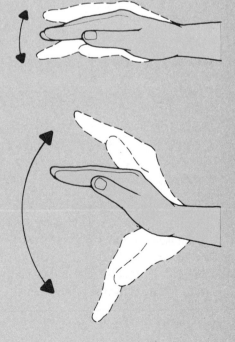

How to wave bye-bye? No. How to prevent the development of CTS. *Top right,* As much as possible, keep your wrists nearly straight. *Bottom right,* Too much flexing could eventually bring on problems.

CHOKING

Jason and Tiffany gaze into each other's eyes, their faces softly bathed in candlelight. They toast their happiness, they joke, they laugh, they savor the most sumptuous steaks they've ever eaten. Just when everything seems perfect, Jason gasps, his skin turns pale, and an expression of panic washes across his face. As he reaches for his throat, Tiffany realizes that he is choking.

Choking is the sixth leading cause of accidental death in the United States, claiming as many as 3,000 lives a year. The tragedy is that most of these deaths could be easily prevented. In the scenario above, Jason's fate hinges on whether he or Tiffany is familiar with the Heimlich maneuver.

"You can't wait for an ambulance, a doctor, or anyone else when someone is choking," says Henry J. Heimlich, M.D., president of the Heimlich Institute in Cincinnati, a man whose name has become synonymous with first aid for choking. Whatever is lodged in the victim's throat cuts off the air supply, he explains. Without air, brain damage occurs in about 3 minutes, death in 4.

When someone is choking, experts say, the only appropriate reaction is the Heimlich maneuver. *Do not* slap the victim on the back! Although vigorously thumping the back was once taught as the proper course of action, there is virtually unanimous agreement among doctors today that the back slap on an adult can drive a foreign object even deeper into the throat.

You can also administer the Heimlich maneuver to yourself. Had Elizabeth Wyllie known the technique, she might still be alive. "It was such a tragedy. My mother didn't know that she could have saved herself using the back of a chair, the kitchen counter, or a railing to perform the Heimlich maneuver," says her daughter, Katherine Wyllie Mansoor. Today, ten years after the death of her mother, Mansoor works as an associate of Dr. Heimlich. "It's too late for my mother, but the Heimlich maneuver can save others," she says.

Protect Children from Choking

Among young children, whose teeth cannot grind food as well as an adult's, choking is an even greater danger. Children choke most often on hot dogs (accounting for one out of six fatal chokings), grapes, popcorn, nuts, sourballs, and vegetables cut into coin-shaped slices. Peeling grapes and hot dogs and cutting all such foods into small pieces before feeding them to a young child will reduce the risk of choking. Nuts should never be given to any child under five, says Dr. Heimlich.

One food that both children and adults need to take caution with is peanut butter. "No one should ever eat peanut butter from a spoon," says Dr. Heimlich. Once lodged in the throat, the gooey treat is about the only thing that the Heimlich maneuver cannot remove, because it gets into the lungs.

Russell Wild

133

CHOKING

The Heimlich Maneuver

Have 3 minutes to spare? That's all it takes to learn how to save a life, says Henry J. Heimlich, M.D., the Ohio physician whose method for aiding choking victims has become a standard first-aid procedure. Anyone can learn to do it, he says. How? All you need to know is here on this and the following two pages.

The first thing you'll learn is how to recognize when someone is choking. Then you'll learn to perform the Heimlich maneuver on other adults, on children, and even on yourself. The next 3 minutes may prove to be the best investment you'll ever make!

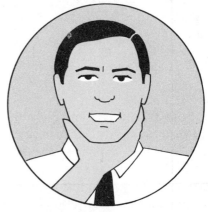

If you see someone bring his hand to his throat, he is probably a choking victim. Go ahead and ask, "Are you choking?" A person who is choking won't be able to speak, but he may nod. People who are choking will rapidly turn pale or blue, lose consciousness, and collapse.

Positioning the Fist

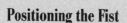

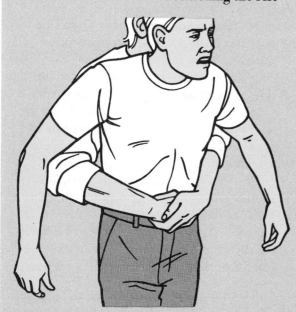

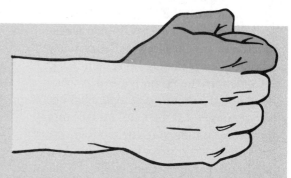

It's important to act quickly when someone is choking. Assuming the victim is still conscious and standing, stand behind him and wrap your arms around his waist. *Left*, Next make a fist with one hand and place the thumb side of the fist against the person's abdomen, slightly above the navel and below the rib cage. *Above*, Note the shaded area of the hand. This is the part of your hand that should be making contact with the person's abdomen. Now place your other hand on top of the fist.

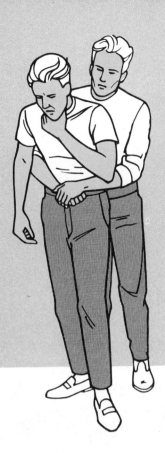

Helping an Adult

Once you have your fist positioned properly, grasp your fist with your other hand, and with a quick upward thrust, press the fist into the choking victim's abdomen. Bend your arms sharply at the elbows, but don't "bear hug" the victim—you don't want to squeeze his rib cage. It may be necessary, says Dr. Heimlich, to repeat the thrust several times to clear the airway. Continue until the obstruction is cleared or until the victim loses consciousness. You'll know the obstruction has cleared when the victim starts to breathe again and his normal skin color begins to return. If the choking victim is a woman in the late stages of pregnancy, thrusts to the abdomen could be dangerous. You should instead perform the maneuver with your fist on the middle of her breastbone. Be gentle.

Helping Yourself

Performing the Heimlich maneuver on yourself isn't as difficult as it may sound. Place your hands in the same position as you would if you were saving someone else. *Right,* That is, stick your fist, thumb side in, directly against your abdomen, slightly above the navel but well below the rib cage. Press upward and inward with a quick motion. Repeat, if necessary. *Far right,* You could also use the firm horizontal edge of a chair back, a table, or a railing. Position yourself against the edge, then press your abdomen against it with a quick movement. You may have to repeat the movement several times before the object in your throat becomes dislodged.

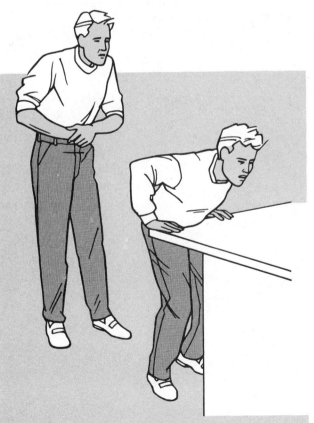

CHOKING

Helping an Infant

An infant found unconscious with no signs of injury or other illness is probably a victim of choking, says Dr. Heimlich. A variation of the Heimlich maneuver may save that infant. *Top,* Hold the baby in your lap. *Bottom,* Or lay him on a firm surface with his feet toward you. Place the index and middle fingers of both your hands on the infant's abdomen, just above the navel and well below the rib cage. Press with a quick upward thrust. You may need to repeat several times to expel the object. Of course, it's best to protect the child from choking in the first place: Never allow your baby to play with any object small enough to be swallowed and do not leave such objects in the crib or carriage.

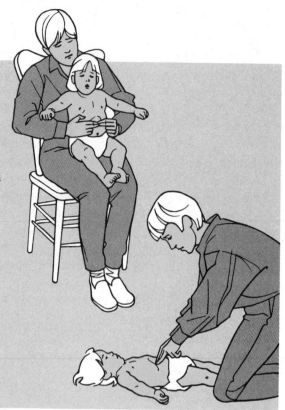

Victim Lying on Ground

The following technique, performed with the victim lying on the floor, is a lifesaver. *Left,* Children, who may not be able to reach around an adult, can use this technique on an adult much larger than themselves. *Bottom,* Kneel astride the victim and use your own body weight to achieve sufficient force for the thrust. Make sure the victim's head is straight and facing up; a turned head twists the throat, which can make it hard to dislodge the object.

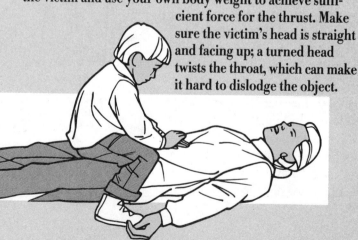

CHOLESTEROL

What's soft and gooey on the outside, tough and gritty on the inside, and can have the effect of a seven-car pileup in rush hour traffic? Give up?

The answer is plaque, an artery-clogging mass of fat, calcium, cellular waste, and that troublesome substance you've been hearing so much about—cholesterol.

Every minute of every day, your heart pumps approximately 4 to 6 quarts of blood throughout your entire body. The blood travels through a miles-long network of smooth, hollow tubes, carrying vital oxygen and food to billions of your body's hungry cells. This network of tubes, or blood vessels, is known as the cardiovascular system.

Unlike the body's muscular system, the cardiovascular system runs pretty much on automatic. That is to say, you don't have to do anything in order to get your blood flowing. There is, however, a whole lot you can do to make sure your blood doesn't *stop* flowing. You can—and you should—watch your cholesterol level.

There's nothing evil about cholesterol in and of itself. Your body even needs it to help manufacture new cells, produce hormones, and form digestive acids. The problem is your body manufactures all the cholesterol it needs to get these jobs done. When you eat a diet rich in cholesterol-boosting foods, your body can't use the surplus.

Too much cholesterol leads to the formation of plaque, which clings to your artery walls and clogs your bloodstream, much like ice jams your household plumbing on a cold day. When this condition develops, doctors say you have what is known as atherosclerosis.

Severe atherosclerosis makes you a good candidate for a heart attack or stroke. Fortunately, this is one candidacy you can avoid. Preventing atherosclerosis is largely a matter of keeping the level of cholesterol in your blood as low as possible.

Do You Need to Be Concerned?

To find out whether you have too much cholesterol in your blood, your doctor will have to give you a blood test. According to guidelines set by the National Institute of Health, you're in the safe zone if your level is below 200 milligrams of cholesterol per deciliter of blood (commonly expressed as 200 mg/dl). The ideal range is below 180.

Don't be surprised, though, if you find that your level is above 200. More than half of all Americans have cholesterol levels over the 200 mark. People whose cholesterol level is between 200 and 240, experts tell us, have "borderline high cholesterol" and are at twice the risk of heart disease compared to folks in the safe region.

Your doctor will fill you in on some other valuable information from your blood test results. First, he can tell you what your low-density lipoprotein, or LDL, level is. LDL is often called the bad cholesterol. This is the stuff that plaque is largely made of.

137

CHOLESTEROL

According to government guidelines, your LDL level should be *below* 130 mg/dl.

Next, your doctor can tell you what your high-density lipoprotein, or HDL, level is. HDL cholesterol is considered good. This is the stuff that picks up excess cholesterol and carries it to the liver, where it can be removed from the body. Your HDL cholesterol level should be *above* 35 mg/dl, according to government guidelines.

Because many other factors figure into your risk of developing heart disease (smoking habits, weight, fitness level, etc.), you should discuss your cholesterol level with your doctor. He can then help you, if necessary, to make adjustments in your lifestyle, aimed at reducing this level.

Lower Your Fats, Lower Your Cholesterol

The most obvious place to begin your lifesaving, cholesterol-lowering program is with your diet.

While it is true that your body makes its own cholesterol, you also consume it, almost entirely in the form of animal fats—meat and dairy products and especially egg yolks. If your cholesterol level is high, you need to cut down on these foods.

Eggs head the list of foods chock-full of cholesterol. One measly egg yolk contains more than 200 milligrams—that's nearly your recommended limit for the entire day! In other words, if you eat one soft-boiled egg for breakfast, you've almost blown your quota for the day.

If you're like most Americans, between 35 and 40 percent of all the calories you consume come from fat. The liver just can't dispose of that much fat, and it ends up—where else?—hung up on the artery walls.

Most doctors say that a healthier diet would derive no more than 30 percent of its calories from fat.

But not all fats are created equal. The fat most linked to high cholesterol levels is the saturated kind, found in meat and dairy products and certain tropical oils such as palm oil, palm kernel oil, and coconut oil. Try to replace these fats with the polyunsaturated kind found in vegetable oils, such as safflower, sunflower, corn, and soybean oils. Or switch to monounsaturated fats, found in olive, canola, and peanut oils.

Choose low-fat and nonfat milk over whole milk; select low-fat yogurt and evaporated skim milk instead of heavy cream. Substitute part-skim ricotta and mozzarella and low-fat cottage cheese for high-fat havarti and cream cheese.

Trade in sour cream for yogurt to top your baked potato. Try fruit ices or delicious sorbets for dessert instead of ice cream. Trim the fat off red meats and the skin off poultry.

Avoid frying your foods. Instead, try steaming, baking, broiling, and grilling. If you must fry, grease the pan with a nonstick spray or use nonstick pans.

Fabulous Fish, Fabulous Fiber

Eskimos, who eat enormous amounts of animal fat such as seal meat, are known to have very low rates of heart disease. How can that be? Scientists say it's largely due to the protective power of fish oil, also abundant in

138

Four Ways to Trim Fat from Your Diet

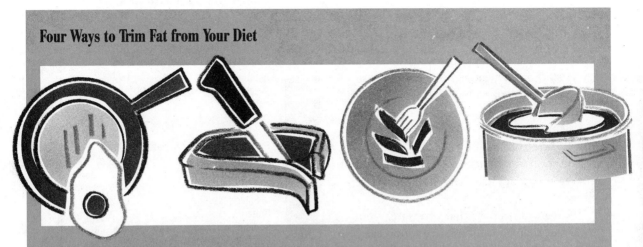

Use a nonstick pan or spray. Miss the taste of butter or margerine? Switch to a sprinkle-on butter substitute. Try using a little water or low-sodium broth instead of oil.

Buy only the leanest cuts of meat. Be sure to trim and discard any visible fat before *and* after the meat is cooked. Remove chicken and turkey skin before cooking.

Serve smaller portions of meat. Make meat a part of a larger dish like a stir-fry or wholesome stew. Cut the meat into thin strips, suki-yaki-style, for the illusion of a larger serving.

Before making a stew or soup, chill the broth for a few hours. The fat will rise to the top and harden. Then you can easily skim it off and start your dish with low-fat ingredients.

the Eskimos' diet. Fish oil contains a special kind of fatty acid called *omega-3*. Although no one can say for sure how it works, ample evidence shows that omega-3 can somehow help to lower cholesterol levels and keep the blood from clotting. Many doctors now recommend at least two fish meals a week, preferably of cold-water fish such as bluefish, salmon, or mackerel.

Fats and cholesterol are the most important dietary factors when it comes to determining your blood cholesterol level, but fiber may also play a role.

You're probably familiar with the hubbub about oat bran. Grocers can't keep oat bran products on their shelves. The reason?

Researchers have found that if you eat foods like oat bran and beans as part of your daily diet, you can reverse the bad effects of eating fatty foods. They work by either escorting cholesterol out of your body or by simply replacing the usual American fare with healthier foods. Either way, you can't lose.

One study done at the University of Kentucky, for instance, found that people who ate oats and beans, in addition to their normal meals, were able to lower their cholesterol by an average of 19 percent in less than a month—a better reduction than most people get using fat restriction and medication.

Try 1/3 cup of oat bran cereal for breakfast

instead of eggs and buttered toast. An oat bran muffin or two makes a great snack. You can also replace meat as your main course with a cup of cooked beans. And be sure to drink at least eight glasses of water daily so that you can keep all that fiber moving through your body.

And don't forget to eat lots of fruits and vegetables. They are also a valuable source of fiber.

Doctors also advise that you watch your total calorie count. Obesity can increase your blood cholesterol level and is linked to other risk factors for heart disease, such as high blood pressure.

Up with Exercise, Down with Smoking

A number of studies show that exercise can help to increase your level of HDL—the protective kind of cholesterol. Exercise also wards off obesity and high blood pressure—two other risk factors for heart disease.

You don't have to sweat through intensive workouts to gain these benefits, either. Studies have shown that walking briskly for one half hour, three or four times a week, can boost your good cholesterol and keep the excess from choking your arteries.

The same research showing that exercise can raise your level of good cholesterol also shows that if you smoke, you can forget about those benefits. Smokers who quit, however, have been shown in one study to experience significant increases in good cholesterol levels in only two weeks.

Russell Wild

Krunchees Potato Chips

Ingredients: Potatoes, cottonseed oil, salt.

Nutritional Information Per Serving:

Serving size	1 oz.
Servings per container	7
Calories	150
Carbohydrates	13 grams
Cholesterol	0 mg
Fat (60 percent of calories from fat)	10 grams
Monounsaturated	2 grams
Polyunsaturated	5 grams
Saturated	3 grams
Protein	2 grams
Sodium	130 mg

Percentage of U.S. Recommended Daily Allowances (RDA)

Calcium	*
Iron	2
Niacin	6
Protein	2
Riboflavin	*
Thiamine	2
Vitamin A	*
Vitamin C	10

*Contains less than 2 percent of the U.S. RDA of these nutrients.

Deciphering Food Label Hieroglyphics

"No Cholesterol!" That's what it says on that tempting bag of potato chips. Great. But does that mean you can just dig in? It can get a bit confusing, but doctors say that dietary cholesterol is *not* the major culprit when it comes to causing high cholesterol in the blood. That dubious honor goes to saturated fats. It's easy to see here that these potato chips are loaded with fat, including saturated fat. Watch out especially for palm oil, palm kernel oil, and coconut oil—they are highly saturated fats commonly used in processed foods. (Cottonseed oil, used in potato chips, is about 30 percent saturated.)

COLDS

Before you sniff at the cold remedies we're about to offer, pretend you're a Roman living 1,900 years ago. That know-it-all Pliny the Younger tells you the latest cure for the even-then common cold is "kissing the hairy muzzle of a mouse." He wasn't trying to be funny.

In more modern times, humorist Robert Benchley's first rule for avoiding the common cold was "Don't breathe through your mouth or nose." Benchley *was* attempting to be funny, but considering the fact that the average American adult gets as many as three colds a year, no one's laughing.

The common cold is so . . . well, common, that to prepare yourself for the annual cold wars you'll have to be well armed both with preventive strategy and (alas) some battle plans should a bug manage to breach your lines of defense.

Know (and Avoid) Your Enemy

First, it's important to know what a cold is and what causes it. Any 1 of at least 100 viruses can cause the common cold. Symptoms are actually produced by your immune system's effort to eradicate the cold virus. By-products of the four-day to one-week battle can include sneezing, sniffling, watery eyes, sore throat, coughing, headache, and a slight fever.

The virus enters your body mainly through the nose and eyes. Like a can of hair spray, a sneeze spreads the virus through the air. A person with a cold is walking around in a virus cloud. His hands are especially contaminated from blowing his nose and rubbing his eyes. Do yourself a favor and red-flag his handshake, any doorknob he touches, his steering wheel, his telephone, his box of tissues.

Keep your distance from people with colds, wash your hands with soap and water after touching things they've touched, and try to avoid touching your face with your hands if you've been in contact with a cold sufferer.

And by the way, a quick rinse of your fingertips under a trickle of cold tap water won't do. A more vigorous scrub may be in order to discourage cold germs and break the chain of infection. Lather well and wash each hand with the other under a steady stream of warm running water. Remember to scrub the backs, as well as the palms of your hands, and pay attention to your fingers and nails. Then rinse your hands thoroughly and dry them well.

There is no medical evidence, by the way, to indicate that cold weather alone will make you catch a cold. The reason most colds occur between September and May is that we spend more time in close quarters (with persons carrying cold viruses)—often in poorly ventilated rooms where colds spread fast.

Keeping toasty makes matters worse: Heating dries the air, as well as the protective mucous membranes in the nose and throat, making us more susceptible to infections. The solution: Keep room humidity high enough with a *steam* vaporizer. Cold-air humidifiers can lower room temperature and may harbor bacterial growths.

You'll have a better chance of avoiding colds if you don't smoke. Smoking stuns the tiny hairlike projections known as cilia, whose job it is to keep airborne invaders from entering the lungs. Studies leave little doubt that smokers suffer more colds and that their colds are more severe.

Battling the All-Too-Common Cold

Science is at a standstill in its efforts to defeat the common cold, but that doesn't mean we can't negotiate for less discomfort from the pesky foe. Here's a roundup of what modern science has determined to be the most effective ways of dealing with the bothersome bug.

Get plenty of vitamin C. In doses of 500 milligrams, four times a day, vitamin C has been shown to diminish a cold's symptoms and length by half. Supplements can help you get enough C: 500 milligrams is the amount found in 6 cups of grapefruit juice from concentrate, 5 cups of cranberry juice cocktail or orange juice from concentrate, or 4 cups of raw chopped broccoli or green peppers. The Recommended Dietary Allowance (RDA) for vitamin C is 60 milligrams. Check with your doctor before taking supplements.

Keep your diet light. Stay away from fats, meats, and dairy products, which are harder to digest than fruits and vegetables. Drink plenty of liquids to replace those lost through your running nose and sweating body. And do enjoy a bowl of good old chicken soup. The vapors and aroma have been found to help clear a cottony head by increasing the flow of mucus.

Suck zinc lozenges. This can also cut the symptoms and duration of a cold. One study showed that zinc gluconate taken 24 hours before the onset of cold symptoms can reduce your cold symptoms by one-third— something to keep in mind if you're in a crowded elevator and someone sneezes before you can escape being contaminated. The suggested dose is one zinc gluconate lozenge every 2 hours during the daytime until the symptoms are gone. Check with your doctor before trying this treatment. It is generally recommended that it not be continued for more than one week. Don't take zinc supplements on a regular basis, though. In moderate amounts zinc helps your immune system, but too much can damage it.

Take it easy. Avoid your usual hard workout and swinging nightlife. Stay home from work, but feel free to take a half hour's brisk walk to get your virus-killing white blood cells circulating.

Stop smoking. When you have a cold, smoke irritates the throat and increases chances of infection invading your lungs.

Gargle for a sore throat. One half teaspoon of salt per 8 ounces of warm water remains a state-of-the-art gargle, experts agree. Sucking on hard candy or specially formulated throat lozenges can also bring sore-throat relief. (You should consult a physician, however, if swallowing becomes a problem or if you find your sore throat is accompanied by a fever higher than 101°F with no other cold symptoms. That sort of tortured throat could be due to strep.)

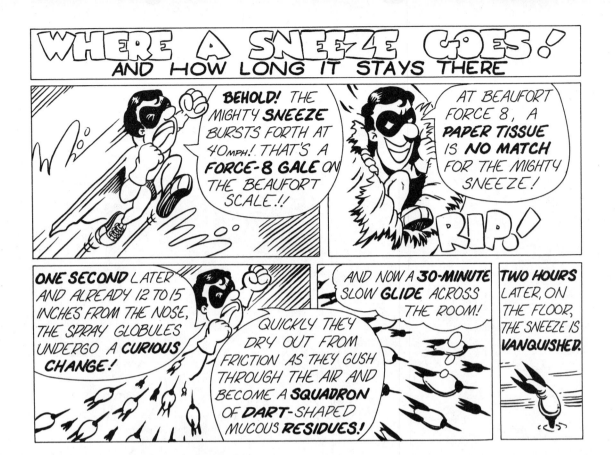

Avoid antihistamines. They usually won't work to unclog your nose because a cold doesn't raise your histamine levels. You can relieve stuffiness with an oral decongestant, but if you have high blood pressure, thyroid disease, or diabetes, avoid using decongestants. Nasal sprays may be used for a short-term effect, but can cause rebound stuffiness when used too often. A dab of petroleum jelly inside each nostril can relieve the rawness caused by nose-blowing.

Try aspirin. Aspirin can help relieve aches and pains for adults, but don't give it to children with colds unless directed to do so by your physician because it is associated with a rare, sometimes fatal disease known as Reye's syndrome. The multisymptom remedies contain doses of various drugs for every symptom you might have. But you may not want to be medicated for symptoms you don't have, especially since these remedies are often loaded with alcohol.

Keep bundled up. To combat the "chills" that can accompany a cold, give your body's defenses the advantage of keeping as comfortably toasty as possible.

Don't drug yourself. Antibiotics can have dangerous side effects and should not be taken for a cold unless there is a secondary bacterial infection such as sinus or ear infection. Decongestants in nose drops or sprays contain potent drugs that constrict blood vessels. If used for more than four days, they can cause a rebound effect.

Rest. The best prescription for a cold, besides getting plenty of liquids and fresh air, seems to be plenty of R and R.

William LeGro

143

COLDS

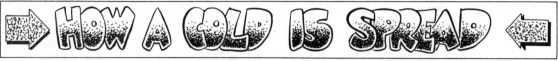

COLIC

He opens wide his little mouth and screams. His round little face turns bright red. He pulls his little legs up to his round little belly and passes gas. His howling may go on for hours, frightening, tiring—even angering—his anxious parents.

Theories about what causes colic abound: Gas is trapped in the baby's digestive system; the baby has an overly sensitive nervous system; mother is overanxious; the baby is allergic to cow's milk or reacts badly to formula; the baby is being breastfed by a mother who smokes. But the cause—if indeed there is a single cause—is unknown. Still, there are some remedies that seem to work, mostly those based on the excess gas theory. But your first step is to get the baby a physical examination to rule out illness. And don't blame yourself—the "anxious-parent" theory has been discarded by most doctors.

If the colic carry (see page 146) doesn't work, try burping the baby frequently while he's nursing, or after each ounce if he's on the bottle. Be sure he's feeding in an upright position to keep the air at the top of his stomach, where it's readily released by burping. Try rolling up a cloth diaper or a towel and putting it under his tummy when he's lying face-down.

Again going on the assumption that gas causes colic, doctors recommend you insert a suppository or a well-greased thermometer in baby's bottom and gently stimulate the rectal area. Then stand back.

Massaging the baby's tummy may help, especially combined with rectal stimulation.

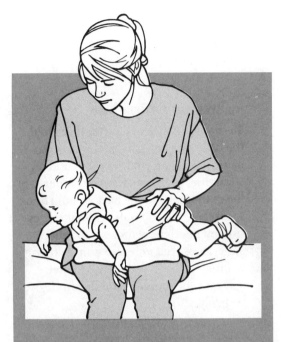

Give Your Baby a "Bottle"

Sometimes it takes more than a reassuring touch or cuddling to relieve a colicky baby's distress. Here's a strategy that many parents have found helpful. You may want to give it a try yourself and see if it does the trick. Hold the colicky child firmly on your lap and place a baby-sized hot water bottle underneath the baby's stomach. (Remember to make sure the hot water bottle is securely capped and make certain the water isn't so hot that it might burn either one of you. As an extra precaution, test the water on yourself first and wrap the hot water bottle in a towel.) While the water's warmth works its soothing magic, sing or hum to the baby.

145

COLIC

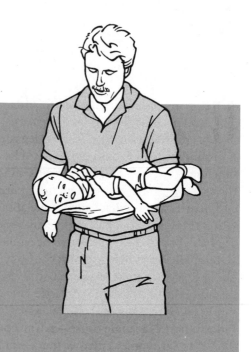

Or try putting the baby in a warm bath for 15 to 20 minutes.

Whether diet causes colic is still a mystery. But if your family has a history of allergies, your breastfed baby may be allergic to the cow's milk you've been drinking. Such an allergy is usually accompanied by other symptoms, such as diarrhea, wheezing, or rashes. Try avoiding cow's milk for a while. Or the baby may be lactose intolerant; another symptom of this inability to digest milk sugar may be watery diarrhea. If you are nursing and suspect your child has lactose intolerance, experiment by drinking an enzyme-treated cow's milk like Lactaid or bottle-feeding the baby with it. If your bottle-fed baby is drinking cow's milk, try switching to soy formula.

An altogether different theory, however, says colic doesn't involve abdominal pain at all. This theory sees "colic" as parents' misinterpretation of their baby's cries for attention. He wants to be cuddled or fed or jiggled or sung to or rocked. Maybe he wants a pacifier, or the sound of the vacuum cleaner, or the vibration and hum of the clothes dryer beneath his infant seat. Several studies showed parents who tried these various remedies had more success in reducing "colic" than those who tried switching their babies' diets. So pick baby up as soon as he starts to cry and don't worry about spoiling him, doctors say. Just give him what he wants and experiment until you find out what that is. Usually it's his mommy or daddy. The result is not a brat, but a baby who trusts you and the world and who learns to communicate.

William LeGro

CONJUNCTIVITIS

Your eyes look as red and bleary as a pair of car taillights in a rainstorm. You feel as though you have road salt trapped under your eyelids. Chances are you have some form of conjunctivitis, an inflammation of the silky-smooth membrane that lines your eyelids and covers the whites of your eyes.

If your eyes itch, burn, and secrete a gummy, yellowish discharge that leaves your eyelashes glued together when you wake up, you may have pinkeye, a painful, contagious type of conjunctivitis sometimes caused by bacterial infection.

These infections of the eye can be serious and in children can even lead to loss of sight, so if you have symptoms, see a doctor.

For temporary relief from the symptoms of infectious conjunctivitis, apply a warm, wet washcloth to your eyes for 5 or 10 minutes, three times a day. The moist warmth will help relieve pain and irritation. Launder washcloths and towels after each use. Wash your hands before applying any medicines to your eye. And to avoid reinfection, be sure not to touch any part of your eye with the applicator.

William LeGro

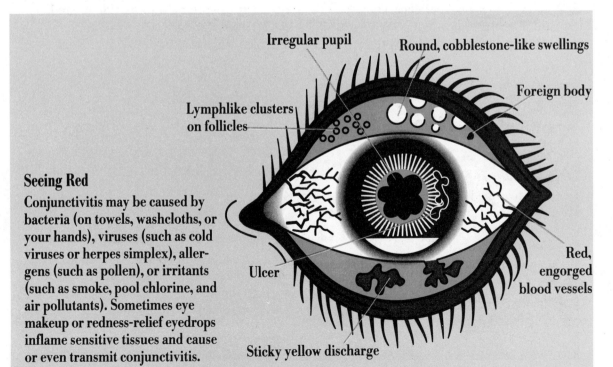

Irregular pupil

Round, cobblestone-like swellings

Foreign body

Lymphlike clusters on follicles

Red, engorged blood vessels

Ulcer

Sticky yellow discharge

Seeing Red

Conjunctivitis may be caused by bacteria (on towels, washcloths, or your hands), viruses (such as cold viruses or herpes simplex), allergens (such as pollen), or irritants (such as smoke, pool chlorine, and air pollutants). Sometimes eye makeup or redness-relief eyedrops inflame sensitive tissues and cause or even transmit conjunctivitis.

147

CORNS

There's nothing happy about feet afflicted with corns. They interrupt your walking program and keep you in your seat when you'd rather be dancing the night away. Amazing, isn't it, how something as tiny as a corn can make such a big difference in how you feel?

Usually, corns are blamed on faulty shoes, but Elizabeth Roberts, D.P.M., professor emeritus of the New York College of Podiatric Medicine and author of *On Your Feet,* says it's often not the shoe but the foot that is at fault. If there is an imbalance of the muscles of the foot or leg, your foot may slip forward in the shoe and roll inward.

Wherever the foot experiences constant, unnatural pressure, a corn or callus forms. (A callus always forms when the pressure occurs over a much larger area.)

"If you keep rubbing your hand, it gets red. Think of what your hand would look like if you rubbed it as many times a day as your foot rubs against its shoe if you are walking improperly," says Dr. Roberts. The blood drawn to the irritated area stimulates new cell growth, and these cells become the corn. Corns become painful when they press on a nerve.

Curtail Those Corns

You can detect a developing corn by regularly examining your feet for any red, tender areas, the early warning sign that trouble is ahead.

Why Corns and Bunions Form

If each time you take a step, your feet rub against your shoe, then excess friction stimulates blood flow. All that blood nourishes the tissue, stimulating the growth of new skin cells. If the toes rub against the top or sides of the shoe for a long enough time, you get a corn. If your shoes squeeze the toes together, then the joint that connects the big toe to the midfoot often compensates by jutting out. That's likely to aggravate a bunion.

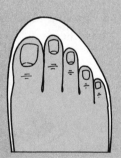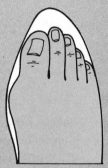

Left, The boxy shoe allows the toes enough room for normal spread. *Right,* But the pointy shoe jams the toes together and is sure to cause corns or aggravate bunions.

To prevent a corn being caused by a shoe, switch to a wider shoe or one with a larger toe box, says Clare Starrett, D.P.M., chairman of the Department of Orthopedics at the Pennsylvania College of Podiatric Medicine. You can also use a moisturizer on the area to decrease friction against the shoe. For the same reason, always wear socks or stockings with shoes, she says.

If the corn has already developed, you can protect the area with a moleskin bandage or wrap the affected area loosely with strands of good-quality lamb's wool. You can relieve a soft corn, the kind you find between two toes, by separating the toes with a little piece of cotton or lamb's wool. Don't try to remove the corn yourself.

Corns should always be removed by a doctor.

"And avoid the corn and callus cures at your pharmacy," warns Dr. Roberts. "All contain a chemical that will break down good tissue more rapidly than the abnormal tissue."

Corns and calluses do serve one useful function. They're your feet's way of telling you there's something wrong with your walk. Maybe your gait is improper, so your feet don't meet the ground as they're meant to. Or maybe one leg is longer than the other.

Walking incorrectly can throw your posture off balance and eventually cause knee problems, night cramping, or lower back pain, in addition to corns. Your podiatrist can help you correct your walk.

Deborah Grandinetti

Smart Tips for a Proper Fit

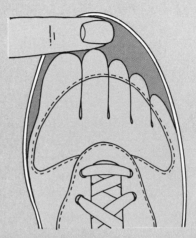

You'll know a running shoe is roomy enough if there is at least ¼ inch between your big toe and the tip of the shoe.

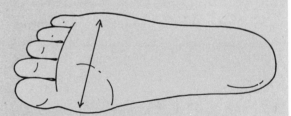

Try shoes on at the end of the day when your feet are more likely to be tired and swollen. Stand on the foot being measured and always fit the larger foot. To determine the shoe width you need, measure across the ball of your foot at the widest part. You'll know a shoe fits properly if, when you are standing, the toe area of the shoe ripples as the salesperson runs a finger across it, the uppers hold the foot securely but without causing irritation, the heel fits snugly, and no part of the foot bulges out when the shoes are laced. Check to make sure that the sole of the shoe bends easily.

149

The Wise Woman's Shoe Wardrobe

There's a lot of wisdom in that old saw: "If the shoe fits, wear it." And if the shoe doesn't fit . . . well, *don't*. Below, we show you how heels of various heights affect your foot and your gait.

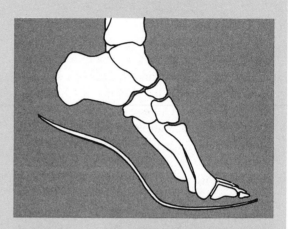

Very high heels throw all your weight onto your toes and the balls of your feet. This leads to corns and other painful growths.

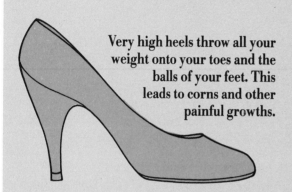

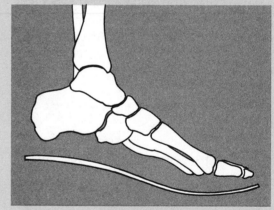

Moderate heels (between 1 and 1½ inches high) distribute weight more evenly between the heels and the balls of your feet. This height allows your feet to flex properly.

When you wear flats, you shift the burden of support to the balls of your feet and your heels, where it properly belongs. Wearing flats stabilizes your gait and allows your toes enough freedom to help you keep your balance.

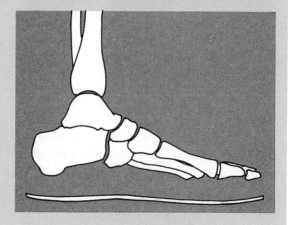

CUTS AND SCRAPES

Awareness lapses for just a moment, and the knife slips. An ankle gives, and a knee scrapes pavement. A finger catches on the crisp edge of a printed page.

The skin, the body's outermost protective layer, tears open. Maybe blood seeps through the opening. Bloody or not, the cut is an open invitation to infectious agents lurking in the area around it.

From your body's point of view, an open wound is a situation to be remedied pronto. In response to a cut or scrape, your body automatically performs a complex series of complex reactions designed to patch up the skin, it's protective armor, according Recia Kott-Blumerkranz, M.D., a Michigan dermatologist.

If your cut is superficial and your blood-clotting mechanisms are in working order, bleeding soon stops. Cuts of any size require treatment, however.

Cleaning the Wound

You can take care of most minor cuts and scrapes yourself. Once the bleeding has stopped, clean the wound gently. You want to remove everything that doesn't belong there without aggravating the broken skin. Pick out any gravel or glass. Double-check to make sure it's all gone. If it's deeply embedded, don't try to remove it yourself. (See "Removing a Foreign Object" on page 152.) Then wash the wound with a mild soap and water or hydrogen peroxide. Now is the time to stop any opportunistic bacteria dead in their tracks.

If you've been cut by a dirty object, you need protection from tetanus. If your shots are not up to date, see your physician.

Left to proliferate, bacteria can deepen a wound and make the skin's repair job tougher. The end result is an increased chance of scarring.

A triple antibiotic ointment—Dr. Kott-Blumenkranz favors Polysporin and Bacitracin—can help zap any lingering bacteria and keep new bacteria from gaining entrance.

Dressing the Wound

The other secret to speedy healing is to keep the area moist.

"Many, many studies show that if you let a wound dry out, you are inhibiting healing," says Dr. Kott-Blumenkranz. "Scabs actually slow things down. That's why it's good to cover a wound, so you can retain that moist surface."

After you clean the wound, cover it. Dr. Kott-Blumenkranz recommends regular plastic bandages or gauze and tape. You might also try the new breathable plasticlike bandages, designed to re-create the skin's natural barrier, but these are quite expensive. Ask your pharmacist about bandages designed to keep the skin moist while it heals.

One final thing you can do to help your body recover quickly from cuts is to eat right. Adequate protein is crucial. So are vitamins C, E, and the mineral zinc.

Deborah Grandinetti

CUTS AND SCRAPES

THE RIGHT WAY TO BANDAGE A WOUND

You probably keep a box of adhesive bandages in the medicine cabinet, right? But there are times when they just can't do the job; if the cut is an odd shape or in an awkward place, for instance.

That's why it's a good idea to also keep on hand a supply of sterile gauze pads and rolls of cloth bandages. It's also okay to use a large, clean piece of cloth.

Any cloth dressing you use should be large enough to extend at least an inch beyond all edges of the wound. To place a dressing on, hold it directly over the wound. Then lower it into place. If you have to slide the dressing around to get it to the right place on the skin, you'll contaminate the wound. If you miss on the first try, throw the dressing away and start with a fresh sterile one. And if you bleed through the first dressing, apply a second one directly on top of the first.

Never use fluffy material like absorbent cotton directly on a wound because the fibers can stick. Cotton wool covered with gauze is a better choice.

Use a bandage to hold the dressing securely in place. Make sure it is as clean as possible. It doesn't have to be sterile.

Don't make the bandage too tight because you could cut off circulation and cause serious tissue damage. Remember, too, that an injured limb might swell, making the bandage even tighter.

Monitor possible swelling or skin discoloration by leaving the toes or fingertips exposed when you bandage the foot or hand. This way, if circulation is shut off or limited,

you can see it. Should swelling, discoloration, a sensation of tingling or coldness occur, loosen the bandage immediately. If the abnormal condition of the skin persists, consult your doctor.

Bandaging a wound the right way can help speed healing. It's also important to change the bandage on a daily basis, says Recia Kott-Blumenkranz, M.D., a Michigan dermatologist.

No matter what you're bandaging, always place the bandage down at a slight angle over the dressing, then wrap around that first piece a few times to anchor it.

Removing a Foreign Object

If you have something other than easily removed bits of dirt or gravel embedded in the wound, you need medical attention. You can follow these emergency procedures when medical help is not immediately available, or even on the way to the doctor's office. Don't try to remove the object. That's the doctor's job. To slow bleeding, elevate the area and apply pressure right next to the wound on the side closest to the heart.

Place the first layer of bandage loosely around the object. Then continue to bandage *around* the object so the entire area is protected. At no time should you place anything directly on top of the object. Next, bandage the wound by wrapping the roll gauze around it in diagonal strips. Make sure the strips do not go over the embedded object or press it further into the skin. Go directly to the hospital.

Elbow

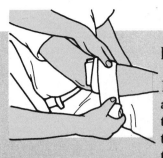

1. Always bandage a limb in the position in which it is to remain. Bend the elbow at a right angle.

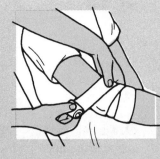

2. Start with two or three turns below the wound. Finish with two or three turns above it, fold in the end, and fix with tape.

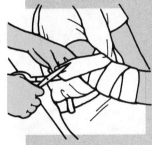

3. If you don't have tape or a pin, leave a length of bandage free and cut it down the center for a tie.

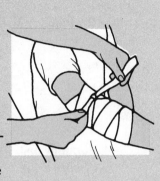

4. Join the two strings with a single knot, pulling tightly just above the cut edge.

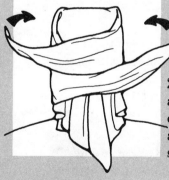

5. Take the two ends around the limb again and tie them.

Head

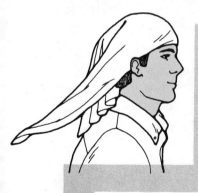

1. Place the center of the triangle base across the forehead so that it lies just above the eyes.

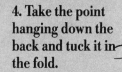

2. Bring the ends above the ears and cross them snugly at the base of the skull.

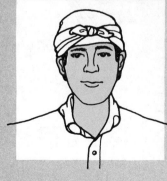

3. Now bring the ends around to the front. Center a knot on the forehead.

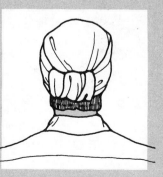

4. Take the point hanging down the back and tuck it in the fold.

CUTS AND SCRAPES

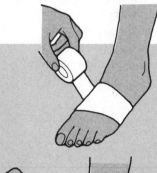

Ankle

1. Anchor the bandage with one or two circular turns around the foot.

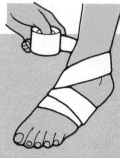

2. Bring the bandage across the top diagonally around the back of ankle.

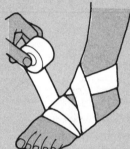

3. Bring the bandage over the foot and down under the arch.

4. Continue making figure eight turns, following the established pattern.

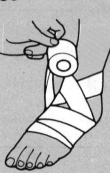

5. Bandage the foot, ankle, and lower leg.

Finger

1. Anchor the cloth bandage at the base of the finger with several circular turns.

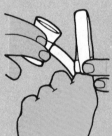

2. Hold the bandage in place. Then bring it up to the fingertip, up over, and back down.

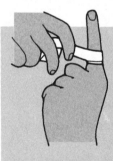

3. Wrap up and down the length of the finger until several layers cover the finger.

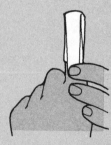

4. Now make circular turns up the finger and back.

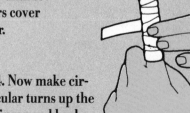

5. Apply tape up one side of the finger and back down.

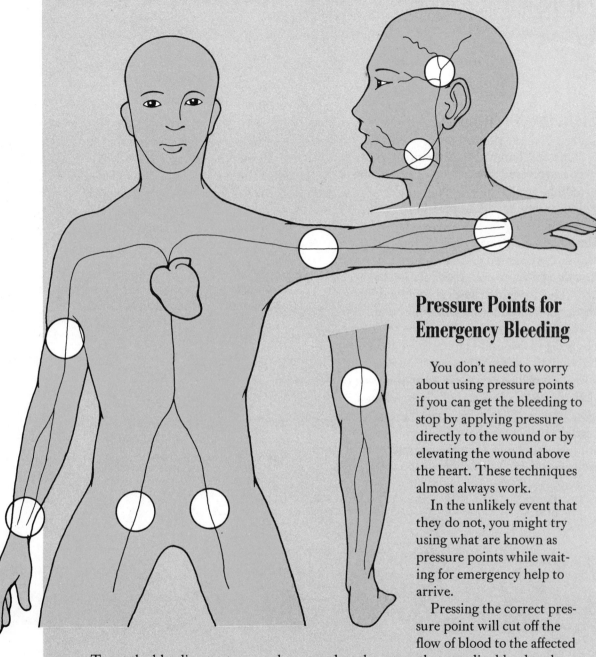

Pressure Points for Emergency Bleeding

You don't need to worry about using pressure points if you can get the bleeding to stop by applying pressure directly to the wound or by elevating the wound above the heart. These techniques almost always work.

In the unlikely event that they do not, you might try using what are known as pressure points while waiting for emergency help to arrive.

Pressing the correct pressure point will cut off the flow of blood to the affected area. To get the bleeding to stop, you have to select the artery that supplies blood to the wound and press it down against the underlying bone. If possible, raise the wounded area above the heart before you press. Apply heavy pressure for no more than 5 minutes. Then apply light pressure for 5 minutes. Continued heavy pressure can cut off circulation to the limb and cause damage.

155

CUTS AND SCRAPES

Stem the Bleeding

Accidents happen. If you happen to be the only person available to help a person who is bleeding, do you know what to do?

If bleeding doesn't stop within a few minutes on its own, put a clean cloth or your clean hand on the wound and apply pressure. But *don't* make that cloth into a tourniquet. You don't want to cut off circulation to the area. Don't remove the cloth. If blood soaks through, apply another cloth on top of it.

If direct pressure doesn't do the trick, try elevating the wounded limb above the heart, but only if you don't suspect a fracture. Elevation will reduce pressure on the wound, slow the bleeding, and make it easier for a clot to form. If the bleeding won't stop, seek medical help immediately. See a doctor if the wound was caused by a foreign object, or if redness and swelling occur.

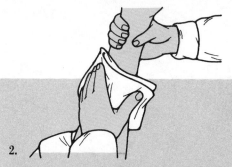

2.

Make sure the wound is clean. If it is, place a thick, clean compress such as sterile gauze directly over the entire wound. Press the cloth down firmly on the wound with your palm.

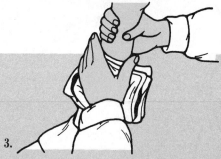

3.

Be careful not to disturb any blood clots that form. If blood soaks through the compress, don't remove it. Simply apply another one on top.

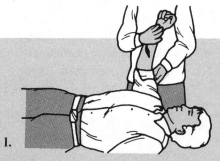

1.

Have the person who is bleeding lie down. Remove clothing from around the wound if you can do so easily. Apply pressure while elevating the affected area above the heart. But don't elevate the wound if you suspect a fracture.

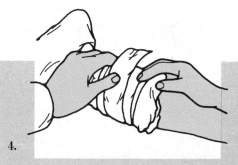

4.

Once the bleeding stops or slows, place a large absorbent cloth over the wound and the dressing. Bandage it firmly with a scarf or strip of clean cloth. Get medical help immediately.

DIVERTICULOSIS

Like junk mail, beeping watches, and sirens, diverticulosis is one of the plights of modern society.

Doctors say the condition, characterized by the presence of little pockets along the walls of the lower intestines, stems from a lack of fiber in the modern diet.

How do they know that?

Largely, they know from population studies. Diverticulosis is found in one-third to one-half of all North Americans and Western Europeans. On the other hand, in most of what we call the "underdeveloped" world, the condition affects few people. In fact, it didn't bother very many people in America and Western Europe until this century.

Studies have found a possible link between diverticulosis and our diets. It seems we don't get nearly as much fiber as we used to, or as we need to.

The High-Fiber Protection Plan

Getting more fiber shouldn't be a problem. Add increasing amounts of fiber to your diet as your digestive system gets accustomed to the extra bulk.

Bran is an excellent source, whether in breakfast cereals, muffins, or sprinkled raw over whatever else you are eating. Vegetables and fruits are good sources. Dried fruits, such as prunes, figs, raisins, and dates, are excellent sources.

Other good sources include whole grains and beans. You might also consider a fiber supplement, such as psyllium seed (Metamucil).

You should also drink six to eight glasses of liquid a day. Fluids are particularly important when adding fiber to your diet, for the two combine to run your stool smoothly through the system and keep your intestines in good condition.

The Quiet Condition

What if you already have diverticulosis?

Relax. Considering how horrible it sounds, it may surprise you to know that you can have diverticulosis without even knowing it. In fact, an estimated one in three Americans over the age of 60 is thought to have the condition, but only a fraction of these are aware of it.

Often when the little pockets become inflamed and start to bleed, people run to their doctors.

If this is your condition, then you are said to have not only diverticul*osis* but also a complication known as diverticul*itis*.

If you are unlucky enough to get diverticulitis—you'll recognize it by the fever, sharp abdominal pains, and possible bleeding—get yourself to a doctor. Once the condition is under control, he will likely prescribe rest, a special diet, and antibiotics.

For the rest of us, the best way of avoiding diverticulitis is to avoid diverticulosis, or, if you have it, to keep it from worsening.

Russell Wild

157

DIVERTICULOSIS

The Ins and Outs of a Common Disease

If you've wondered what diverticulosis looks like, wonder no more. The balloonlike pouches that you see attached to the colon are the diverticula. They occur where the colon wall is weakest, at those points where the blood vessels that supply nutrition and oxygen to the colon enter the bowel. While one in three Americans over the age of 60 is thought to have the condition, only a fraction may even be aware of it.

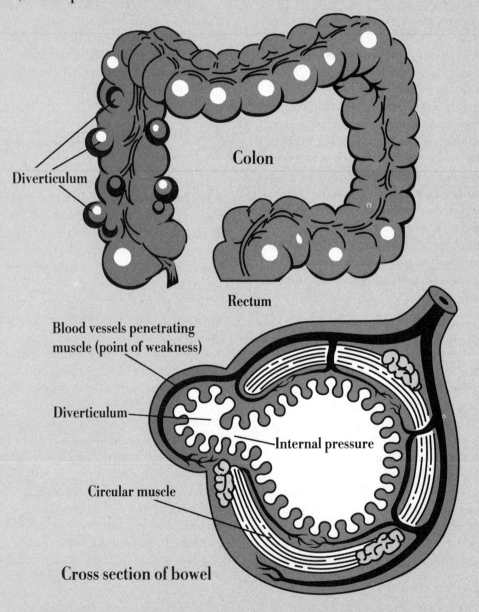

Diverticulum

Colon

Rectum

Blood vessels penetrating muscle (point of weakness)

Diverticulum

Internal pressure

Circular muscle

Cross section of bowel

DRY SKIN

Having skin like an alligator is no reason to shed crocodile tears or any other kind. Unless, of course, your dry skin happens to be on your cheeks, in which case a little watering might help. Dry skin is usually nothing more than skin that lacks water.

Water? Not oil?

That's right. It's a common misconception that dry skin lacks oil. And that isn't the only misconception about dry skin. Let's clear up a few: First, neither wrinkles nor a tight or "dry" feeling after you wash are necessarily signs of dry skin. Wrinkles come with aging. A tight feeling after washing is normal.

Why then are so many people convinced they have dry skin? Perhaps we've been subjected to too much advertising, says Thomas Goodman, M.D., coauthor of *Smart Face: A Dermatologist's Guide to Saving Your Money and Your Skin.* "The cosmetic and skin-care industry simply has the female public so thoroughly indoctrinated toward thinking 'dry' that it seems very few women are able to look at their faces with any objectivity," says Dr. Goodman.

How can you know, objectively, whether or not your skin is dry? One simple test is to put a strip of cellophane tape on your arm or leg. Pull the tape off and transfer it to black construction paper. Viewing the tape on the paper, you will see a pattern of skin cells. The more the cells clump together, the drier the skin. If the cells appear evenly distributed, the skin has adequate moisture.

The Art of Washing

Let's say you take the tape test and you "fail." What next? Dermatologists suggest a number of strategies. Start with using soap sparingly and be sure to rinse yourself extremely well. Overwashing and underrinsing contribute to dry skin.

If you can, postpone washing or shaving exposed areas in the morning before facing the elements. The natural sebum (skin oil) offers some protection from the wind and cold. Avoid long, leisurely baths or showers and stay out of hot water (including hot tubs). Go for short cool showers.

When it comes to washing your face, make sure you check out the tips on page 160.

Adjust Your Thermostat

Aside from improper washing, dry air is another major cause of dry skin. Dry air is usually the result of overheating the house in the winter. For moister skin, keep your house cool. And if turning down the thermostat still leaves you with dry air, consider installing a humidifier. The best place for one is in the bedroom—where you spend most of your time.

Another tip for winter skin care is to apply a creamy sunscreen before extended outings. It not only protects the skin from the drying effect of the wind and cold, it will shield you from the drying effect of ultraviolet light.

Russell Wild

DRY SKIN

A BEDTIME TREAT FOR YOUR MOISTURE-STARVED SKIN

After a long day beating around the hot, dusty city, your face deserves a good wash before you retire for the night. You do want to be careful, however, that you don't wash out the skin's moisture along with the dirt and grime.

If you tend to have dry skin, consider giving up soap in favor of a mild cleansing lotion designed especially for dry and sensitive skin (check with your pharmacist). Or, if you prefer a bar of soap, choose a mild soap that contains cold cream, coconut oil, lanolin, or cocoa butter.

Possible choices are Basis or Neutrogena brands.

A moisturizer also helps. By applying it after washing, you seal in the moisture. In fact, it should be applied only to damp skin. If you apply a cream or oil to dry skin, the skin underneath stays dry.

Saving Money

Many dermatologists feel that any product that can hold in moisture—including petroleum jelly, mineral oil, or any vegetable oil—may work just fine as a tool against dry skin.

You may want to use a special moisturizing cream, however, because it is less greasy than petroleum jelly. But don't believe in any supermiracle (and superexpensive) commercial creams that promise to chase away wrinkles and make you look generations younger. They don't exist.

Saving Face

Finally, establish order to cleaning your face at the end of the day. Your nightly skin-care routine should consist of four steps.

- Removing your makeup
- Cleansing
- Applying a toner
- Moisturizing

Follow the steps as illustrated, and you will be on your way to beating the dry skin problem.

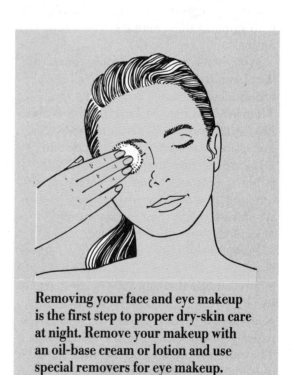

Removing your face and eye makeup is the first step to proper dry-skin care at night. Remove your makeup with an oil-base cream or lotion and use special removers for eye makeup.

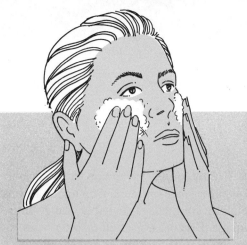

Choose a mild soap or cleansing lotion designed especially for dry skin. Look for a cleanser that contains cold cream, coconut oil, lanolin, or cocoa butter. You want to lather up your face and neck using *warm,* not hot, water.

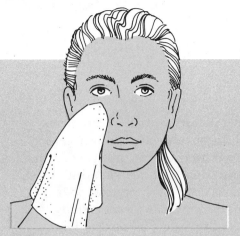

Now pat dry with a soft towel. If your skin is very dry, consider blow-drying rather than using a towel. Flip the dryer from warm to cool.

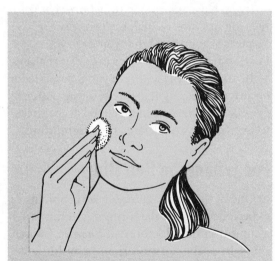

Choose an alcohol-free toner for its mild ingredients, usually water mixed with menthol or camphor. Saturate a cotton pad and smooth the toner over your face and throat using upward strokes.

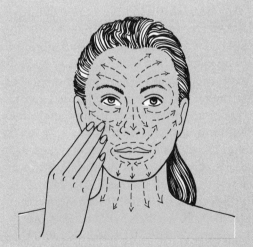

Moisturizers help by sealing in moisture, so you want to apply them while your skin is still moist from the toner. Dab the moisturizer on lightly and stroke gently away from the center of the face toward the sides.

EAR PROBLEMS

Consider the ears. Sensitive instruments that help you tune into your environment, your ears bring you the splash of rain on the roof, the whine of the dentist's drill, the crunch of boots on virgin snow, your neighbor's blaring radio, a lover's tender whisper . . . But you get the picture. Or rather, thanks to the complex anatomical marvel of your ears, you pick up on a whole world of sound. It is a world you want to protect and preserve.

The way you treat your ears over a lifetime influences their long-term health. When it comes to safeguarding your hearing, noise is public enemy number one.

Any noise that is loud can cause damage to the delicate hair cells of the inner ear responsible for transmitting sound vibrations. But how loud is too loud? You can't really be sure without sound-sensing equipment, but you can take a pretty good educated guess.

Hearing experts measure sound in decibels, commonly abbreviated dB. The very lowest sound the human ear can detect is measured at 0 dB. The higher the decibels, the more intense the sound, increasing in units of 10. So 10 decibels is 10 times more intense than 0 decibels, 20 decibels is 100 times more intense than 0, and 30 decibels is 1,000 times more intense than 0. Eighty decibels is the point at which noise can become dangerous, but that depends on how long you listen to it. How can you tell when noise has reached this danger level?

As a rough guide, something is too loud if you have to raise your voice or shout to be heard. Any sound that makes you wince, or later experience dullness, ringing, or a stuffy feeling in your ears is probably doing some damage. Because noise can do long-term damage to your hearing, it makes sense to take steps to protect your ears.

If you work in a noisy place, wear commercially available hearing protectors—ear plugs. Rolled-up cotton is inadequate. If you are a home craftsperson who frequently uses power tools, you should wear hearing protectors, too. The same applies if you are a hunter. And if you are a music lover, keep the stereo volume at a reasonable level.

If you have any reason to believe that your hearing has diminished, see your doctor. Experts recommend that you have your hearing tested at least once between the ages of 40 and 50. This will give you a baseline for evaluating hearing loss due to aging. After age 50, hearing should be tested every three to five years even if there are no symptoms.

For Whom the Bell Rings

One of the more common ear problems experienced by adults is ringing in the ears, a condition that doctors call *tinnitus*. Causes range from the not-so-serious (a buildup of wax) to the rather serious (a middle ear infection, a hole in the eardrum, high blood pressure, or thyroid problems). Because these more serious causes deserve medical attention, you are advised to see a doctor.

If the cause is high blood pressure, work with your doctor to get it under control.

162

Caffeine is a more common culprit than many tinnitis sufferers realize, hearing experts say. Aspirin can also cause ringing in the ears.

That Fishy Feeling

An infection of the outer ear canal is often referred to as swimmer's ear. But don't think you have to be a swimmer to get it. Sometimes water from the shower can get stuck in the ear, bringing with it bacteria and fungi, which tend to enjoy the warmth and darkness that your ear provides.

Swimmer's ear starts off with a feeling that your ears are blocked and itchy. At this point, experts advise that you apply antiseptic eardrops, sold under various brand names at your pharmacy. Or, you can make your own eardrops out of rubbing alcohol, which helps to dry the ear and may kill the bacteria and fungi. Dripping a bit of alcohol into your ear whenever you leave a swimming pool or shower is a good preventive measure.

Also recommended for swimmer's ear is a mixture of equal parts of alcohol and white vinegar. Dropping the mixture in your ears may be more effective than the alcohol alone in killing whatever is lurking within.

It's time to see your doctor if the infection has gotten to the stage where the ear is painful to touch, or a thin, clear liquid starts

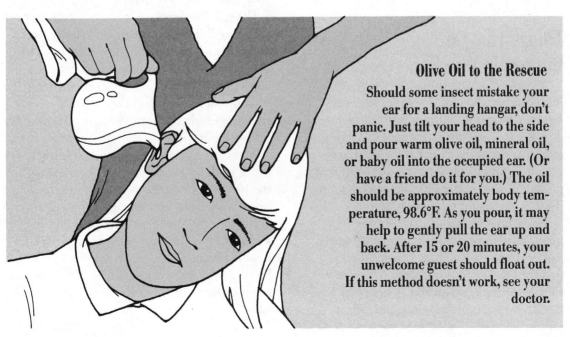

Olive Oil to the Rescue

Should some insect mistake your ear for a landing hangar, don't panic. Just tilt your head to the side and pour warm olive oil, mineral oil, or baby oil into the occupied ear. (Or have a friend do it for you.) The oil should be approximately body temperature, 98.6°F. As you pour, it may help to gently pull the ear up and back. After 15 or 20 minutes, your unwelcome guest should float out. If this method doesn't work, see your doctor.

EAR PROBLEMS

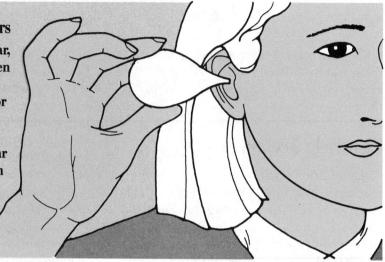

Three Days to Wax-Free Ears

To remove wax from your ear, place a few drops of hydrogen peroxide or mineral oil into your ear canal twice a day for two or three days. This will soften up the wax. Then a gentle rinsing using a soft ear syringe filled with lukewarm water should clean out the wax. Do not use cotton swabs or pointed objects.

to appear. Also, if you have ever had a perforated or ruptured eardrum, you should consult your doctor before you administer your own eardrops.

Things That Go Buzzzzz in Your Ear

It may not be anything quite so microscopic as a bacterium that gives your ear trouble. Certainly every summertime jogger or biker has had the experience of a flying gnat mistaking his ear for some kind of air terminal. Occasionally, these little kamikazes get tangled up in the wax and can't get out. This is no fun for either one of you.

Experts recommend that you wash the gnat out with warm water from a rubber bulb syringe. For an insect larger than a gnat, such as a moth or roach, you want to fill the ear with mineral oil. That plugs the breathing pores of the insect and kills it within minutes. Then, if the varmint doesn't

float out of its own accord, see your doctor for help with the eviction.

Ear Care in the Air

What if the problem with your ears isn't anything flying into them, but simply flying itself? For some airplane travelers, the change in atmospheric pressure can bring the discomfort and pain of ears that refuse to pop.

Popping is the process by which the pressure inside the ears is equalized with the pressure outside.

You can help your ears pop and bring a quick end to your discomfort. Experts say the best way to do this is to pinch your nostrils shut and suck in a mouthful of air. With your mouth closed, use your cheeks and throat to force air into the back of your nose as if you were trying to blow your fingers away from your nostrils. If this proves painful, stop immediately. Swallowing and yawning may also provide some relief.

Russell Wild

Let's Hear It for the Ears

The old expression "what you see is what you get," certainly does not pertain to the ear. The part you see is but a relatively small part of the whole. The part of the ear visible from the outside, as well as the ear canal, make up what we refer to as the outer ear. But you also have a middle ear and an inner ear. The middle ear consists of three tiny connected bones called the hammer, anvil, and stirrup (so named for their shapes), the eardrum, and the eustachian tube. The inner ear consists of the vestibule, semicircular canals, and snail-shaped cochlea.

Each part of the ear has an important role to play. The outer ear scoops up sound waves and directs them into the middle ear. The middle ear passes them on to the inner ear. The inner ear converts these sound vibrations into nerve impulses and transmits them to the brain.

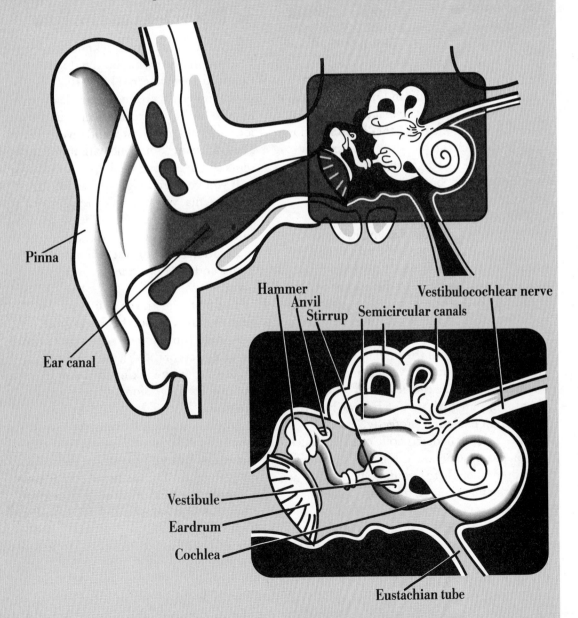

Pinna

Ear canal

Hammer
Anvil
Stirrup

Semicircular canals

Vestibulocochlear nerve

Vestibule
Eardrum
Cochlea

Eustachian tube

EMPHYSEMA

If you have emphysema, chances are good that you and your doctor know where it came from. "I'd say 90 percent of all emphysema is caused by cigarette smoking," says Norman H. Edelman, M.D., a specialist in pulmonary medicine at the University of Medicine and Dentistry of New Jersey—Robert Wood Johnson Medical School in New Brunswick and a consultant for scientific affairs for the American Lung Association.

Emphysema is a disease that slowly destroys the fine tissue of the lungs that is essential for oxygen to reach the bloodstream. Just how cigarette smoke wreaks such havoc is not fully understood, but doctors have some pretty good ideas.

The process seems to work like this: Smoke enters the lungs, causing irritation and inflammation. The body automatically releases destructive enzymes to fight what it perceives as an invader. In theory, the body should also release other protective enzymes to buffer the lung so it is not injured by the body's own defenses.

But in the lungs of the smoker with emphysema, the protective enzymes seem to go on strike—while the destructive enzymes are running amok. "There's a balance between the amount of natural protective enzyme and the amount of destructive enzyme that a person has. If somehow this balance gets disrupted, then there's going to be destruction of the fine tissue in the lung," says Dr. Edelman.

And so the lung is damaged—both by the cigarette smoke itself and by the body's own defenses called into service to fight off the smoke.

An Illness You Can Live With

It's all well and good to know what causes emphysema, but what do you do about it once you have it? First, know that even if your lungs are damaged, your life doesn't have to be. "Emphysema occurs in all forms—mild, moderate, and severe," says Dr. Edelman. "Someone with mild emphysema can live a long life."

If you've been diagnosed as having emphysema, you've already seen a doctor. And that's essential. For while emphysema can't be cured, your doctor can provide medications and suggest rehabilitation programs and lifestyle adjustments to help you cope.

The first adjustment in lifestyle you'll need to make, in fact the single most important thing you can do, is *quit smoking*. Some aspects of the disease cannot be reversed, but by kicking the habit today, you can slow its progession and prevent new problems.

Tobacco is an addictive drug, so quitting is not easy. The most successful quitters are those who join well-organized professional programs, says Dr. Edelman. Either your doctor or the local office of the American Lung Association can assist you in finding such a program.

Russell Wild

166

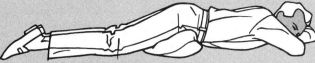

Positions to Clear Congestion

There are many positions that may help a person who has emphysema clear mucus from the lungs. Before you try these, check with your doctor to find out which positions are best for you. *Above,* In the first position, lie facedown with a pillow under your pelvis. *Right,* In the second position, lie flat on your back with your knees bent. The pillow goes under your hips. *Below,* In the third position, lie on your side. Rest your head on your arm and drop your free arm behind you. Again, position the pillow under your hip.

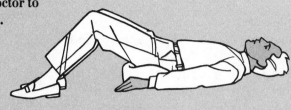

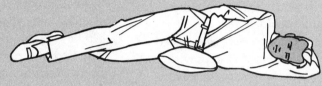

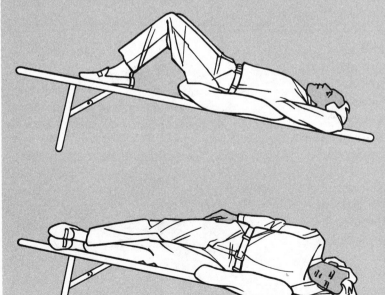

You may find a slant board helpful for clearing your lungs. Once again, check with your doctor to find out if these positions, or others, are likely to be helpful for you. *Top left,* In the first position, you lie on your back with your arms under your head and your knees bent. *Bottom left,* In the second position, you lie on your left side, and then repeat on your right side. Cough vigorously while holding these positions for 3 minutes.

167

EMPHYSEMA

EXERCISE FOR EMPHYSEMA

People with emphysema—like anyone else, only more so—should make every effort to be in good physical shape.

Walking is one of the most useful and enjoyable ways to strengthen the body, say experts at the American Lung Association. Start with a short daily walk and try to walk a little farther each day. Breathe slowly and deeply. Walk with your arms hanging loosely and your chest and shoulders relaxed.

As you walk, strive for an easy, even speed. Try to take the same number of steps with each breath. Try, for example, to take two steps while you're breathing in and four steps while you're breathing out. Experiment to find the number of steps that works best for you.

Take caution as you venture outdoors, however. Outdoor air pollution is an irritant that is all-too-easy to find these days. Avoid highly polluted areas. If you live in a city, consider perhaps walking indoors at a local mall on days of smog alerts. And if you have allergies, the same advice holds true for days when the pollen count is high.

Cold weather can be anything but a breeze to those with emphysema. Cold itself can be a trigger that tightens the bronchial airways. Take special care to dress warmly.

The following exercises were developed by the American Lung Association. Its experts say the best time to do them, or any exercise, is in the morning and the evening after you've cleared your lungs of mucus. Remember, the secret to success is doing some exercise *every* day.

168

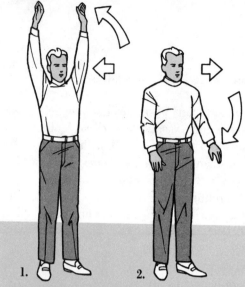

(1) Raise your arms and breathe in deeply, filling your lungs completely. *(2)* Lower them slowly as you breathe out. Repeat three times and gradually increase the number of repetitions as it becomes easier for you.

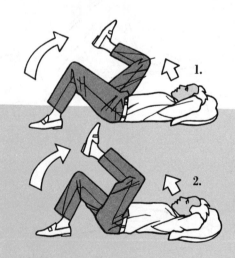

(1) Lie on your back with your knees bent. Raise your right knee toward your chest as you breathe out. Breathe in as you lower your leg. *(2)* Repeat three times, then switch legs.

(1) Lie on your back, bend your knees, and place your hands behind your head. Breathe in. *(2)* As you raise your head and shoulders as far as you can, breathe out. Feel your stomach muscles tighten. You don't have to sit all the way up. Start with three repetitions and gradually increase.

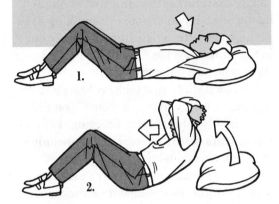

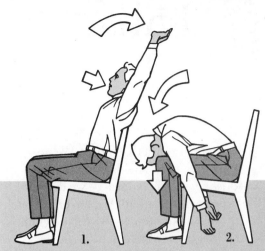

(1) While sitting in a chair, lean back, and raise your arms as you breathe in. *(2)* Then lean forward slowly, tucking your chin into your chest and letting your head fall to your knees as you breathe out. Repeat three times.

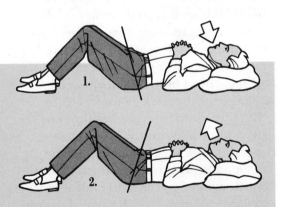

(1) Lie down with your knees bent and relax as you breathe in. *(2)* Tighten your stomach muscles and buttocks as you breathe out. You should feel the small of your back press toward the floor. Repeat three times.

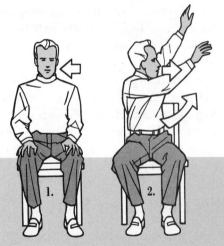

(1) Sit in a straight-backed chair, relax your shoulders, and inhale. *(2)* As you slowly exhale, turn your trunk to the left and reach your arms up over your left shoulder as if reaching behind you. Bounce your arms a few times. Rest a moment, then repeat on the other side.

EXERCISE

Life in the twentieth century. We no longer work the fields from dawn to dusk for our daily meals—we drive to the supermarket instead. We no longer pitch coal to warm our homes—we flip a switch. We no longer even have to hoist ourselves from our easy chairs to change channels on the television—we push buttons on the remote control.

This is the age of automatic door openers, electric drills, gas mowers, power-this and power-that. Elbow grease has been replaced by industrial lubricants. This is life in the twentieth century. The good and easy life.

Or is it? Humanity is now realizing that there's a flip side to all this switch-flipping. There is a litany of ailments directly linked to our increasingly mushy lifestyles.

But combating a lazy lifestyle doesn't mean you have to plow fields and shovel coal. On the contrary. The remedy for our modern life of ease is to incorporate regular exercise into life—*fun* exercise, be it swimming, biking, tennis, volleyball, hiking, ballet, or tending a garden.

Active Body, Happy Heart

What does exercise have to offer? Well, we *could* start with more energy, greater self-confidence, a trimmer body, more energy, reduced irritability, or a sounder night's sleep, but let's not. Let's start with America's number one killer: heart disease.

When the Centers for Disease Control in Atlanta reviewed 43 studies that link inactiv-ity with heart disease, they concluded that lack of exercise has the same bad effects as having high blood pressure or smoking a full pack of cigarettes a day. But while only one in ten Americans has high blood pressure, *six in ten* lead a sedentary life.

One such study that looks at heart disease and the "couch potato syndrome" comes from the Honolulu Heart Program. Following 12 years of study, researchers concluded that men over 64 who exercise regularly reduce their incidence of heart disease by half. A middle-aged man who exercises can expect a 30 percent drop in his odds of developing heart disease.

At the University of North Carolina at Chapel Hill, another study compared the effects of aging and exercising. Reviewing the health of 3,100 men, the researchers concluded that the right kind of exercise can offer more heart protection than would pushing back the clock *19 years.*

Exercise contributes to a healthy heart in many ways. Most directly, it increases the size of the heart and the efficiency of the heart muscle. It also reduces the amount of oxygen required by the heart both at rest and during exercise (which is why if you're fit, you'll have a slower pulse rate). Exercise also may widen the arteries, helping to keep them free of dangerous plaque.

In addition, exercise benefits the heart by combating several factors that often contribute to heart disease: high cholesterol, triglycerides, stress, and obesity.

Take cholesterol, that dietary culprit that

is to one's cardiovascular system as clumps of hair are to a bathtub drain. Perhaps the most important determinant of whether your arteries plug up with cholesterol-laden plaque is the amount of fat you eat. But it appears that exercise is also a factor. One survey of more than 1,000 men revealed that the more active had higher levels of HDL cholesterol (the good kind that is thought to partially counteract the effects of the bad). The active men also had lower levels of triglycerides, cholesterol's nasty pals that help cause heart problems.

As for stress, another risk factor of heart disease, there are a large number of studies which show that exercise can be an enormously effective tool for calming the body and mind. Some doctors say that exercise releases endorphins, a natural tranquilizer produced by the body.

And when it comes to weight control, for either your heart or your vanity, experts agree that exercise can make the difference between a body that's good and a body that's great. Beyond the mere fact that exercise burns up calories, it also affects a person's metabolic rate, that is, the rate at which the body consumes energy. Active people tend

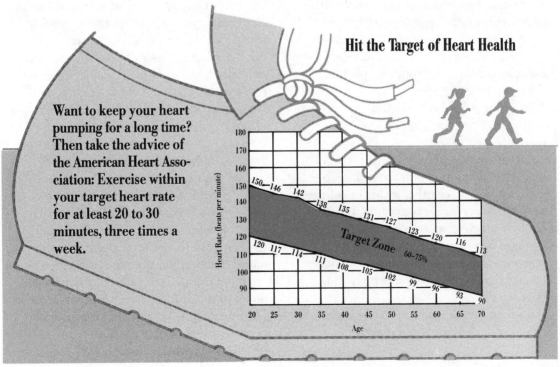

Hit the Target of Heart Health

Want to keep your heart pumping for a long time? Then take the advice of the American Heart Association: Exercise within your target heart rate for at least 20 to 30 minutes, three times a week.

Heart Rate (beats per minute)

Target Zone 60–75%

150—146 142 —138 135 131—127 123 —120 116 113
120 117—114 111 108—105 102 99 —96 93 90

Age: 20 25 30 35 40 45 50 55 60 65 70

180 170 160 150 140 130 120 110 100 90

to develop higher metabolic rates, allowing them to burn more calories at play or at rest than inactive people.

A Wealth of Positive Effects

It may not be headline news to you that exercise is good for weight control, but the many other benefits of exercise may surprise you.

Did you know, for instance, that exercise can strengthen not only your muscles but your *bones?* Doctors at the University of California at San Francisco measured the mineral density in the spinal bones of 46 young men. Some exercised regularly. Others spent all their free time watching soaps and playing cards. The doctors found that bone density was 14 percent greater in the group that exercised regularly. (Previous studies showed similar results.) So what good are mineral-dense bones? For one, they are less likely to fracture, a common problem among the elderly.

Exercising may also beef up your immune system, and by so doing, prevent certain kinds of cancer. Researchers at Harvard found that women who had been active in basketball, swimming, tennis, track, gymnastics, volleyball, or other sports in college later had a lower incidence of breast cancer than their inactive peers. Their sedentary classmates had twice the risk for breast cancer—as well as 2½ times the incidence of cancer of the uterus, ovaries, cervix, and vagina.

And then there's colon cancer, the second biggest cancer killer of both men and women. Three large population studies have found that men with physically active jobs, such as carpenters, plumbers, gardeners, and mail carriers, are much less likely to develop colon cancer than accountants, lawyers, bookkeepers, and other workers whose physical activity consists of shuffling paper and pushing pencils.

The connection between exercise and careers doesn't end with colon cancer, either. One survey found that executives who regularly participate in sports like running, basketball, and swimming, annually earn $3,000 more than their less athletic counterparts. One theory is that active people exude confidence, competitiveness, and energy— qualities for which employers are willing to pay a premium.

And if greater income won't lure you into an exercise program, consider the following: Physical activity fights aging. People who remain active throughout their entire lives can gain as much as a *25-year* advantage in performance ability over people who retire to their easy chairs. A study at Brown University looked at 4,500 middle-aged and elderly people and found that active 70-year-olds could typically perform physical tasks as well as inactive 50-year-olds.

The physically active are also far less likely to suffer from depression. Scientists can't say why for sure, but many studies show that exercise beats the blues. One large study by the National Institute of Mental Health found that depressed men who don't exercise are more than *12 times* as likely to remain down in the dumps as men who do exercise.

Some doctors believe the reason active people experience fewer cases of the blahs is because of chemical changes that occur in the body during exercise. In particular, exercising may tend to lower the amount of adrenaline in the blood. And, as we mentioned when discussing stress, physical activity also causes the body to release endorphins, the body's natural tranquilizer.

A Minimal Investment, a Big Payoff

Perhaps the best finding from the Brown University exercise study is that it takes just *moderate* activities, such as walking and gardening, to bring about all the benefits of exercise.

Doctors, in fact, are in general agreement that you can remain fairly fit with an exercise investment of little more than 20 minutes, three times a week.

So how do you get started in an exercise program? Experts say the most important first step is to make a commitment to yourself—one that you will keep. Next, you must set aside the time. Remember, you need at least 20 minutes of aerobic exercise, plus a few minutes to warm up and cool down, three times a week.

You probably don't need a medical examination before starting a modest exercise program, although it wouldn't be a bad idea, especially if you're over 35 and have never exercised before. Of course, if you have a history of heart and lung disease, high blood pressure, or any other serious medical condition, you ought to talk to your doctor before getting geared up.

But even if you are in perfect health, start out slowly and cautiously. A good rule of thumb is to increase the amount of exercise you perform by no more than 10 percent each week. So if you walk briskly for 20 minutes, three times a week, and cover a mile each time, you can press yourself to cover 1.1 miles the following week. At the end of ten weeks you'll be covering 2 miles, every 20 minutes—more of a *run* than a walk—so keep in mind that "rules of thumb" have definite limits.

Think of your exercise routines in three parts. Each should include a warm-up period of about 10 minutes, in which to rev up your blood flow and warm and stretch your muscles. Then, begin your aerobic exercise, that is, the 20 minutes or more in which you shoot for your target heart rate (see the chart on page 171). When you're done huffing and puffing, spend at least 5 minutes stretching and cooling down.

Of course, once you start, you'll want to stick with your exercise program. Experts say there are a number of factors essential to sticking with it. Among them, you need to establish realistic expectations, use reliable equipment, establish a specific time and place to work out, vary activities (to fight off boredom), and enlist the support of your friends and family.

Keep in mind that the first six months of a regular exercise program are really the test—most people who drop out do so within this period.

If you have any questions, find yourself a good teacher in the physical activity of your choice. The illustrations on the following pages should also serve as a helpful guide.

Now get on your mark . . . Get set . . . Go!

Russell Wild

Walk Your Way to Greater Health

The first step in your new exercise program may be learning how to walk. No kidding. David Balboa, sports psychotherapist and coauthor of *Walk for Life: The Lifetime Walking Program for a Healthy Body and Mind*, and his wife Deena run The Walking Center of New York City. It's a clinic that teaches people how to walk in a fashion that provides not only good exercise, but relaxation, greater self-esteem, and a sense of inner balance and harmony.

What's wrong with the way you may be walking now? "In this culture, people are taught to walk without moving their hips," says Balboa.

Men who move their hips may well be afraid of being labeled effeminate, and women who sashay are afraid of looking coquettish.

Stiff hips are only the beginning of our awkward walking styles. Many of us try to alter our walking styles to look like our favorite movie stars, such as John Wayne. So we swing our shoulders forward, turning side to side as we walk. Others make like prizefighters, cocking their arms and shrugging their shoulders. Still others flail their arms.

The end result is that what *should* be the most natural thing in the world becomes wholly unnatural. And instead of feeling relaxed and energized at the end of a walk—the way you should—you end your walk feeling tense and fatigued.

The Natural Way to Walk

Walking should be "fluid and effortless,"

says Balboa. A first step (no pun intended) is to make certain that both feet are pointed in the direction you are going. Don't allow your toes to veer off in opposite directions. It may help to visualize yourself walking along a narrow path.

Allow your shoulders and arms to swing naturally. Your arms will swing faster as you walk faster. Keep your shoulders relaxed and dropped, trying not to hang your arms as if you're carrying shopping bags. Take note that your arms are swinging as far back as they are forward.

Pull your shoulders back only slightly. Keep your body perpendicular to the ground and walk tall. Your walking not only *reflects* the way you feel, says Balboa, your walking *affects* the way you feel. If you walk in a confident manner, you will gain confidence.

With each step, land on your heel. Flex your foot and allow it to roll from heel to toes. Try to push off lightly from the back foot with each stride.

Let your hips loosen a bit more than they usually do. Feel your center of movement coming from an inch above your belly button. Breathe deeply as you walk and "think rhythm," says Balboa.

He recommends that novice fitness walkers attempt to put in at least 20 minutes a day, three or four days a week.

Done properly, walking can get your heart beating fast, says Balboa, "but there's more to life than reaching your target heart rate." Above all, he believes, walking should be fun—and part of your life.

174

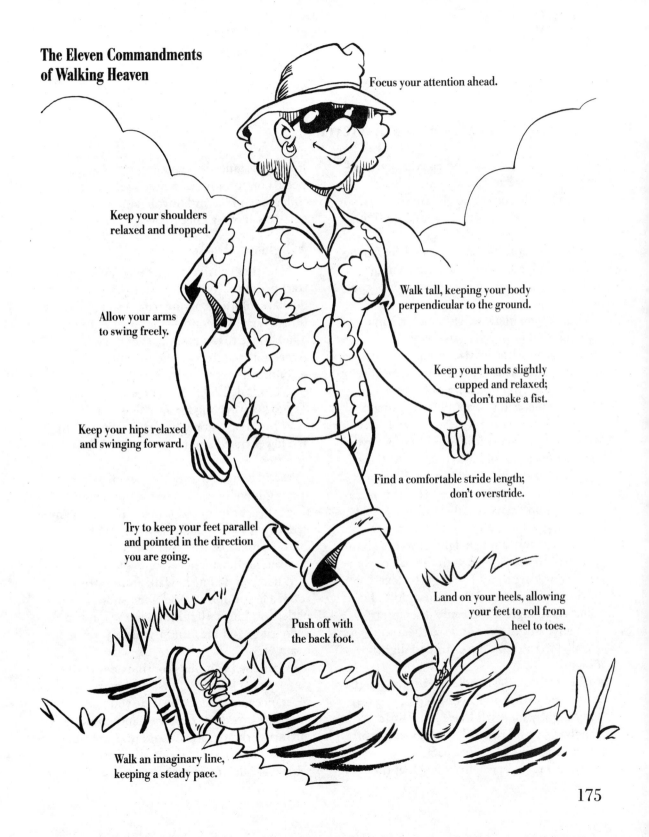

The Eleven Commandments of Walking Heaven

Focus your attention ahead.

Keep your shoulders relaxed and dropped.

Walk tall, keeping your body perpendicular to the ground.

Allow your arms to swing freely.

Keep your hands slightly cupped and relaxed; don't make a fist.

Keep your hips relaxed and swinging forward.

Find a comfortable stride length; don't overstride.

Try to keep your feet parallel and pointed in the direction you are going.

Land on your heels, allowing your feet to roll from heel to toes.

Push off with the back foot.

Walk an imaginary line, keeping a steady pace.

175

EXERCISE

Getting the Most from Your Exercycle

It's the one exercise you can do anytime—even in a blizzard. Exercycling. It's a great way to burn calories and elevate your heart rate right in the comfort of your own living room.

No wonder stationary bikes are by far the most popular form of fitness equipment sold—outnumbering sales of all other types put together.

But do you know what to look for in such a bike? And how to best use one?

Fitness experts say you should start by making sure the exercycle you pick is the right size for you. If it isn't, you won't feel comfortable, and you could hurt yourself. Start with the saddle. Check the width by sitting on it. The saddle should support your pelvic bones, not dig into your flesh. If the saddle does dig into you, have a bike dealer show you some wider ones. If you're using a gym bike and can't readily change the seat, cushion it with a pad.

Then check saddle height. If you push the pedal all the way down with the ball of your foot, your knee should be slightly flexed.

Next, adjust the angle of the saddle. If the front is too high, it can cause discomfort. Remedy: Adjust the saddle so the front is parallel to the top tube or tipped slightly down.

Next, check the handlebar. Set the height and angle so that when you hold it, you lean only slightly forward. Place just a little weight on your arms. That way, you're not likely to strain your lower back.

Take it easy, especially at first. Set the bike's resistance low enough so that you can pedal comfortably. Too much resistance can inflame tendons and hurt ligaments and cartilage in your knee.

A Beginner's Workout

Now that your bike is set to go, it's time to start pedaling. When first starting out, try to do 40 revolutions per minute—10 revolutions every 15 seconds—for 3 to 5 minutes. Then move to the main part of the workout. Accelerate to 60 rpm: one revolution per second. An easy way to estimate this is to count "1,001, 1,002 . . ." with each revolution. Try to keep cycling for a total of 20 minutes.

When you're done, cool down by pedaling at a lower speed and resistance for 3 to 5 minutes.

You may need to modify the intensity of this regimen, of course, to maintain your target heart rate or to ensure comfort. In any event, you should end this workout after the 20 to 25 minutes are up or you feel you've done enough, whichever comes first.

When you do finish, walk around the room a few minutes. And don't shower or bathe for at least 10 minutes after you stop exercising. You may unduly stress your heart.

When the beginner's routine doesn't tire you, try tougher workouts. Add more resistance and extend the time you pedal, but don't overdo it. Change hand positions during workouts. Also, stand up from time to time and pedal for about 30 seconds to relieve saddle pressure and stretch your legs.

176

Ten Tips for Better Biking

Place just a little weight on your arms
so as not to strain your lower back.

With pedal all the way up, your knee shouldn't bend
above your hips; if it does, adjust the seat higher.

Back should be flat,
not hunched
over.

If saddle pressure is
too much, stand up and
pedal for a while.

With pedal all the way down,
your knee should be slightly flexed;
if not, adjust the seat lower.

Set handlebar so that you are
straight or leaning forward
only slightly.

Change hand
positions during
workouts to reduce
soreness.

Saddle
should
be firmly locked in
place to avoid
slipping or falling.

Set the bike's resistance
on low when first
starting out.

Make sure
the angle
of the seat
is comfortable, either
parallel to the top
tube or with the
front slightly
tipped down.

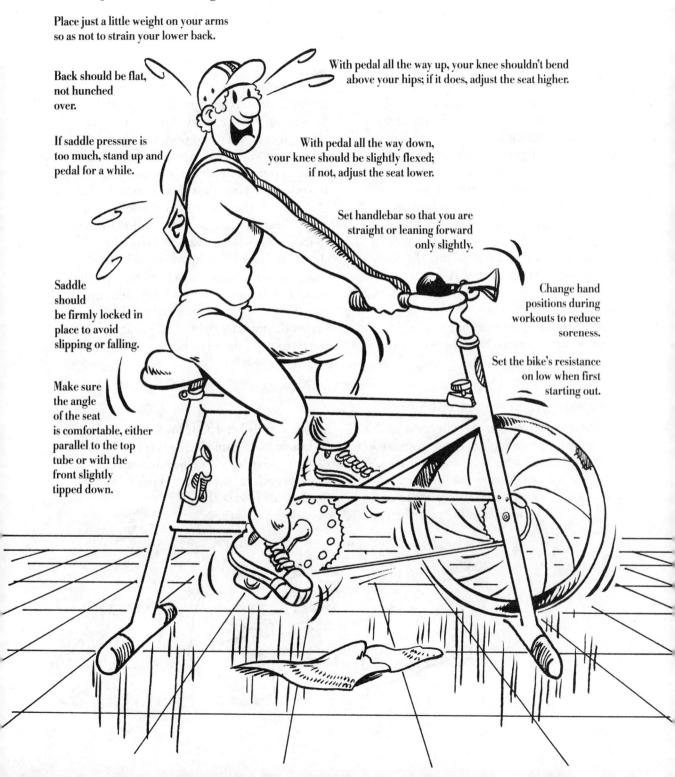

EXERCISE

STRETCHING YOUR MUSCLES

You have your new sneakers on, and they feel *fantastic*. You take a deep breath of the cool, fresh morning air, and every inch of you feels alive. You figure you have enough energy to do a 3-minute mile.

Haven't you forgotten something?

You sure have. Jumping cold into hard exercise is a major cause of athletic injuries. A warm-up readies your body by raising its temperature and making the muscles more supple and easier to stretch. A good warm-up might include easy calisthenics, or perhaps a brisk walk or slow jog.

After 5 minutes of warming up, you're ready to stretch. Stretching the body loosens, limbers, and further warms cold muscles. Stretching is also a good idea when you're through exercising and want to cool down. After your workout, stretching helps your muscles remain flexible and allows your heart to slowly readjust to its normal beat.

As you do the stretches on the following pages, keep in mind at all times that the way to loosen muscles is *slowly*. All stretches should be held for *at least* 5 seconds. You should never bounce into a stretching postion. Jerky movements trigger a reaction in the muscles known as a *stretch reflex,* which makes the muscles tighten and counteracts the purpose of the stretch.

Shoulders, Upper Arms, Chest

Grab a rolled-up towel to help you with this stretch for the shoulders, upper arms, and chest. *(1)* Start with your arms overhead, elbows straight, holding the towel in both hands. *(2)* Lower your left arm, allowing your right arm to slightly bend. *(3)* Slowly lower your right arm to the same level as your left. *(4)* Now move both arms downward as far as feels comfortable. Hold this position for several seconds, then raise both your arms.

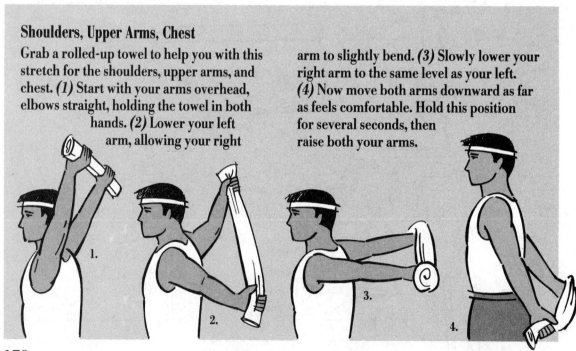

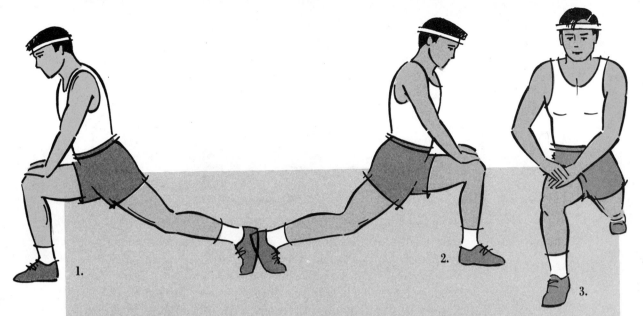

1.

2.

3.

Upper Thigh, Hip

This stretch works primarily the upper thigh and the hip. *(1)* Position both your hands on your knee, then press forward and downward. Hold for several seconds. *(2)* Twist your body and turn to the other side (no need to move the feet). Repeat on each side several times. *(3)* Do not allow the knee of your forward leg to get in front of the ankle. In other words, keep your shin perpendicular to the ground. This will allow for the greatest stretch of the back leg.

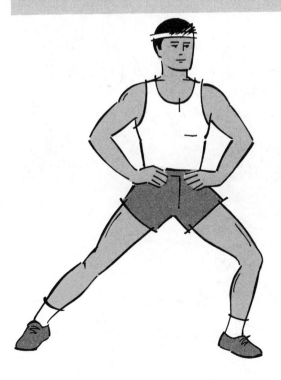

Inside of Thigh

Your adductor muscles are the muscles on the insides of your thighs. To give them the stretch they deserve, keep your back straight, spread your legs, tighten your buttocks, and lean sideways until you feel the pull in the groin. Hold the position on one side for several seconds, then move to the other side. Repeat several times. As you progress, bend your knee farther to give your adductor a greater stretch.

179

EXERCISE

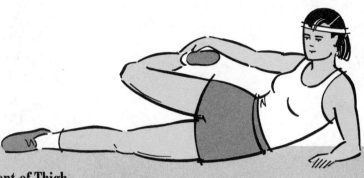

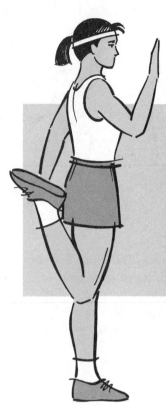

Front of Thigh

Your quads are the large muscles at the front of your thighs. For this stretch, *above*, you can either lie on your side or, *left*, stand. Standing, lean against a wall with your right hand for balance. Bend your right leg behind you and grab it with your left hand. Slowly pull your foot toward your rear end. When you just feel the pull at the front of your upper leg, hold it for several seconds. Repeat a few times on both sides.

Back of Thigh, Lower Back

This is a healthy stretch for the back of your thigh, as well as your lower back. *(1)* Sit with your right leg out straight and the left leg bent, knee toward the floor. Rest the sole of your left foot on the inner thigh of your right leg. *(2)* Bend your torso slowly forward from the hips toward your right foot until you feel a slight stretch. Hold for several seconds. When you no longer feel the stretch, try to go a tad further. Switch legs and stretch to the other side.

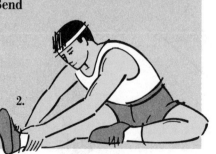

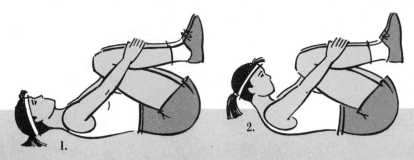

Back

One of the most common and painful injuries among weekend warriors is pulled back muscles. Protect your back by giving it a little stretch. Start by lying on your back with your knees bent and your feet flat on the floor. *(1)* Next, hug your knees and slowly pull them up to your chest. Hold for about 10 seconds, then slowly return your feet to the floor, first the right, then the left. *(2)* To loosen up your stomach muscles, remain in the back stretch position and curl up your shoulder blades.

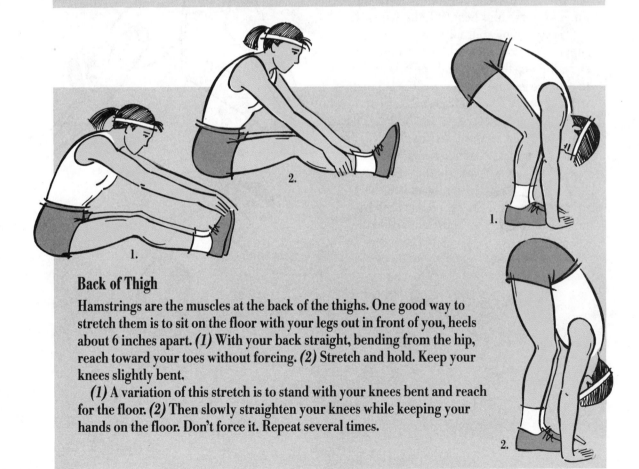

Back of Thigh

Hamstrings are the muscles at the back of the thighs. One good way to stretch them is to sit on the floor with your legs out in front of you, heels about 6 inches apart. *(1)* With your back straight, bending from the hip, reach toward your toes without forcing. *(2)* Stretch and hold. Keep your knees slightly bent.

(1) A variation of this stretch is to stand with your knees bent and reach for the floor. *(2)* Then slowly straighten your knees while keeping your hands on the floor. Don't force it. Repeat several times.

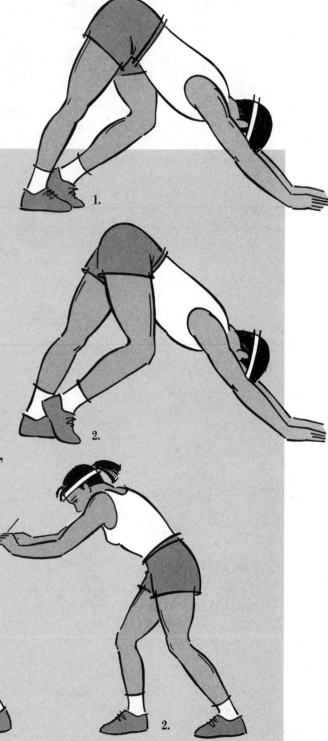

1.

2.

Achilles Tendon

Achilles, the mythological warrior, wasn't the only one vulnerable at the heel. You have a tendon there that needs to be stretched to avoid injury. *(1)* With your hands flat on the floor and your back straight, straighten one leg, pressing the heel downward, while the other knee remains bent. *(2)* Alternate sides.

(1) Or, leaning your forearms against a support, stretch your right leg behind you, straightening the knee while pressing your heel to the ground. Keep your toes pointed straight ahead. The left leg remains bent. Keeping your back straight and both feet flat, move your hips forward. Switch sides. *(2)* For another kind of stretch, start in the same position, but bend your back leg so that both legs are bent. Hold the stretch. Reverse position of legs and repeat.

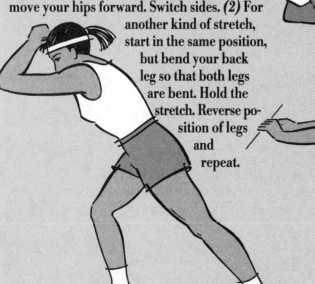

1.

2.

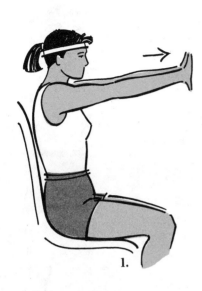

1.

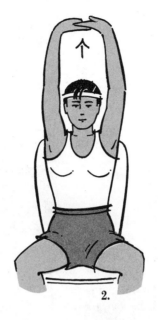

2.

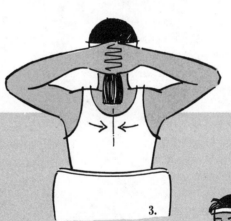

3.

Arms and Shoulder Blades

(1) Lock your fingers together and straighten your arms in front of you, palms facing out. Hold for several seconds, then repeat. *(2)* With your fingers again interlaced, turn your palms up and stretch your arms overhead. Hold and repeat. *(3)* Now, lock your hands behind your head, keep your elbows straight out to the sides, and try to pull your shoulder blades together. Hold for several seconds, then release, and repeat. *(4)* With your left hand, hold the right arm just above the elbow. Pull your elbow toward your left shoulder and look over the right shoulder. Do the other side.

4.

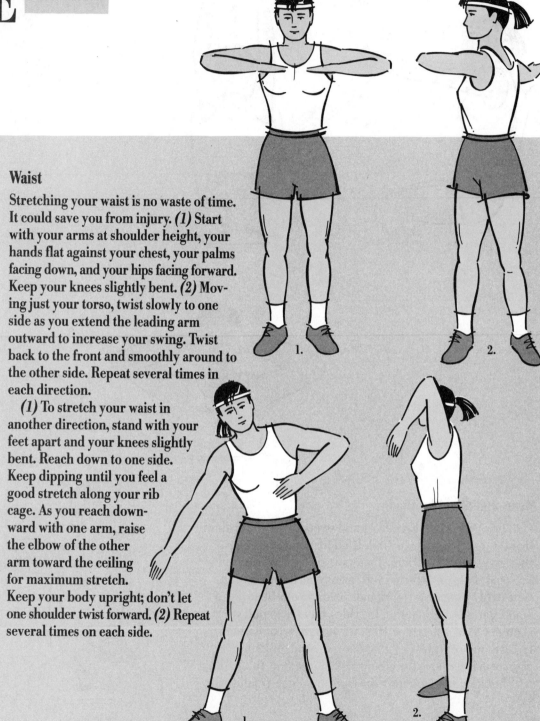

Waist

Stretching your waist is no waste of time. It could save you from injury. *(1)* Start with your arms at shoulder height, your hands flat against your chest, your palms facing down, and your hips facing forward. Keep your knees slightly bent. *(2)* Moving just your torso, twist slowly to one side as you extend the leading arm outward to increase your swing. Twist back to the front and smoothly around to the other side. Repeat several times in each direction.

(1) To stretch your waist in another direction, stand with your feet apart and your knees slightly bent. Reach down to one side. Keep dipping until you feel a good stretch along your rib cage. As you reach downward with one arm, raise the elbow of the other arm toward the ceiling for maximum stretch. Keep your body upright; don't let one shoulder twist forward. *(2)* Repeat several times on each side.

1.

2.

1.

2.

Back

Here's a good back stretch, whether you're about to exercise or you've just been sitting in an uncomfortable chair for too long. *(1)* Start by grabbing a pole, such as a broomstick, placing it behind you, and hooking your arms around it. *(2)* Standing with your feet about shoulder width apart and your knees relaxed, turn to one side as far as you can without straining. Allow your hip to move with you and turn your head in the direction you are turning. *(3)* Twist several times in each direction.

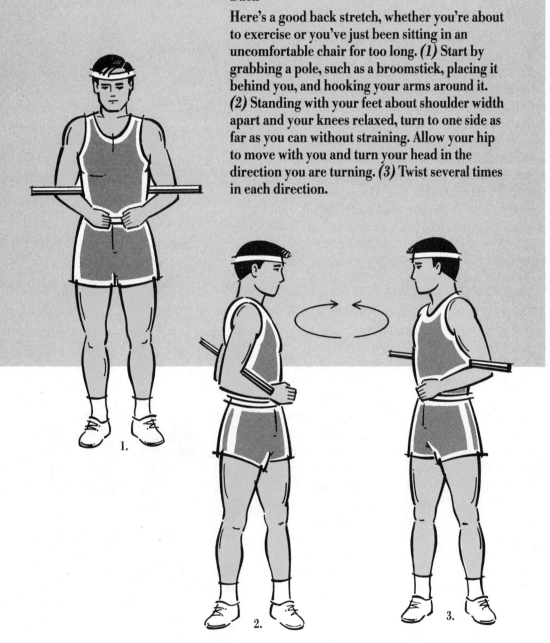

1.

2.

3.

EYE PROBLEMS

Your eyes are two of your body's most valuable parts. And two of its most vulnerable. Accidentally drop a heavy box on your toe or jab your finger with a kitchen knife, and chances are you will sustain only a minor injury. But catch the tiniest speck of coarse dust in your eye or inadvertently point the spray nozzle of an aerosol can toward your face, and things could get serious really fast. Damage control for eye problems must be fast and efficient. Unless your problem is a harmless foreign object that you can successfully remove yourself, head for a hospital emergency room *pronto*. In general, eye injuries should be treated by a medical professional. There are, however, a few things you can do for yourself to treat your eyes and protect your vision.

If you accidentally splash a harmful substance—like household cleaners, bleach, garden chemicals, or paints—into your eyes, run for the water faucet. Tilt your head so that your injured eye is closest to the bottom of the sink, hold your eyelids open with your fingers, and flush the eye with running water until the chemical has been washed out. You can also put your face in a basin of water to clean your eye. When the chemical is removed, cover your eye lightly with a clean pad, such as a handkerchief, and seek medical treatment.

Treat a cut eye by securing a clean, dry pad over it. If you've been dealt a swift blow to the eye, cover it with a piece of cloth soaked in cold water or ice cubes. In both situations, seek medical care.

Judith Lin

186

Removing a Particle from Your Eye

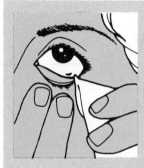

Remove a stray eyelash or speck of dirt floating on the white of your eye by gently dabbing it with the moistened corner of a clean handkerchief.

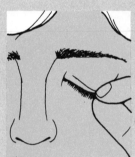

Locate a wayward particle by pulling your upper lid down over your lower lid. This should dislodge the particle.

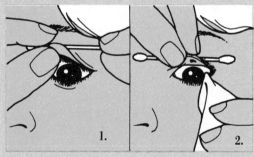

1. 2.

Remove a particle from someone else's eye by placing a cotton-tipped swab or match over his upper lid. Then hold onto the lashes of his upper lid and fold it back over the swab. If you find the particle, remove it with a moist handkerchief or wet swab. See a doctor if you still can't spot the speck.

EYESTRAIN

Eighty percent of your awareness of the world comes to you through your eyes. You check your watch for the correct time, look both ways before crossing the street, read books, watch movies, admire artwork, or gaze affectionately into the eyes of a loved one. All day long you use your eyes. It's no wonder that sooner or later they get tired. Or worse. Do your eyes ache, itch, or burn? Is your vision blurry? Do you get headaches or feel tired or irritable? Do you have times when you make more mistakes or feel dissatisfied with your job? You may be suffering from eyestrain.

Close Encounters

Eyestrain occurs most commonly among people who engage in tasks requiring that they focus on objects up close for an extended period of time. A homemaker cross-stitching a handkerchief, a child building a model, and the zillions of adults who work at computer video display terminals (VDTs) are prime candidates for eyestrain.

What exactly is getting strained when you experience eyestrain? Each of your eyes is hooked up to six muscles that manipulate its movement from right to left and up and down. When you stare at something close (3 feet or closer) for a long time, the muscles responsible for side-to-side motion can become fatigued.

Your iris, the round colored part of your eye surrounding the pupil, also can become strained. Your iris is actually a muscle that opens and closes to regulate the amount of light entering the pupil. An iris's work is never (or hardly ever) done. You may be relaxing in a movie theater, for instance, but your iris is continually adjusting your pupil to varying degrees of light.

Your ciliary muscles may also become fatigued. These muscles push or pull your eyes' lenses into different shapes to enable you to shift focus when viewing objects at varying distances. These muscles can sometimes "lock into" close-up focus—when you've spent a couple of hours reading a book, for example.

Fortunately, there are things you can do to prevent eyestrain. Taking your eyes off close-focus and giving them a long-distance break is one of the best remedies, says Lowell Glatt, O.D., a New York optometrist who helps businesses create visually healthy work environments. He suggests, for instance, that each time you turn a page of this book, you gaze over the top of it into the distance. If you have a job that's hard on your eyes, take a break every hour or so. Stand up and stretch, Dr. Glatt suggests, and for a few moments aim your eyesight at something at least 20 feet away, whether it's across the room or out the window.

People with desk jobs are not the only ones who suffer from eyestrain. People who spend a lot of time outdoors often experience eyestrain because of glare from the sun. A good pair of polarized sunglasses will effectively cut glare.

Judith Lin

Light Up Your Life

Do you tire easily while reading or working? You may need to throw some light on your problem. Literally, two out of three interior designers in a recent survey reported that poor lighting was the most common complaint among their clients' office workers. Getting the optimum amount of light is an important factor in preventing eyestrain, whether we spend our days shuffling paperwork or knitting a pair of mittens. Too little light makes clear eyesight a struggle, while too much light can make you tense and fatigued. You may need to experiment somewhat to find the level you're most comfortable with.

In addition to direct lighting on your work, you should also have general illumination that is soft and indirect. This type of lighting is best because it creates soft shadows and mild contrasts between the task you're working on and the surrounding area, experts say. Your best bet is the diffuse illumination of a ceiling light. Make sure the light is not too bright: The lighting in any room should be two or three times dimmer than the lighting aimed at the task you're working on.

Two ideal arrangements for lighting the material you're working on are shown in the illustration at the right. Don't use lamps at eye level—they create too much contrast and glare. Also avoid high intensity lamps, which cast intense light that can be intensely fatiguing.

Work surfaces and background colors also affect your eyes. A light, natural wood desktop with a clear, nonglaring finish is best. Background colors on the floor, ceiling, and walls—especially a wall you're facing—should be warm or grayish white. Too much color can strain your eyes.

Watching Television

Proper lighting, as well as proper positioning, can help television watchers to easier viewing, too. The American Optometric Association recommends the following:

- Avoid reflective glare from the television screen by placing your set in the room away from lamps, windows, and other sources of light.
- Adjust the set's brightness and color to your individual comfort.
- Place the set at approximately eye level so you don't have to look up or down at the picture.
- Watch from a distance at least five times the width of the screen.

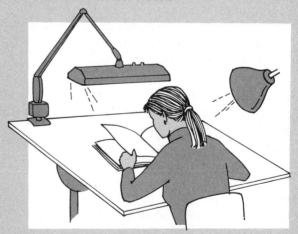

An ideal way to illuminate your work or reading is with either a light behind you, placed so that it does not cast a shadow on the work, or a shielded lamp in front of you.

The Right Light for Your Desk

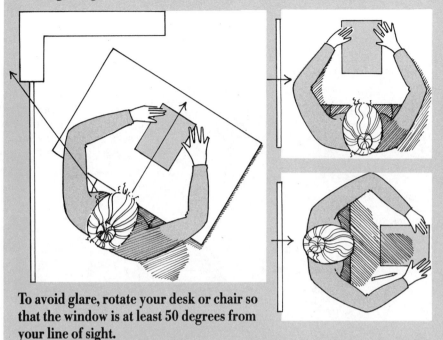

To avoid glare, rotate your desk or chair so that the window is at least 50 degrees from your line of sight.

Do not sit parallel to a window. Sunlight is pleasant, but it can stress your eyes. If you're especially sensitive, draw the blinds and use artificial light.

Do not sit with your back to the window, or, like the proverbial groundhog, you'll be seeing your own shadow. Watch out for shadow-casting lamps, too.

"Palmistry" That's for Real

Refresh tired eyes with a technique called *palming*, developed by ophthalmologist William Bates, M.D. Sit in a comfortable position, your elbows resting on a table or a pillow in your lap. Rub your hands together briskly and form the palms into hollow cups. Place them over your eyes, gently lifting the weight of your eyebrows up from your eyes as you do so. Do not place any pressure on the eyeballs themselves. The bony part of your hand above your wrist should rest on your cheekbones. Open your eyes briefly to make sure they are enveloped in darkness. Then close your eyes and visualize pleasant, relaxing scenes. Perform this technique about once a day for 15 minutes, or as often as you need to for relief.

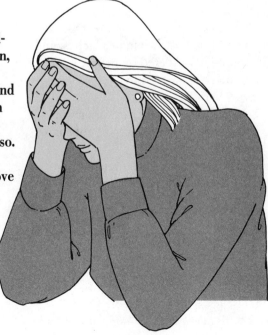

EYESTRAIN

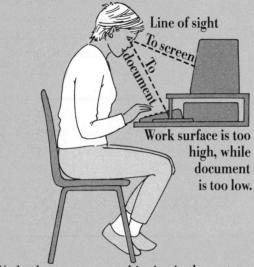

Keyboard is too high, arms are too high, and there's no support for wrists or forearms.

Line of sight
To screen
To document

Work surface is too high, while document is too low.

No back support or cushioning in the seat

Screen is at a good height and is adjustable.

Document is close to the screen and in easy view.

Line of sight

Wrist support

Keyboard and table allow arms to be more appropriately placed.

Adjustable chair

Eye-Friendly VDT Use

Computers are great. Not so great are the burning eyes, blurred vision, headaches, and fatigue frequently suffered by people who work at video display terminals, otherwise known as VDTs.

The American Optometric Association offers these guidelines to help prevent such problems:

Your VDT should have a screen large enough to display letters of normal size, should present sharp, solid letters with a minimum of flicker, have brightness and contrast controls, and a screen that can be turned and tilted.

You should light the room indirectly with a lamp that doesn't reflect directly into the screen. Use less light than usual. Try a 60-watt bulb in a small room or remove half

the bulbs from ceiling light fixtures. Keep the VDT away from the glare of sunlight.

Adjust the VDT's brightness so that it is three to four times higher than the overall room lighting. Then adjust the contrast: Screen characters should be five to ten times brighter than the background.

Place material you're reading at the same height and distance as the VDT screen, eliminating the need to radically shift your focus from one to the other.

Remember to blink, something you may actually forget to do for as long as a minute or two while focusing on a VDT. Practice blinking for a minute or so before you sit down to work.

Take a 10- to 15-minute rest break for every hour you spend at the VDT.

Apply a Little Pressure

You don't have to be Chinese to appreciate acupressure. This ancient technique employs the application of firm yet gentle pressure to strategic points along the body—in this case, near the eyes—to bring about pain relief and healing.

Neither do you have to be Chinese, let alone ancient, to locate these special points. "Most of us rub our eyes in those exact same spots," says David Molony, a Pennsylvania acupuncturist. (Acupuncture uses the same map of points that acupressure does, but entails the insertion of thin needles rather than the application of pressure.)

According to Chinese medical theory, Molony explains, acupressure relaxes the eyes by restoring the circulation of blood and *chi*, the body's essential life energy. *Chi* makes its way through the body along pathways called meridians, three of which originate in the eye. Eye tension will cause either a stagnation or deficiency of *chi*. By applying acupressure to points along these meridians, the flow of *chi* is restored and your eyes invigorated.

Acupressure can prevent eyestrain as well as relieve it, Molony says. "Using acupressure as a preventive method starts you out in a relaxed state. This can actually lengthen the amount of time it takes for your eyes to get tired."

Try it first thing in the morning, before and after you do anything strenuous with your eyes, and once again in the evening. To perform acupressure, lean your elbows on a table and allow your head to fall forward very slightly. The required pressure will be provided by the weight of your head. Being careful to keep fingernails away from your eyes, press on each of the points until you feel a heavy sensation around it—this should take about 10 seconds—and then move on to the next point.

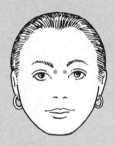

Place your thumbs just under the inside edge of your eyebrows while your elbows are resting on a table. Massage in one direction.

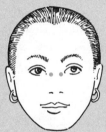

Place your thumb and index finger of your left hand at the inner corners of your eyes. Massage upward and then downward.

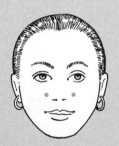

Place your middle and index fingers just to the sides of your nose. Lift your middle fingers and massage with your index fingers.

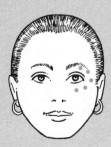

Place your thumbs on your temples and use the side of your index finger to rub the points outward, first over your eyes, then under.

EYESTRAIN

Helping Both Eyes Focus on One Object

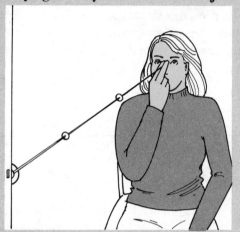

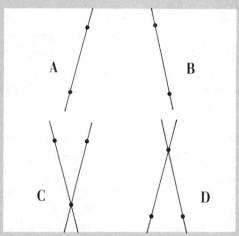

Help your eyes focus at the same time: Tie a 7-foot-long string to a door handle and put two beads on it. Pull the string to your nose and look at the first bead.

You may see *a* or *b* if only one eye is seeing. Try blinking your eyes, shaking the beads, or moving the string until you see *c*. Then focus on the far bead and try to see *d*.

Improving and Strengthening Overall Focus

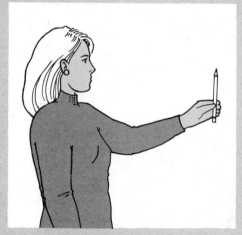

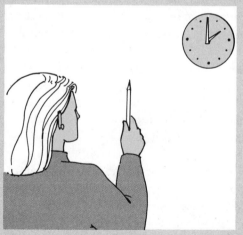

Look at the tip of a pencil about 20 inches away. Bring the pencil toward you until the tip blurs, then push it away. Repeat several times.

Hold a pencil tip at the point where it just blurs and is in line with an object about 20 feet away. Alternate your focus between the pencil and the distant object.

FAINTING

There's something so "feminine" about fainting. In old movies, damsels in distress were forever collapsing into the arms of handsome leading men. Heroines in romance novels invariably succumb to stupor when their beloved is thrown off a horse or is kidnapped by Colombian drug lords.

In reality, however, men do their fair share of fainting, too. In one medical survey, 25 percent of all adults reported that they had fainted at least once in their lives. A condition known to the medical profession as *syncope* (pronounced SIN-ko-pe), fainting occurs when your body's reflexes suddenly slow your heart rate and dilate your blood vessels, causing a quick drop in blood pressure and an inadequate blood supply to the brain.

During a fainting episode, you'll probably feel dizzy, light-headed, or physically weak. Your face may grow pale or your vision dim. You may sweat, yawn, burp, or feel sick to your stomach. The situation reaches a dramatic climax when you lose consciousness and keel over.

Fortunately, the problem is short-lived. Unless there's some deeper underlying disorder, you will revive within a minute or two, and all will be well. Just don't jump suddenly to your feet, an action that could make you faint all over again.

People actually do faint as a response to terror, intense pain, sudden emotional stress—even the sight of blood. Why? A nerve that helps to control breathing and blood pressure—the vagus nerve—can become overstimulated by stress, pain, or fear. Some people faint when they give blood, at the sight of blood, or even the medical instruments used for drawing it.

Low blood sugar levels from going without food for too long also may cause fainting. So can long periods of resting in bed or standing.

Certain medications, including some diuretics, tranquilizers, and drugs for high blood pressure, have been linked to fainting episodes, as have certain diseases.

Other Common Causes

Diabetes is also associated with fainting because of the effect it has on the nervous system that controls blood pressure and pulse.

People who suffer from migraines are more prone to syncope at all ages. These people are especially susceptible to fainting while drinking alcohol, standing up quickly, or when in a hot room.

Speaking of hot, everyone is more susceptible to fainting spells when he spends time in the hot sun, a sauna, or whirlpool, or when he becomes dehydrated. It's very important to drink plenty of water if you are exerting yourself outdoors.

All of these activities may particularly affect the elderly. As we get older, the nervous system becomes more delicate and slower in its ability to react to changes in the environment.

Judith Lin

FAINTING

What to Do When You Feel Faint

Feeling faint? *Right,* To keep from losing consciousness, plant yourself in the nearest chair, lean forward, and hang your head between your knees. This position will supply your brain with fresh blood.

   If someone has already fainted, first lay the person on her back. Check carefully for breathing and pulse. Don't be surprised if the pulse is weak and slow, as this often occurs right after fainting. If you can't detect breathing or find a pulse, get emergency medical treatment.

   Below, If you do find a pulse, raise the person's legs above head level. The increased blood flow will help revive her more quickly—usually within a minute or two. Loosen her clothing and make her comfortable. Make sure she has plenty of fresh air, but keep her out of hot sunlight.

   When the person revives, she'll probably feel weak. Have her lie or sit quietly for a while before she stands up. Don't splash cold water on her face or give her anything alcoholic to drink. A glass of orange juice, a small snack, or a cold compress on the forehead might help her feel better.

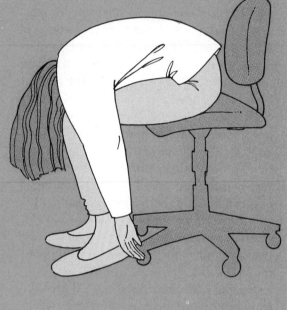

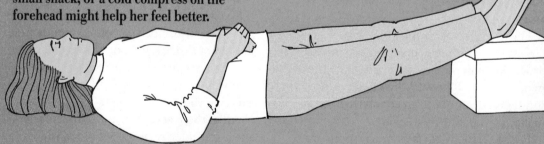

FATIGUE

Winston Churchill handled fatigue like a true statesman: He came, he saw, he napped. Even while Nazi tanks rumbled across Europe, Churchill would retire for a quick snooze, claiming it allowed him to work late into the night.

That was then. Now, in addition to napping, our society has mastered a number of instant relief alternatives to beat fatigue. Americans spend billions a year on caffeine and sugar to jolt themselves into activity.

But once the heady, blood-pumping rush is over, there's no mistaking it: We're tired. According to one expert, fatigue is the seventh most common complaint that doctors hear—between 21 and 24 percent of all adults say it's a "major problem."

In some ways all this yawning is to be expected. We don't get enough sleep. In fact, between 15 to 20 percent of all Americans have chronic insomnia. As a nation we don't eat right. We eat sugary breakfast cereals, if anything, in the morning; huge calorie-and fat-laden meals at lunch; ditto for dinner. We don't exercise: Walking to the refrigerator doesn't count. And don't forget stress—in recent years, the S word has become part of the job description for most employees. All of these things can contribute to fatigue. In fact, 20 to 45 percent of all cases of fatigue may be attributed to physical conditions, 50 percent to psychological factors.

For most people, some relatively minor changes in diet, behavior, and even attitude can put pep back in their steps. Above all, remember that fatigue is not a natural part of growing old. In fact, it's sometimes a sign that something else may be wrong. If you're suddenly feeling unexplained fatigue—particularly if your schedule isn't as hectic as it used to be—see your doctor. Fatigue often accompanies serious illnesses like heart problems and even cancer.

But if you're simply feeling run down, try some of the home remedies listed below. You have nothing to lose but your lethargy.

If you feel drained of energy, chances are you won't have to look far to find out what pulled the plug.

Some likely suspects in the energy theft line-up include caffeine, nicotine, and sugar. They give energy for a while, artificially forcing the adrenal glands into overdrive, but after the joyride, our body is out of gas. Alcohol and lack of sleep also rob their victims of zest.

Eat for Energy

To beat the blahs, it's not enough to know your enemy. You have to take action. What you eat makes all the difference in whether your body is zooming along at full throttle or stuck in idle.

Nutritional experts recommend a diet of high-energy foods that have undergone a minimum of processing, foods such as fresh fruits and vegetables, whole-grain products and cereals, dried beans, fish and chicken. The bottom line: This diet, rich in complex carbohydrates, maintains blood sugar at a more even level. It helps you avoid the energy peaks followed by the valleys of fatigue that are the common lot of people who rely on sugary snacks to fuel them through the day.

For a high-energy treat that beats candy, try protein bars, says Vicky Young, M.D., assistant professor in the Medical College of Wisconsin's Department of Preventive Medicine. They contain some sugar, but during digestion the protein provides a more even source of fuel, she says. A tip for added energy in the evening: Eat your largest meal for lunch, says Dr. Young.

One final note on diet. Iron deficiency can lead to anemia, which in turn can lead to fatigue. Women need to be especially careful to get enough iron. The Recommended Dietary Allowance for adults and adolescents is 10 to 15 milligrams. Among the best food sources of iron are beef liver, dark meat turkey, broiled lean ground beef, boiled lima beans, dried sunflower seeds, prunes, cooked broccoli, and cooked spinach. If you're supplementing, stick to the RDA unless your doctor tells you otherwise.

Being Upbeat Beats the Blahs

There may be more to Gene Kelly's rain-soaked solo than just a memorable moment in the cinema classic, *Singing in the Rain*. Gene's upbeat attitude, researchers are discovering, may have been as important as the latest dance step in keeping him light on his feet.

In fact, some researchers believe that the most powerful predictors of exhaustion are not physical, but psychological. Case in point: A Maryland study that detailed

patients' medical histories, psychological profiles, and frequency of fatigue, found that people who reported feeling depressed were seven times more likely to be fatigued than people without emotional problems.

But getting happy takes a plan of action. Even something as simple as keeping a journal can give your attitude a lift. One study, involving college students, found that writing 20 minutes a day, four days a week, about the things that concerned them helped improve their outlook.

Weekend getaways can do wonders for a flagging spirit, says Benjamin Natelson, M.D., professor of neurosciences at the New Jersey Medical School. "You've got to give yourself the opportunity to relax," he says. "Show me someone who's in the office late, and I'll show you at least an hour a day that's being wasted," he says.

Frazzled executives, Dr. Natelson says, should perform at least one selfish task a week, like visiting a friend. He also stresses practicing time management.

Perhaps most important, try to maintain a positive attitude. But even when you're down, remember: You don't have to stay there. Katherine Ferrari, president of the International Laughter Society (no joke) in Los Gatos, California, says listening to a comedy tape "loaded with wholesome, positive humor" can quickly lift your spirits. She also says it's important to cultivate friends with healthy outlooks. Avoid whiners, especially when you're feeling depressed: They'll just make you feel worse, she says.

Exercise is probably the last thing you feel like doing when you're tired. But what if exercise made it easier for your body to handle daily physical and emotional stresses? What if exercise wiped out weariness and revved up your energy and enthusiasm?

Remove Fatigue with Movement

If your body isn't exercised regularly, it probably doesn't use oxygen very efficiently. Your muscles need that oxygen, or they won't work as long or as hard as they can. The result of all this sitting around: When you need muscle power, you don't get it, and you tire easily.

What's more, even as your muscles sag, so, too, does your self-image. Your emotional state can become a mirror image of your physical condition, adding to your fatigue.

But you don't have to go to a gym and pump iron to get physical. Boosting your daily calorie expenditure a mere 300 calories a day for about 300 days could enable you to lose 25 pounds a year, according to Bernard Gutin, Ph.D., professor of applied physiology and education at Teacher's College, Columbia University. You'll not only look better, you'll have more energy. His suggestion: Burn the calories through natural activity. Instead of cranking up the Chrysler to run an errand or go to work, walk. Forego the claustrophobic environs of the elevator for a jaunt up or down the stairs.

Soothing Pick-Me-Ups

Deep breathing and massage can supplement your antifatigue exercise routine. A foot massage that focuses on the bottom of the foot, just under the big toe, takes advantage of an important acupressure revival point, according to Michael Reed Gach, founder of the Acupressure Institute in Berkeley, California. Massaging this point is a source of energy for the entire body and provides a quick way to pick yourself up from a state of fatigue.

Progressive relaxation can also soothe fatigue. Sit in a comfortable chair and then alternately tense and relax all the muscle groups of the body, from the toes and legs up to the neck and face. Bring the tension up to a high level in each group of muscles, hold it for several seconds, and then release. Relax for 10 to 20 seconds, feeling the tension drain from your body. Repeat. This technique, which lasts about 20 minutes, should result in a relaxed state.

The Fine Art of Napping

After everything is said and done, on some days a nap could be just what the doctor ordered. The ideal nap time may be between 2 and 3 P.M., when your body naturally yearns for sleep, says Wilse Webb, Ph.D., professor of psychology at the University of Florida and one of the country's leading authorities on naps. Allow yourself no more than an hour's rest, or else your nap may interfere with your night's sleep. The urge to nap comes naturally midway between the time we wake and the time we go to sleep—although sleep deprivation and fatigue makes the urge even stronger, says Dr. Webb. "Winston Churchill used to cork off during the afternoon because he would stay up most of the night," he says. "If it worked for him, it ought to work for anybody."

Brian Kauffman

197

FATIGUE

EXERCISE EQUALS ENERGY

If you're sick and tired of feeling sick and tired, and an ice storm is preventing you from taking your afternoon stroll, we have just the thing: Energizing exercises that you can perform in your living room or even on the job. The following exercises also provide a mild stretch and help alleviate tension. Best of all, they're fatigue-fighters that you can perform anywhere—to start the day or to re-invigorate your entire system. Some cautions apply, though: Check with your doctor before beginning any exercise program. Avoid any sudden movements. If you experience any pain, stop immediately. While performing these exercises, remember to breathe evenly and keep the knees slightly bent.

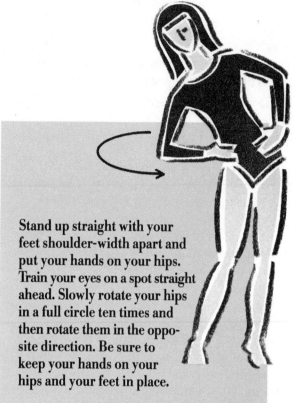

Stand up straight with your feet shoulder-width apart and put your hands on your hips. Train your eyes on a spot straight ahead. Slowly rotate your hips in a full circle ten times and then rotate them in the opposite direction. Be sure to keep your hands on your hips and your feet in place.

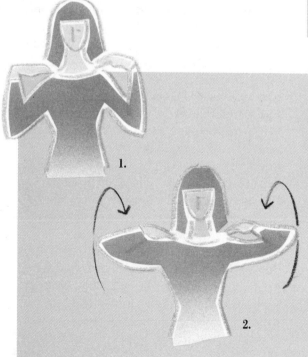

1.

2.

This one will temporarily make you look like a chicken, but it's great for the shoulders. *(1)* Put your hands on your shoulders. *(2)* Slowly rotate your arms ten times so your elbows make small circles in the air. Repeat ten times in the opposite direction.

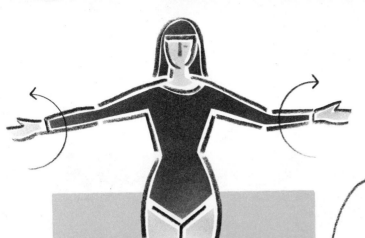

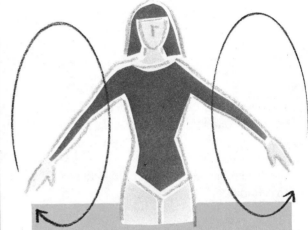

Here's an exercise for the shoulders to help combat the tension and soreness that invariably accompany holding a telephone or driving a car. Stand with your feet shoulder-width apart. Slowly raise your arms to shoulder level with your palms facing up. Rotate your palms forward, down, and back ten times so that your hands make small circles. Repeat in the opposite direction.

Stand with your feet shoulder-width apart. Slowly raise your arms out to the side, parallel to the ground, palms down. Begin making small circles with your arms. With each rotation, make the circles larger until both shoulder sockets rotate. Repeat in the opposite direction.

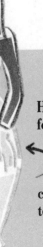

Here's a gentle movement for all you Charleston fans. Stand up straight with your knees touching each other, your feet close together, and your toes facing forward. Crouch over and put your hands on your knees. Now circle your knees ten times in a clockwise direction. Then repeat the circles counterclockwise. Experiment with making the circles a little larger. Stop at once if you feel any discomfort. It's best to skip this particular exercise if you tend to have knee problems.

199

FATIGUE

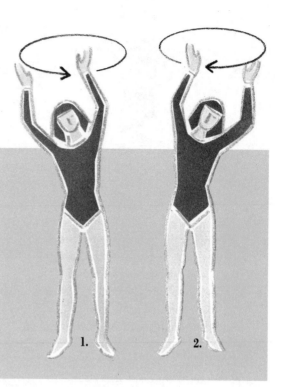

Stand with your feet shoulder-width apart. Slowly raise your hands above your head. *(1)* Pretend you are grasping a beach ball overhead. *(2)* Begin rotating the imaginary ball, ten times in one direction and then ten times in the other direction.

1.   2.

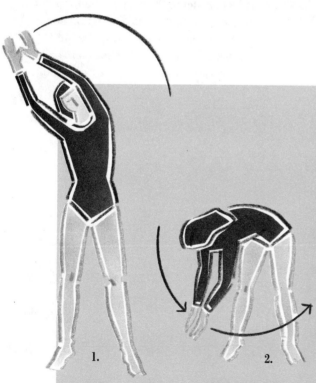

Save this exercise until you're properly warmed up. *(1)* Stand with your feet shoulder-width apart. Raise your hands above your head. Begin making a small circle just as you did in the previous exercise. *(2)* Make the circles larger until you are making gigantic circles with your entire body. Be sure to exhale as you bend over and inhale as you raise your hands above your head. Continue the movement for no more than 3 minutes. If you begin to feel dizzy, stop immediately.

1.   2.

FLATULENCE

He knows he really shouldn't, but life's too short and tonight's dinner special at Tina's Tasty Tortilla is too terrific to pass by. So, throwing caution to the wind, Lenny goes ahead and tells Tina he'll tackle a caldron-size serving of her hot 'n' spicy homemade chili with extra beans on the side. And make that a couple of cold beers, too, he says, to wash it all down.

The chili proves delicious—but predictably odiferous. Prescient of pungent scents to come, Lenny's lower intestine launches into familiar rumblings just as Tina comes by with the check. In a flash, he's on his feet and paying the bill, out the door, into his car and roaring away—heavy on the gas in more ways than one.

If there's anything nice to be said about the unplanned release of cooped-up gas (called flatus), it's that the whole smelly business is not so much a medical problem as a social one. Rarely due to any disease or abnormality, flatulence is perfectly normal. Researchers sniffing around for statistics found that young to middle-aged men pass gas an average of about 14 times a day, releasing a total of about 2½ cups of fumes. Some people are more gaseous than others. Severe cases can involve as many as 140 passages per day.

Excess gas is usually the result of foods not fully digested in the stomach and small intestine. The food makes its way to the colon, where bacteria go to work, ferment-

Yoga Relief

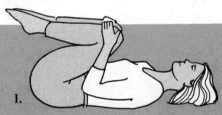

1.

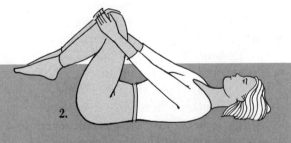

2.

This yoga pose helps ease out excess gas. Lying on your back, bring your knees to your chest as you exhale. Inhale and let your knees fall away. Repeat these movements for 2 minutes.

Now inhale deeply into your lower abdomen, and as you exhale you should find your lower back relaxing and the rectum open for quick relief of your gas symptoms.

FLATULENCE

Getting the Gas out of Beans

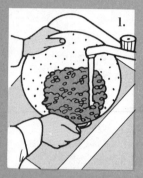
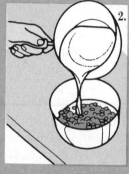
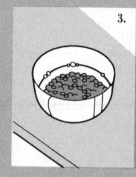
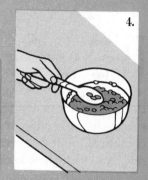

To cut back on the gas-producing substances in beans, *(1)* rinse the uncooked beans thoroughly. *(2)* Boil a pot of water and pour enough over the rinsed beans to completely cover them. *(3)* Allow the beans to soak for 4 hours or longer, depending on the type of bean. *(4)* Remove any beans that have floated to the top during soaking and drain the rest.

To cook the drained beans, add fresh water to the pot until it reaches 2 inches above the beans. Cook for about 1 to 3 hours, tasting occasionally, until the beans are tender. Cooking time depends on the variety of bean; white beans tend to be the toughest and require the most cooking. Wait until the cooking is almost done before you add salt or tomato juice.

ing it. The by-product is a stinky gas containing the chemical hydrogen sulfide, of rotten egg fame. There's only one way out for this gas, and you're sitting on it.

The biggest food culprits are carbohydrates that contain a lot of fiber. Beans are a surefire gas generator for most people, even for unsuspecting animals. Among other foods linked to flatus attacks are apples, bagels, bananas, bread, brussels sprouts, cabbage, carrots, celery, citrus fruits, eggplant, lettuce, onions, pastries, potatoes, pretzels, prune juice, raisins, and wheat germ. Beer and other drinks that contain yeast can get gas going, as can soft drinks and coffee.

Simply avoiding those foods that cause

flatus is your best bet for relief. If you're trying to eat more fiber, increase its presence in your diet gradually over a period of several weeks to allow your body to adjust.

Lactose intolerance also can cause flatulence. Lacking the enzyme lactase, some people can't digest lactose, the sugar in milk. The undigested lactose in the colon then goes through the same stinky fermentation process previously described. Test yourself for lactose intolerance by avoiding all dairy products, wet and dry, for two weeks. If flatus decreases, you have lactose intolerance and need to keep milk and dairy products at a low level in your diet.

Judith Lin

FOOD POISONING

There was something funny about supper tonight at Aunt Velma's, and you don't mean the part where Uncle Louie went into his old "Hey, kids! How's about we construct a lifelike model of Mount Rushmore with our mashed potatoes and gravy?" routine. No, there was something funny about the meal itself—maybe the meat loaf that wasn't cooked quite all the way through or the fruitcake that was past its prime last Christmas. Not one to be rude, you ate everything on your plate. But now that you're home, you have this queasy feeling in your stomach and an awful churning down in your bowels and—uh oh!—you'd better hightail it to the bathroom right now!

Chances are, you have yourself a home-grown case of food poisoning. About two million Americans are struck by food poisoning each year, reports the U. S. Department of Agriculture (USDA). Most cases are due to improper handling of food in the home. Fortunately, the condition probably won't kill you, but don't be surprised if you feel lousy for at least a day or two.

Bacteria Soup

Food poisoning, or foodborne illness as scientists call it, results when you inadvertently eat food that contains large quantities of bacteria or the toxins they produce. These bacteria come in two major classes: the food-spoilers and the food-poisoners.

Molds and yeasts are common food-spoilers. They are happiest at lower temperatures and will flourish in your refrigerator, where they reproduce like crazy in fresh fruits, vegetables, cheese, and tomato products. Eating such food can make you sick, but most of us don't usually make this mistake because rotten food is anything but appetizing.

Food-poisoning bacteria are a lot sneakier. We usually can't see them, smell them, or taste them. They thrive at room temperature, between 60 and 90 degrees, multiplying to potentially dangerous levels in food left out on your kitchen countertops or in grocery bags in the trunk of your car. Refrigerating them effectively cools down their growth.

More than 20 kinds of foodborne bacteria can poison you. Three of them are responsible for most of the trouble. *Staphylococcus aureus,* or staph, is a type of bacteria we all carry, mostly in our noses and on our skin. When food is not handled in a sanitary manner, staph can sneak into it and produce powerful toxins that cannot be destroyed by ordinary cooking.

Salmonella is always present in varying quantities in all animals' intestinal tracts, including our own. Chicken, eggs, meat, and unpasteurized milk are major carriers. Fortunately, thorough cooking can kill it.

Perfringens, sometimes called the cafeteria germs, often lurk in food that is served in quantity and left out for long periods. This bacteria thrives in oxygen-free environments, like the one to be found, for instance, in the middle of a big bowl of Thanksgiving stuffing.

Diarrhea, nausea, vomiting, fever, and gas

FOOD POISONING

pains are all symptoms of poisoning by these bacteria. You may start feeling sick anywhere from 2 to 36 hours after eating and get better anywhere from a day to a week later. If you're basically healthy, the problem probably won't be too serious. Just drink lots of liquids to replace fluids lost through diarrhea or vomiting. See a doctor if your symptoms are more severe.

One deadly form of food poisoning is caused by botulism bacteria, which can produce toxins in canned foods. About a third of its victims die. Fortunately, botulism is quite rare. There are only 10 to 15 cases each year in the United States. Most cases traced to foods that were canned at home. Following proper canning techniques can ensure your safety. Botulism attacks its victim's nervous system, causing double vision, droopy eyelids, and difficulty swallowing or breathing 12 to 48 hours after eating. Immediate medical treatment is essential.

It sounds so simple: "Common sense is normally adequate to prevent your kitchen from being the source of a food-poisoning outbreak," says Gerald Kuhn, Ph.D., professor of food science at Pennsylvania State University. But as Dr. Kuhn also points out, "We all had different standards as we grew up," so what may be common sense to one person may be news to another.

For starters, be a sharp shopper.

"Common sense to me means buying foods smartly," says Dr. Kuhn. Select foods that look fresh, smell good, and are properly packaged. If they're meant to be refrigerated, make sure they're cold. And keep them cold on your trip home from the grocery store, he

says, or bacteria-laden moisture could form on their surfaces. If you drive a long distance to shop, take along a cooler with ice to preserve perishables.

Plan ahead. Buy foods with an idea of when and how much you're going to use, advises Dr. Kuhn, "That way it will still be of a safe, high quality when you do sit down to eat it." Check the packages for a "sell by" or "use by" date and buy only what fits your schedule. Plan to use eggs within a few weeks of purchase. (Don't ever use cracked or dirty eggs, by the way. The dirt could be—ugh!—chicken manure.)

Protect yourself against botulism by not buying cans that are seriously dented or swollen, or jars that are cracked or have loose lids. (If you do your own home-canning, follow sterilization procedures carefully.)

Cool It, Cook It, and Store It

Most foodborne bacteria thrive at temperatures between 40 and 150°F. Keeping food colder puts a freeze on bacterial growth. Get your just-purchased perishables into the refrigerator or freezer as soon as you get home. The cold doesn't actually kill bacteria but forces it into hibernation. When food is returned to a temperature of 40 to 45°, the bacteria revive. For this reason, don't refreeze meat and vegetables that have thawed. Instead, use it promptly or cook it before you refreeze.

When it comes to actual food preparation, get ready for battle. Despite federal food inspections, says the USDA, you must assume that much of the food that comes into your kitchen is contaminated. "Anywhere from

30 to 70 percent of all raw chicken meat you buy will actually contain some salmonella," says Dr. Kuhn. (In fact, he says, *you* undoubtedly contain some salmonella in your intestinal tract.) Raw meat, raw dairy products, and fish are also carriers.

Proper preparation can free your food of bacterial threat. Before you begin, wash your hands, especially after you've gone to the bathroom. The worst bacteria are transmitted by way of feces.

Use clean utensils, cutting boards, and other equipment in your food preparation and continually reclean them between steps to avoid what Dr. Kuhn says is a common cause of food poisoning: cross-contamination. "An example of this," he says, "is the person who carries chicken breasts outside on a plate and puts them onto a charcoal grill with a fork. Then he removes the cooked chicken with the same fork and carries it back into the house on the same plate, allowing the uncooked juices to recontaminate the cooked food with bacteria from its raw stage." Use a clean plate and utensils instead.

The high temperatures of boiling, baking, frying, or roasting food eliminate a lot of poisonous bacteria. Just make sure you cook food thoroughly. Don't interrupt cooking, which invites bacterial growth, but cook it completely at one time. If you're using a microwave oven, rotate meat so it cooks all the way through.

Don't give in to the temptation to taste food before it's done cooking. Some bacteria could still be alive. Taste-testing can also transmit the personal germs you're carrying to your family's meal.

Protective Packaging

What's the best way to repackage food you just brought home from the grocery store? Don't. Meat and poultry should stay in the wrap they came in because your hands will only introduce more bacteria. If the store wrap is torn, however, rewrap the item in wax paper, plastic wrap, or aluminum foil.

Sometimes you'll find mold lurking inside a package of cheese, a jar of jelly, or on the edges of vegetables. Chop it off or scoop it out, then rewrap the remainder in fresh wrap.

Throw out items like hot dogs or lunch meat if the liquid around them becomes cloudy.

If you won't be serving food you've just cooked for awhile, keep it covered and warm—between 140 and 165°. And pack up leftovers promptly. "A lot of foods are nearly sterile after they've been cooked, but the air can easily recontaminate them," says Dr. Kuhn. "Bacteria are carried around on particles in the air, in dust, and on insects. Pop leftovers into the refrigerator quickly so that even if a few bacteria do land on them, they're not going to have a chance to grow rapidly." Meats, vegetables, and anything made with sauces are especially dangerous to leave sitting out. When the time comes to serve leftovers, cover and thoroughly reheat them to kill any bacteria that might have been introduced.

Judith Lin

205

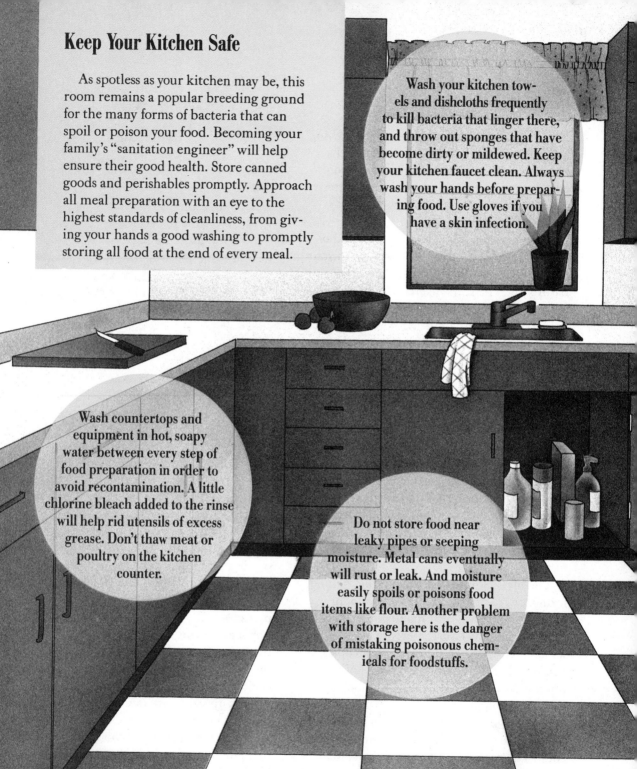

Keep Your Kitchen Safe

As spotless as your kitchen may be, this room remains a popular breeding ground for the many forms of bacteria that can spoil or poison your food. Becoming your family's "sanitation engineer" will help ensure their good health. Store canned goods and perishables promptly. Approach all meal preparation with an eye to the highest standards of cleanliness, from giving your hands a good washing to promptly storing all food at the end of every meal.

Wash your kitchen towels and dishcloths frequently to kill bacteria that linger there, and throw out sponges that have become dirty or mildewed. Keep your kitchen faucet clean. Always wash your hands before preparing food. Use gloves if you have a skin infection.

Wash countertops and equipment in hot, soapy water between every step of food preparation in order to avoid recontamination. A little chlorine bleach added to the rinse will help rid utensils of excess grease. Don't thaw meat or poultry on the kitchen counter.

Do not store food near leaky pipes or seeping moisture. Metal cans eventually will rust or leak. And moisture easily spoils or poisons food items like flour. Another problem with storage here is the danger of mistaking poisonous chemicals for foodstuffs.

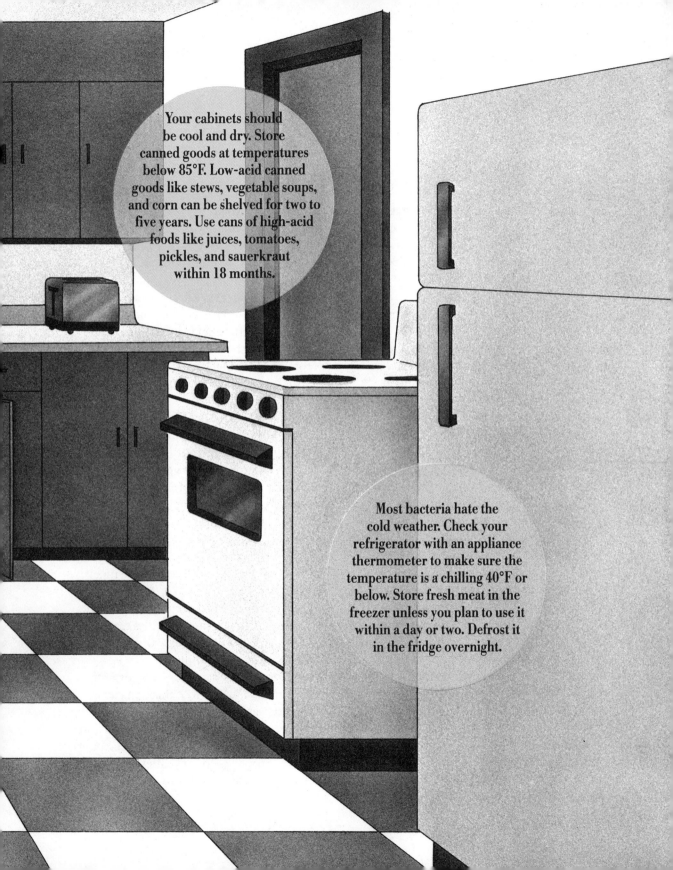

Your cabinets should be cool and dry. Store canned goods at temperatures below 85°F. Low-acid canned goods like stews, vegetable soups, and corn can be shelved for two to five years. Use cans of high-acid foods like juices, tomatoes, pickles, and sauerkraut within 18 months.

Most bacteria hate the cold weather. Check your refrigerator with an appliance thermometer to make sure the temperature is a chilling 40°F or below. Store fresh meat in the freezer unless you plan to use it within a day or two. Defrost it in the fridge overnight.

FOOTACHES

Take off your shoe and look inside. Now consider what you squeeze into that space every day of your life: 28 bones, 33 movable joints, 107 ligaments, and an assortment of fat pads, nerve endings, and blood vessels.

We're talking about your foot. This unassuming body part was designed to sustain, on average, more than 100,000 miles of wear. Can any other vehicle you own claim the same durability? With the original parts?

That's not to say everyone's feet remain problem-free. If yours ache, you may be using your foot and leg muscles in ways nature never intended. Or maybe you wear shoes that fight the natural shape of your foot. (See the chapter on corns on page 148.)

"Most footaches stem from an imbalance in the muscles," says Elizabeth Roberts, D.P.M., professor emeritus at the New York College of Podiatric Medicine.

To judge whether muscle imbalance is your problem, look in the mirror. Can you drop a straight line from mid-knee to your second toe? Or does the line veer off to the side? Neither your knees nor ankles should roll in, says Dr. Roberts.

The only way to treat foot pain caused by a habitual bad gait is to improve your muscle imbalance. A podiatrist can help by strapping the foot, using dressings, modifying your shoes, and teaching you proper walking technique. Meanwhile, here's what you can do for immediate relief from some of the more common causes of foot pain. The problems should be diagnosed by a health care professional.

Plantar fasciitis. The plantar fascia is a broad fibrous band of tissue that attaches to the heel, supports the arch, and helps the foot meet the ground at the right angle. If you tend to roll your feet in as you land on them, you can overstretch this tissue and cause it to tear away from the bone.

For short-term relief from the pain and inflammation, stay off your feet. Ask your doctor about taking an anti-inflammatory drug such as aspirin. Applying ice to the area may also help.

Achilles tendinitis. This is an inflammation of the tendon which runs a third of the way up your calf from your heel bone. The condition is common to joggers and to women who suddenly switch to low-heel shoes after years of wearing high heels. Wearing high heels tends to shorten the Achilles tendon, so if you switch to low-heel shoes, your shortened tendons will really have to stretch to allow your heels to meet the floor.

Regular stretching exercises will prevent this condition. If you have Achilles tendinitis, resting your feet will help ease the pain. Massage can speed healing.

Neuroma. This is a benign tumor of the nerve at the ball of the foot that can cause a burning sensation or a feeling of pins and needles near the affected area. Causes include tight shoes, skates laced too tightly, running on uneven surfaces—or anything that places extra stress on the ball of your foot.

Deborah Grandinetti

The Feel-Great Foot Massage

There are few things in life as luxurious as a good, leisurely foot massage, especially when those poor feet of yours are dog-tired and aching.

While it is possible to massage your own feet, how much better to persuade a friend to indulge you. Follow the step-by-step directions below for a deep foot massage that revives sore muscles. Practice so you can make the movements fluid.

Stroking on a good massage oil first can only add to your pleasure. You might want to add a few drops of an essential oil,—a flower or forest fragrance will make the experience really sensual. Then the feet will smell as wonderful as they feel.

Of course, don't massage chapped, blistered, or broken skin.

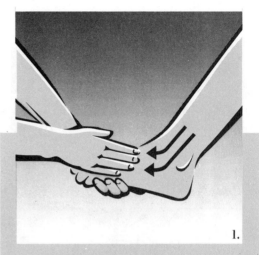

1.

Take the sole of the foot firmly in the palm of your hand and let your palm comfortably support it. Use your other hand to stroke the left side of the instep from the ankle to the toes. Use firm pressure. Move the fingers smoothly over the instep in one continuous stroke. Repeat the stroke on the other side of the instep. Do each stroke twice.

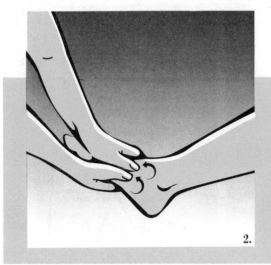

2.

Slide the hand supporting the foot around to one side and bring your other hand opposite to it so your thumbs are just under the anklebone. Trace small circles over the ankle and down to the bottom of the foot. Then use a stroking motion to bring the thumbs back to their starting point. Repeat, making sure to roll the muscles underneath your thumbs.

(continued)

FOOTACHES

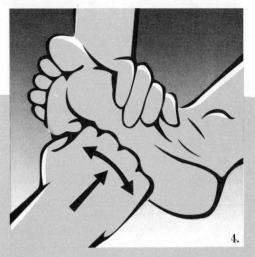

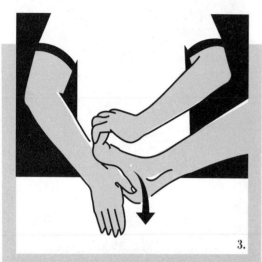

Hold the toes back with your left hand. Make a cup of your right hand. Then place the curled pinky and edge of your palm just below the toes. Stroke firmly down toward the heel. Turn the hand so that it ends the movement with the palm flat on the table. Repeat this movement several times.

Make a fist. Work it into the sole from the toes to the heel with a firm twisting motion. You'll want to brace the foot with your other hand so that the person you're working on won't have to push against your pressure. Work the foot from toe to heel, then reverse. Repeat this several times.

Next, place the pads of your thumbs on the sole so that your fingers lace around the top of the foot. Firmly knead the area from the base of the toes to the heel. Really press in so you'll stimulate the entire sole of the foot. Work from toe to heel, then reverse. Repeat several times. Have your partner tell you how hard to press.

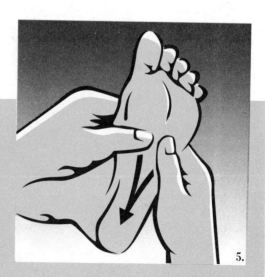

Flex Those Feet

If your tired feet ache at the end of the day, treat them to a little exercise.

"What? Exercise? After standing all day? Exercise?!"

Think of these foot exercises as corrective care, as an apology to your feet for the shoes that scrunch them, the hard running surfaces that jolt them, the poor posture that forces them to work extra hard.

Regular practice of this series of exercises will rev up your circulation. The effort will also impart grace to your walk as your muscles grow stronger and your joints become more flexible.

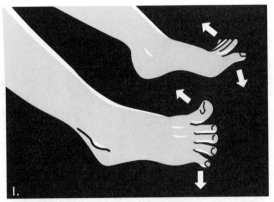

Sit down and raise your feet off the floor. Try to move your toes from the left to the right and up and down. See how far they'll move.

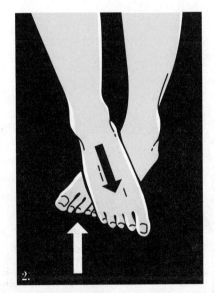

Put one foot on top of the other. Press the top foot down as you try to push the bottom one up. Then reverse feet and repeat.

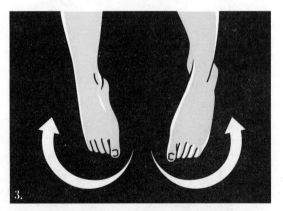

Spread your feet a foot apart. Circle them toward each other, then away from each other. Reverse direction several times, feeling the stretch through your ankles.

(continued)

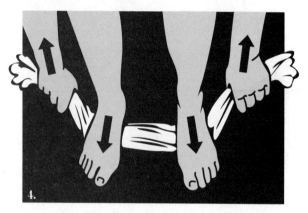

4.

Grab the ends of a rolled-up towel with your hands. Now push down with your feet while you pull up with your hands.

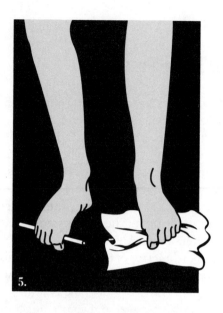

5.

Educate your toes. Try to pick up a towel with one foot, a pencil with the other. Reverse items, then repeat.

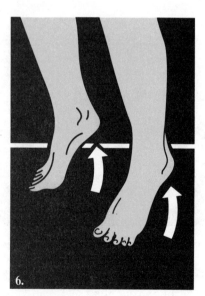

6.

Stand up and position your bare feet so they're inches apart. Slowly raise and lower yourself, using just your feet.

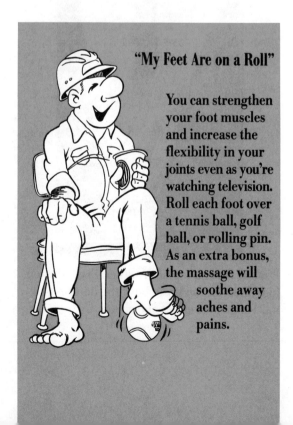

"My Feet Are on a Roll"

You can strengthen your foot muscles and increase the flexibility in your joints even as you're watching television. Roll each foot over a tennis ball, golf ball, or rolling pin. As an extra bonus, the massage will soothe away aches and pains.

FROSTBITE

You don't have to be exploring the Arctic Circle to get it. Waiting on a corner for a bus just about any January morning in Chicago can expose you quite thoroughly to the subfreezing temperatures and blasting winds that set up the ideal conditions for frostbite.

When temperatures drop below freezing, your body's central heating system kicks into high gear to keep precious body parts like your heart, vital organs, and brain nice and toasty. But your hands, feet, nose, and ears are all located in outposts far away from your main furnace, and, therefore, are more vulnerable to frostbite. They can't fend for themselves, either, in the way that your legs or arms can, as they don't possess big heat-generating muscles.

What's more, the lower outside temperatures drop, the more your body hoards heat by decreasing blood flow and by slowing your metabolism down. Blood circulation to your hands and feet may virtually cease in the coldest of cold weather. This lack of blood flow makes them even more vulnerable to frostbite.

Symptom #1: Pain; Symptom #2: Absence of Pain

Pain is a good indicator of frostbite. Be alert to strange aches in your extremities if you've been out in subfreezing temperatures, regardless of how long. Another good indicator is the *lack* of pain. Sometimes your initial pain may go away, leaving you presuming that the frostbite warning you had earlier was a false alarm. But beware: Your tissues may be so thoroughly frozen that they have lost all sensation, including that of pain. In some cases, frostbite sufferers never feel even the slightest tinge of pain. In other cases, the initial pain never lets up. Skin discoloration is another symptom of frostbite. Paleness may be a sign of poor blood circulation. Or your skin may look purple, the result of the dangerous blood clotting that sometimes accompanies frostbite in the hand or foot.

Seriously frostbitten tissue may feel hard when you press down on it, not unlike, say, a chicken drumstick straight from your freezer. And no wonder: Frostbitten tissues are gradually freezing. Ice crystals form between the cells, and in the process suck valuable water out of the cells. The result is dehydration, leaving the cells damaged in both structure and function. Permanent damage will be slight, however, if you thaw out frostbitten tissues soon enough.

A more severe kind of frostbite is caused by touching metal—a crowbar, for instance—that has been outside in subfreezing temperatures. In this case, ice crystals may rapidly form within the cells themselves, destroying them and decreasing the chances for recovery.

Put a Muzzle on Frostbite

Dressing defensively is important in preventing frostbite. Wear clothing in layers

FROSTBITE

that not only insulate against cold but also transmit moisture away from your body. Make sure elastic bands around your wrists or ankles aren't too tight, as they can constrict your circulation. Don't wear boots that are too tight, either. Make sure the circulation to your feet is not constricted by extra socks or socks that are too thick. Wear flexible leather boots that allow your feet to perspire naturally and swell.

Your head and neck lose a lot of body heat. Wearing a nice warm hat that covers your ears and the back of your neck will help retain heat. In severe weather, cover your face as well. Avoid a frostbitten nose or ears by keeping them out of direct, cold winds, whether you're snowmobiling or hiking on a windswept mountain. Even the corneas of your eyes can get frostbitten during an

activity like skiing. Wear protective goggles.

Your hands will stay warmer in mittens than in gloves, because mittens allow less heat to escape from your fingers. Wear mittens or gloves to prevent direct skin contact with cold metal items like tools or car door handles. Metal extracts heat from your tissues rapidly and can produce severe freezing.

Beware of contact with liquids like gasoline that remain liquid when left in freezing conditions, but can cause instantaneous freezing when spilled on skin.

And be especially careful if you smoke. Smokers have a higher incidence of frostbite than nonsmokers, probably because nicotine constricts the blood vessels. Kick the habit before you lose your feet.

Judith Lin

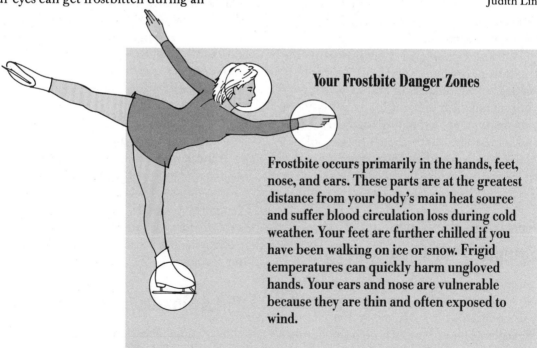

Your Frostbite Danger Zones

Frostbite occurs primarily in the hands, feet, nose, and ears. These parts are at the greatest distance from your body's main heat source and suffer blood circulation loss during cold weather. Your feet are further chilled if you have been walking on ice or snow. Frigid temperatures can quickly harm ungloved hands. Your ears and nose are vulnerable because they are thin and often exposed to wind.

Steps to Frostbite Relief

If you or someone you know has frostbite, begin treatment promptly. Rewarming is essential. You can do this by placing the frostbitten part(s) inside the victim's clothing, next to his body for warmth. Get him indoors quickly. A few don'ts are as important as the dos: Don't rewarm with the direct heat of a heating pad or hot water bottle. Don't place him right next to a radiator or fire. Don't rub the affected parts or try to burst any blisters. And don't give the person alcoholic beverages or allow him to smoke.

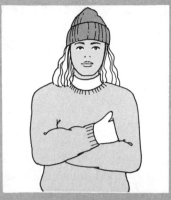

Rewarm frostbitten parts. Use your armpits to warm your hands, someone else's armpits to warm frostbitten feet.

If your toes or feet are affected, lie down and elevate them. Walking on frostbitten feet will only worsen the problem.

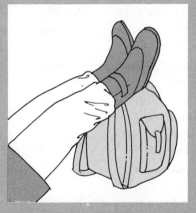

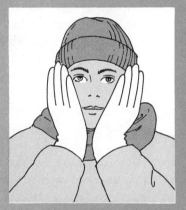

If your face feels frostbitten, warm it with dry, gloved hands until normal color returns.

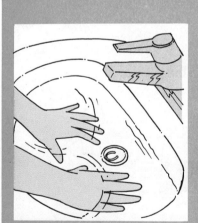

Immersing frostbitten parts in warm (not hot) water is ideal. The water should be 104 to 108°F. Use a thermometer to check the temperature.

When you're all thawed out, put a sterile or clean gauze or cloth over broken blisters and between frostbitten fingers and toes.

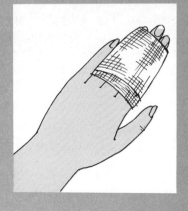

GUM AND TOOTH PROBLEMS

Dental caries, gingivitis, periodontitis, edentulism—they're a mouthful. These maladies can make you ache, bleed, swell, sometimes even make your breath smell. Fortunately, none of them is inevitable as long as you take good care of your teeth and gums.

Not that many years ago, a kid wasn't a kid without a few cavities. Today, thanks to improved dental hygiene, half of America's schoolchildren have no tooth decay at all. Those who do have cavities have fewer than their parents or grandparents did when they were young. Measures such as using fluoride toothpaste and switching to sugarless gum are preventing tooth decay among children.

Dental health is better among grown-ups, too. Adults today are less likely to end up with dentures and without their natural teeth (a condition called edentulism). According to a survey of oral health nationwide, more than a third of Americans still have all their natural teeth, and approximately half have lost just one tooth. Only 4 percent of employed Americans have had all their teeth replaced. That's the good news. What does remain a serious problem, however, is periodontal disease. About 43 percent of adults in the national survey had problems with bleeding gums, and 84 percent had deposits of tartar. Both are signs of gum disease.

Plaque: The Bacterial Barrage

The culprit behind most tooth and gum problems is plaque, a substance that is naturally present in everyone's mouth, day in and day out. Plaque is made of dried saliva, food debris, and bacteria, about 300 different kinds of which call your mouth home, regardless of how clean you may keep it. Most of these bacteria actually serve a protective function, fending off other germs to keep you free of infection. But they can turn on you when their numbers and types get out of balance. And the damage they do pretty much depends on how old you are.

Tooth decay can start as early as infancy. A baby's very first tooth is susceptible. Most cavities occur during childhood and adolescence. When you grow up, decay of your teeth slows down. As an adult, however, you're more vulnerable to decay down in the roots of your teeth and are more likely to

Toothbrushing Techniques

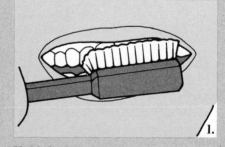

Hold the bristles of your toothbrush at a 45-degree angle to your teeth and scrub along the line of your gums in short strokes. Work gently.

develop gum problems. How can you prevent the bacteria in your mouth from multiplying and doing damage?

Avoid eating a sugary, high-carbohydrate diet, which throws things out of kilter very quickly. The bacteria gorge on sugar and carbohydrates, multiply into sticky masses, and adhere to the surfaces of your teeth. In a healthy mouth, plaque is colorless and virtually invisible.

But you can see the damage it causes all too well. Plaque produces acids that eat away your teeth's protective enamel. The result is tooth decay. If plaque isn't removed from your teeth, it combines with calcium and phosphorus to form more visible white or yellowish deposits called tartar, or calculus. Layer upon layer builds up, wreaking greater

havoc on your teeth and hardening to the point that only your dentist can chip it away.

Plaque can also do its dirty work along the roots of your teeth and beneath your gums, causing periodontal disease. This condition gradually destroys your gums and other structures supporting your teeth.

Most Americans over 40 have some form of periodontal disease. The problem can begin in childhood, though the disease doesn't usually reveal itself until adulthood. One study showed that gingivitis, the earliest form of the disease, affects more than one-third of children aged 6 to 11 and more than two-thirds of adolescents.

If you have gingivitis, your gums will become red and you'll notice swelling around one or more of the teeth, symptoms that will

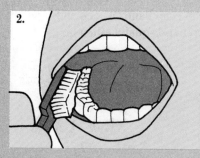

Work over the outer and inner surfaces of your upper and lower teeth. Remember to keep the brush bristles angled against the top of your gum line.

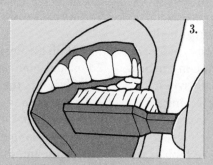

Now give a good scrubbing to the chewing surfaces of your teeth where food debris easily collects. Clean slowly, giving each tooth individual attention.

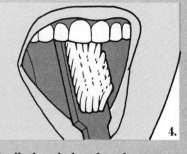

Finally, brush the often-forgotten inside surfaces of your front teeth, top and bottom. Hold the brush at an almost vertical angle and scrub them up and down.

217

time. Eventually, your gums
may ____ to bleed easily, especially while
you're brushing or flossing your teeth.

Gingivitis, if left untreated, can escalate to
periodontitis. Infected pockets form between
the teeth and gums. Your breath smells bad,
but worse yet, the bone that supports the
teeth is destroyed, so that the teeth become
loose and eventually start falling out.

Give Plaque the Brush-Off

The most important point to remember
about both tooth decay and periodontal
disease is that you can prevent them. At
some stage, periodontal disease can even be
reversed. Dentists find that, when properly
treated, inflammation can subside, swollen
gums can shrink and grow firm, and loose
teeth may even become more stable.

The key to proper treatment is plaque
control, a job that is never done. Within
24 hours after removing one layer of plaque,
a new layer begins to glom onto your teeth.
To unglom it, you need to brush your teeth
for 3 minutes at least once or twice a day.
Brushing is especially important at bedtime.
While you sleep, saliva secretion is reduced.

Preventing plaque's formation in the first
place is also important, especially when it
comes to your diet. If there's anything
plaque loves, it's a nice sugary treat like a
candy bar or a can of soda pop between
meals. Plaque uses the sugar to establish a
stickier stronghold in your mouth. What's
more, every time you eat anything, sweet or
not, plaque launches a 20-minute acid attack
with your teeth in the direct line of fire. So
try to limit eating to mealtimes. If you do

snack, eat nondecay-promoting foods like
nuts, popcorn, or raw vegetables. Cheese, by
the way, seems to actually neutralize the
formation of acid. Chewing sugarless gum a
few minutes after a snack appears to help
neutralize acids, too.

See your dentist regularly, at least twice a
year, for a checkup and to have tartar
removed professionally. If you show signs of
periodontal disease, your dentist may recommend more frequent cleaning.

Judith Lin

How To Floss

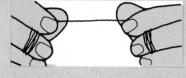

(1) Break off
about 18 inches
of floss and
wrap the ends
around one finger of each hand. Waxed and
unwaxed floss seem to be equally efficient.

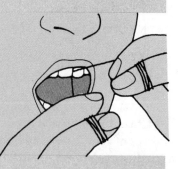

(2) Pull the floss
taut and gently
guide it into the
gap between two
teeth until it
reaches your gums.
In an up-and-down
motion, floss the
sides of each tooth
to remove plaque and food particles trapped
there. Then move on to the next gap, using a
clean section of floss.

HEADACHES

If it hadn't been for Lewis Carroll's bouts with migraines, *Alice's Adventures in Wonderland* wouldn't be half so whimsical. But what seemed like flights of fancy on Carroll's part were—at least part of the time—souvenirs from his flights into pain.

Carroll drew inspiration from the visual distortions he experienced just prior to his attacks—an intriguing phenomenon doctors call the migraine aura.

Few of us have such use for our head pains. In fact, 40 million doctor visits each year are prompted by headaches. An estimated 157 million workdays are lost due to headaches, according to a Louis Harris survey.

Fortunately, this ancient affliction is more manageable than ever. If you suffer from headaches, there's a wide array of effective drug-free methods to combat the pain and discomfort.

Tailor the Treatment to the Cause

There are three basic categories of headaches. Tension headaches are by far the most common, afflicting up to 90 percent of headache sufferers, according to Seymour Diamond, M.D., director of the Diamond Headache Clinic in Chicago and author of *Hope for Your Headache Problem*. The remaining 10 percent include vascular headaches, such as migraine and cluster-style headaches, and those caused by underlying illnesses.

Here's how to tell what kind you have and what to do about it.

Taming the Tension Headache

Typically, the tension headache sails in just when things aren't going so hot. Maybe your work is piling up, and you aren't clearing your desk fast enough to please your boss. Or you and your spouse have just had a spat.

Soon the muscles in your neck, jaw, and face tighten. You feel a dull, aching sensation in your head. The pain is most acute across a narrow band that encircles your head like a hat brim.

"If you can relate the headache to something that's going on around you, walk away from it—even if you have to go sit in the bathroom," says Dr. Diamond. "Try to relax. Think of something pleasurable."

If you're by yourself, try acupressure techniques, applications of heat, then cold, or the brushing method to relieve your pain. (You'll learn all of these effective healing methods on pages 223 to 225.) The earlier you catch the headache, the more successful you'll be in short-circuiting the pain. You might also ask a friend or partner to treat you to the massage sequence described on pages 226 to 227. Healing touch can be remarkably soothing.

Remember, aspirin and aspirin substitutes are fine for relief of occasional headaches, but you may be asking for trouble if you use aspirin more than twice a week. "If you use aspirin more than that, you can actually promote chronic muscle tension headaches," says Lee Kudrow, M.D., director of the

HEADACHES

California Medical Clinic for Headache in Encino.

If you've unwittingly come to depend on over-the-counter pain relievers for daily relief, stop immediately. There's a good chance your daily headache will disappear, says Dr. Kudrow.

Dr. Diamond and Dr. Kudrow agree that stress, anxiety, frustration, depression, and repressed hostility can all bring on simple tension headaches. But the chronic tension headache—near-constant unrelieved pain—is another matter.

"The chronic tension headache really has nothing to do with tension," says Dr. Kudrow. Rather, it results from fluctuations in the levels of two chemicals your body manufactures: norepinephrine and serotonin.

"We know that a chronic tension headache can be initiated by physical or emotional trauma, by illness or high fever," says Dr. Kudrow.

Biofeedback Releases Tension

Learning how to consciously relax the muscles can be of tremendous help in relieving a chronic headache. One system that will help you learn how is biofeedback, a technique Dr. Kudrow says is effective for 80 percent of people who suffer from tension headaches. Ask your physician to refer you to a biofeedback trainer.

Usually, people need six to ten lessons to really learn the technique, says Dr. Diamond. When you get the knack of it, you practice the technique at home every day until you're confident about being able to relax instantly, at will. "I use it on all my hospital patients very successfully," says Dr. Diamond.

Outmaneuvering the Migraine

Migraine headaches are one of the nastier tricks your genes can play on you. If both of your parents are prone to migraines, there's a 70 percent chance you'll be affected, too. If one parent is affected, you have a 50 percent chance that migraines will torment you. The problem is likely to show up when you are in your early twenties and disappear sometime around the age of 50. Some unfortunate individuals are afflicted with migraines in childhood, however.

Fluctuations in levels of serotonin are also thought to be a factor in migraine headaches. Changes in serotonin level can cause the blood vessels around the brain to constrict. This cuts off oxygen, leading to sensory disturbances—such as distorted vision or strange odors—that are part of the migraine aura. Typically, another change in serotonin level releases the constriction and causes the blood vessels to swell. At this point, the aura leaves and the pain sets in. Migraine pain can last for hours or days. Nausea and vomiting often accompany this condition.

Curiously enough, migraines affect four times as many women as men. Some women suffer migraines only around the time of their menstrual period.

To help head off an attack, you can try to constrict the blood vessels by placing a cold gel pack against your forehead.

Migraine sufferers have also found great relief from a technique known as hand-warming. The idea is to consciously relax yourself and direct the blood flow into your hands by imagining that your hands are getting warmer and warmer. It is especially easy to learn this technique with the help of biofeedback, because the measuring instruments will let you know without a doubt when you've succeeded. Many people learn to raise their hand temperature at will by 10 to 15 degrees, says Dr. Diamond.

The hand-warming technique was discovered, almost by accident, during research on biofeedback at the Menninger Clinic in Kansas. A follow-up study, involving headache sufferers only, found it successful in reducing or eliminating headaches in a majority of the people who tried it.

When to See the Doctor

If you're getting a headache every day, or nearly every day, you need to consult your doctor. The problem might not be tense muscles or throbbing blood vessels, but inflammation stemming from an underlying disorder.

You should also consult your doctor if your headaches are interfering with your work or social activities, if you've never had headaches before and you've just started getting a lot of them, or if they begin after a bout of coughing or from exertion, says Dr. Diamond.

If you decide you'd like to see a headache specialist or if you want more information about headaches, you may contact the National Headache Foundation, 5252 Northwestern Avenue, Chicago, IL 60625.

Pain Prevention

Once you learn to foil your headaches, you can take steps to ensure that they won't return. That may require a little detective work on your part. There are certain common headache triggers, but unless you want to live an unduly restricted life, it makes sense to sleuth until you find those that affect you. You may find you need to try several strategies at once.

A headache diary can help you detect whether there's a pattern to what sets off your headaches. For every headache, write down what you were doing just before its onset—what you ate, where you were, what was happening emotionally, and what the weather was like. (For some people, changes in barometric pressure or wind conditions can trigger a migraine, says Dr. Kudrow.)

Some of the more common headache triggers are listed below. Although they are particularly applicable to the migraine sufferer, sufferers of chronic tension headaches may also recognize some of them. Chronic tension headaches actually have more in common with migraine headaches than they do with the occasional tension headache, according to Dr. Kudrow. If you can figure out from your diary what may be triggering your headaches, a few simple changes in your lifestyle may be all it takes to banish headache pain from your life.

Food sensitivity. The culprits are tyramine and similar substances that are found in red wine, chocolate, nuts, navy beans, and dairy products such as aged cheese, sour cream, and yogurt; nitrates, which are found in cured meats such as ham and cold cuts; and monosodium glutamate, an ingredient in many processed foods and a flavor enhancer in Chinese cuisine. Experiment with eliminating these foods from your diet.

Drugs. Daily use of certain migraine-relief drugs, such as Cafergot, Wigraine, and

H EADACHES

Ergostat, can increase your chances of getting recurring headaches. Other potential problem drugs include decongestants, nasal sprays, appetite suppressants, certain diuretics, and medications for arthritis and hearing problems. If you suspect that one of these products is triggering your migraines, consult your pharmacist or physician. You may be able to substitute another drug that won't cause headaches.

Oral contraceptives and supplemental or replacement estrogen drugs are problematic, too. Dr. Kudrow finds that 85 percent of migraine attacks are associated with hormonal changes. Women who switch to the nonestrogen minipills don't have a problem, he says.

Irregular habits. If your system is sensitive, something as simple as an irregular sleep schedule or erratic eating habits can cause migraines. Dr. Diamond asks his patients to wake at the same time every day, even on holidays and vacations, and to be careful not to skip meals.

Light. Even bright light or looking up at the sun can trigger headache attacks. Tinted glasses can help, says Dr. Diamond.

Altitude changes. If you plan to vacation in the mountains or someplace where the elevation is higher than you're accustomed to, ask your doctor about taking a diuretic the day before you go.

Unresolved emotional trauma. Continuing anxiety about unresolved emotional trauma is often at the root of chronic headaches, says Dr. Diamond, who has found short-term psychological therapy beneficial for his patients.

Deborah Grandinetti

222

What Kind of Headache Do You Have?

You'll feel pressure between your eyebrows and above and below your eye sockets if you have a sinusitis headache. Migraine pain is more severe and covers a larger area. A sharp, stabbing sensation on one side of the head, especially around the eye, usually indicates a cluster-style headache. Tightness around the scalp or neck points to a tension headache.

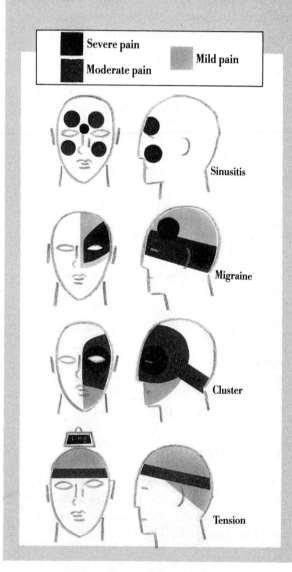

Severe pain

Moderate pain

Mild pain

Sinusitis

Migraine

Cluster

Tension

Hot and Cold Relief

A steamy hot towel and a gel cold pack are sometimes all you need to knock out headache pain. Always apply heat at the first sign of a tension headache. A cold gel pack against your forehead may help banish a migraine. You might boost the effect if you imagine your hands becoming warmer at the same time you apply the pack. If the headache progresses, apply the gel pack or a washcloth-covered ice pack to the spots where you feel pain.

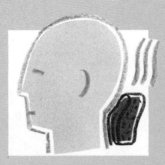

If you use a hot water bottle, position your head so that your neck isn't burdened by its weight.

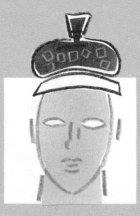

If heat doesn't do the trick, try applying a soothing cold pack to the top of your head.

Give Your Headache the Brush-Off

To keep headaches at bay, brush your scalp daily to improve blood circulation, says biophysicist Harry Ehrmantraut, Ph.D. The technique can also help you banish headache pain. Use a good natural-bristle hairbrush or shower brush with rounded-tip bristles. Beginning at your temples, move the brush in half-inch circles and work your way down. Then do the opposite side. Next, bring the brush just left of the center of your scalp and work down, using half-inch circles. Finish by brushing the area just right of the center of your scalp.

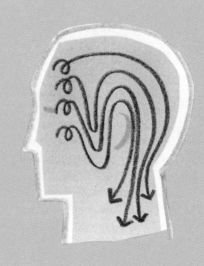

HEADACHES

Press Here for Headache Relief

If you can catch a headache-in-the-making, acupressure can serve you well. Experiment with each of these points so you can discover which ones work the best for you. Although some of these points are not on or near the head, they can be equally effective, say acupressure experts.

In the beginning, you may find that the specific "headache points" are very tender, so start gently. Don't press hard enough to hurt yourself. Keep the pressure steady for about 20 seconds and let up gradually. Most points have a partner on the opposite side of the body. Be sure to work both.

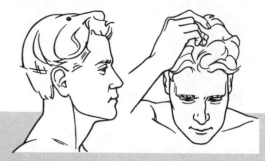

Top of Head

Above left, Find the center of your head, in line with your ears. *Above right,* Press firmly on that spot, using a circular motion.

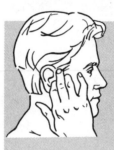

Side of Head

Bring your finger in front of the upper part of the ear and feel for the depression in front of the jaw muscle attachment.

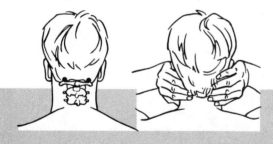

Back of Head

Above left, Bring your fingers level with your earlobes and feel for two "bumps" as shown. *Above right,* Lower your fingers about an inch until they are just under the bumps. Then rock your head back until you feel the muscles relax. You can either pull your elbows forward and vigorously massage this area of muscle with your fingertips or pull your elbows back and use your thumbs.

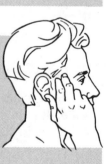

Front of Ear

Feel for a depression in the skull, in line with your eyebrows. Use your middle fingers to press firmly, using a circular motion.

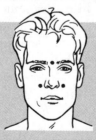

Sinuses

One sinus point is located between the eyebrows. The other two are located on each side of the nose, alongside the nostrils.

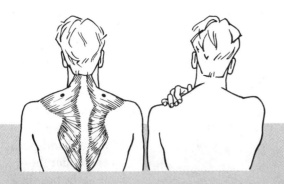

Shoulder

Rest the heel of your right hand on your left collarbone so that your thumb presses against your neck. *Above right,* Curve your fingers over your shoulder. *Above left,* The tip of your middle finger is now over the "shoulder point." Press in deeply as you vibrate your fingers rapidly.

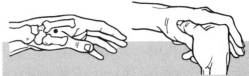

Hand

Above left, To find this point, stretch the thumb away from the other fingers until you can see the web of skin. *Above right,* Now place your other thumb into that bony triangle between the thumb and index finger. The point you want to press is on the bone of the index finger.

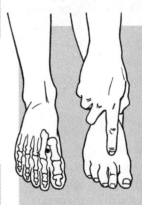

Top of Foot

Left, Find the depression between first and second toes. *Right,* Bring your finger about an inch above the web between the toes.

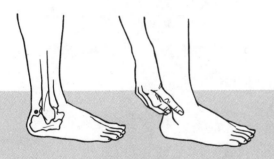

Achilles Tendon

Above left, To find this point, feel for the depression behind the ankle bone on the outside of your leg. One way to give yourself enough leverage to press hard here is to sit down and then bend forward as if you were going to touch the floor with your hand. Bring your right arm down and press the elbow against the inside of your right thigh. *Above right,* Reach around the right leg and use your middle finger to press the point.

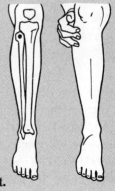

Shin

Place your finger on the outside of your kneecap, then slide it down to the head of your shinbone. *Right,* Slide it another inch down to the sensitive spot. *Left,* That's your point.

HEADACHES

Rub the Trouble Right Out

Massage can be an enjoyable addition to your arsenal of headache fighters. The massage should be deep enough to stimulate circulation in the arteries and capillaries of the scalp muscles. You can reach the main artery that supplies the scalp by working the point just in front of where the upper ear attaches to the scalp. You can also focus on the trapezius muscle, a triangle-shaped muscle that begins behind your neck and drapes over your shoulder blades. If you're on your own, knead and squeeze the muscles behind your neck. Or talk a partner into following the sequence below.

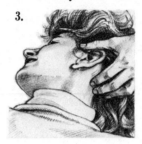

Turn your partner's head to the side. Let it rest comfortably in one hand. Using the fingertips of your free hand, push up and under the bone at the base of the skull. Hold, letting pressure build, then release. Work right along the rim, searching out tense spots. Repeat on the other side.

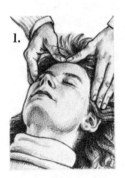

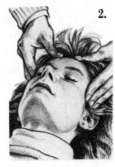

Rest your thumbs just above the eyebrows. Draw them up and out toward the temple. Again, draw them out toward the temple, working in strips until you cover the entire forehead.

Stand behind your partner. Ask her to relax, lean back, and rest her head against your body. Cup your hands and then spread your fingers apart. Place them at the top of her forehead. Now use the tips of your fingers to massage the scalp right along the hairline. Begin at the top of her forehead and work your way down to the base of the skull. Take your time and ask your partner to tell you how much pressure to use.

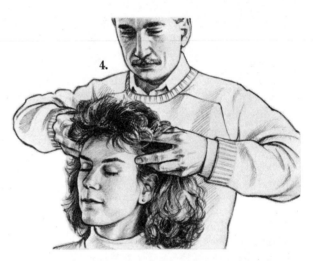

Use the fingertips to press on your partner's temple for 10 seconds. Slowly release pressure and make slow circles over both temples. Ask your partner how much pressure she prefers.

Have your partner clench and unclench her teeth, so you can locate the jaw muscles.

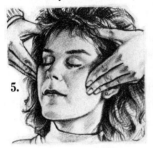

Massage these muscles thoroughly by pressing in, in circles, with the pads of your fingers. Rest your thumbs on the scalp for support.

5.

Have your partner focus on her breathing. Place your fingertips as shown, above the middle of the eyebrows. Imagine that you are drawing energy from deep inside you and sending it out through your fingertips.

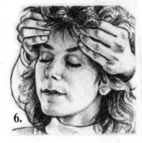

6.

Center your middle and ring finger on your

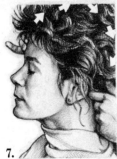

partner's forehead. Rest the fingers of the other hand in the hollow at the base of her skull. Now lightly draw the top fingers down the scalp to the base. Repeat several times.

7.

Bring the fingers of both hands to the center of the forehead, just above the brows. Lightly draw your fingers up to the top of the head. Here, separate your hands. The left hand moves down over the left ear, over the left shoulder, and off. The right hand follows suit on its side. Repeat the movement several times.

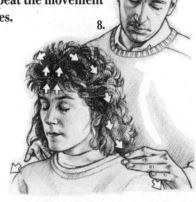

8.

Start as before, by resting your fingers on your partner's forehead. Stroke up to her hairline, separate your hands, and let each trace the hairline on down. Continue the stroke behind the ears and around the rim of the skull to the center. When your hands meet at the center, pull them away from the skull.

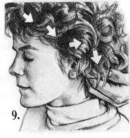

9.

HEARTBURN

Not since you left the old neighborhood have you tasted Italian food like this. Antipasto replete with shimmering red peppers, spicy pepperoni, and black olives straight from the barrel. Thick hunks of bread and butter. Mounds of spaghetti and chunky, homemade sausage drowning in tomato sauce. And for dessert, a chocolate liqueur-laced cannoli. Mmmm, hits the spot! But moments later, the spot getting hit is hitting back—smack-dab in the middle of your chest. You have yourself a good old-fashioned case of heartburn.

Heartburn is one of the most common problems seen by gastroenterologists.

Actually, if it weren't for a muscle called the lower esophageal sphincter (LES), located at the point where your esophagus and stomach connect, you would probably have heartburn after every meal. This one-way valve opens, dropping food down into your stomach, and then closes, keeping digestive stomach acid from coming up. Sometimes, however, the valve opens at the wrong time or doesn't close completely, allowing acid from your stomach to squirt into your esophagus. The pain you feel is your tender tissues' way of yelling "ouch!" as they recoil from their acid shower.

Eating at regular times slowly and in a relaxed atmosphere can help assure that the LES does its job efficiently. And smaller meals, which leave your stomach more quickly and produce less acid than large meals, are a help.

What you eat can also make a difference.

A diet high in fat encourages the secretion of heartburn-causing hormones. These hormones increase acid production, delay stomach emptying, and get right in there and flip your esophageal sphincter open. After-dinner chocolates, peppermints, and alcohol can have the same effect, as can smoking.

Coffee, tea, and citrus and tomato juices have all been linked to heartburn. Water, on the other hand, can cool things down.

If you're overweight, keep track of how much you eat, too. Shedding excess weight seems to take a load off your digestive system and reduces heartburn as well.

Trying to sleep with a case of heartburn is an invitation to insomnia. A "backwash" of stomach acids is more likely to occur when you're lying down with a full stomach, so try not to eat for at least a couple of hours before going to bed. If you do go to bed right after eating, try raising the head of your bed 6 inches or so (use blocks of wood under the bedposts). Tilting your bed helps gravity keep acid down in your stomach.

Antacids are effective in neutralizing stomach acid. Liquid antacids, which do a better job of spreading themselves across the surface of your esophagus, are preferable. They can interfere with your body's absorption of other medications, such as aspirin or the antibiotic tetracycline.

If heartburn persists, see a physician, as your symptoms may signal a more serious problem.

Judith Lin

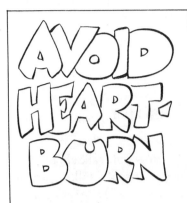

AVOID HEART-BURN

AVOID FATTY FOODS, ALCOHOLIC BEVERAGES, COFFEE, CHOCOLATE, MINTS, AND LYING DOWN AFTER DINNER.

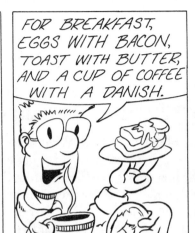

FOR BREAKFAST, EGGS WITH BACON, TOAST WITH BUTTER, AND A CUP OF COFFEE WITH A DANISH.

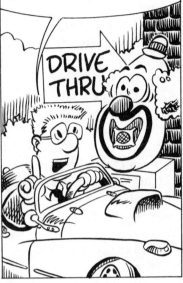

FOR LUNCH, I'D LIKE A BACON CHEESEBURGER WITH FRENCH FRIES AND A CHOCOLATE SHAKE.

DRIVE THRU

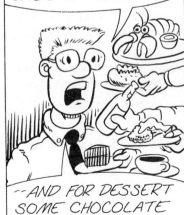

AH, WAITER, I'D LIKE WINE, LOBSTER WITH BUTTER, A BAKED POTATO WITH SOUR CREAM, BROCCOLI WITH CHEESE SAUCE---

---AND FOR DESSERT SOME CHOCOLATE MOUSSE AND A CUP OF COFFEE.

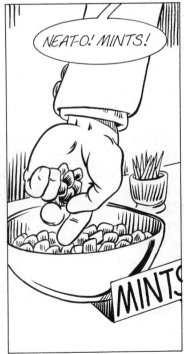

NEAT-O! MINTS!

MINTS

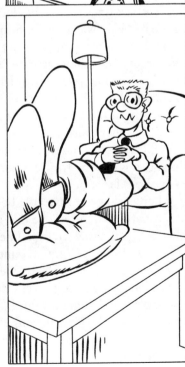

229

HEART DISEASE

The heart is an amazing living instrument that beats about 100,000 times and pumps nearly 2,000 gallons of blood every day of your life.

"The heart is what provides the fuel and oxygen that keeps the whole body going," says Laurence Watkins, M.D., a cardiologist who is a committee member of both the National Heart, Lung, and Blood Institute and the American Heart Association (AHA). But the best argument for keeping your heart healthy is this: If you don't, you risk a heart attack.

If you were to have a heart attack, you'd be far from alone. A person who survives a heart attack finds that he has lots of company in the recovery ward, in the hospital's rehabilitation program, and in the doctor's office receiving follow-up care. The lucky ones become members of this far-from-exclusive club. The unlucky ones . . . well, more Americans die from heart attacks than from any other cause.

While America has no monopoly on heart disease, it is extremely rare in some countries. Why should that be?

There is no great mystery about the causes of our nation's number one killer. We can blame it on the way we live. The good news concealed in this gloomy statement is that you can use the scientific knowledge of what causes heart disease to prevent it. How? By making a few changes in your lifestyle. And you won't have to give up your all-American pleasures to go live on nuts and berries in the Indonesian rain forest, either.

The Heart of America

What exactly is *heart disease?*

"In America, when people talk about 'heart disease,' they are usually talking about ischemic heart disease," says Dr. Watkins, who practices cardiology in Plantation, Florida. Ischemic heart disease, also known as coronary artery disease or coronary heart disease, is caused by a narrowing of the arteries, which results in decreased blood flow to the heart muscle.

However, a large number of disorders can affect the heart. Sometimes it is not the arteries that are affected but the heart valves or the muscle. The reason most people think of heart disease as primarily a disease of the arteries is because that is the most common thing that goes wrong with hearts in America, says Dr. Watkins.

Heart experts say that there are several factors well within your control that will help to determine whether or not you develop any kind of heart disease. The three biggest ones, according to the AHA, are cigarette smoking, high blood pressure, and high blood cholesterol.

When Smoke Gets in Your Veins

If you had to pick just one thing to do —right this moment—to most decrease your chances of a heart attack, what would it be?

"That's easy," says Dr. Watkins. "Quit smoking."

If you smoke a pack of cigarettes a day, you have more than twice the risk of heart attack than do people who have never smoked. And if you smoke two or more packs, you are carrying a risk of heart attack three times greater, say the experts at the AHA.

If you quit today, however, your risk of heart disease will immediately start to decrease. And guess what? Ten years after quitting, your risk of death from heart disease will be almost the same as if you'd never smoked at all!

Just what the numerous toxic ingredients in tobacco smoke do to your heart and blood vessels could fill volumes. Smoking tends to make your blood gooey, narrow your blood vessels, deprive your heart of oxygen, and put added pressure on the heart, to say nothing of what smoking does to your lungs.

Saying good-bye to tobacco isn't easy. Smoking is addictive—both psychologically and physically. If you need help quitting, talk to your doctor. You can also turn to the American Heart Association, the American Cancer Society, or the American Lung Association. There are a wide variety of stop-smoking programs—something to fit every personality. If it's been years since you tried to quit, you may be pleasantly surprised.

The Cholesterol Culprit

The level of cholesterol in your blood also plays a significant role in determining your risk of developing coronary heart disease, says Dr. Watkins. Cholesterol is the major component of the plaque that can clog arteries. Everybody has some cholesterol in his blood—it's only when the levels get too high that you put your heart and blood vessels at risk.

The high level of blood cholesterol among Americans is largely due to the American diet. We eat too much fat, particularly saturated fat, the kind found in meat and dairy products and in foods made with coconut or palm oils. Many foods high in saturated fat are also high in dietary cholesterol, another troublesome factor. Foods exceptionally high in cholesterol include egg yolks and organ meats.

But here is some exciting news. Even if years of having high cholesterol has caused considerable accumulation of plaque in your arteries—you may be able to actually *reverse* the damage simply by modifying your diet.

"The body has a great capacity to heal itself if we give it a chance," says Dean Ornish, M.D., director of the Preventive Medicine Research Institute in Sausalito, California. "But if three times a day we're putting more fat and cholesterol into the body than it can metabolize, then it never gets a chance to heal itself."

To prove his point, Dr. Ornish assembled 12 volunteers with coronary-artery blockage and put them on an extremely low-fat, no-cholesterol diet. In addition, he had them exercise regularly and practice stress-reducing meditation. Also, those who smoked quit. The results? In one year, the group's average blood cholesterol readings dropped by more than a quarter, and their coronary-artery blockages decreased almost 10 percent.

Have your cholesterol level checked if you don't know what it is. And do something about it if it's too high. Diet is the best place to start. Your doctor can discuss other measures with you. (Turn to the chapter on cholesterol on page 137, for more information.)

Hypertension Harms Hearts

Hypertension, or high blood pressure, is an indication that the heart is working harder than it should and that the arteries are under undue strain. If untreated, hypertension can make it progressively harder for your heart to pump enough blood to meet your body's needs.

Hypertension is often called the silent killer. It is silent because many people who have it don't know it, and it is a killer because it is a contributing factor to fatal conditions such as heart attack, stroke, and kidney failure.

What can you do about high blood pressure? Plenty. Although doctors aren't sure what causes it, they do know that several factors can make it better or worse. By watching your weight and your consumption of salt and alcohol and by getting regular exercise, you'll be heading in the right direction.

You may also need medication. In any case, you won't know you have high blood pressure unless you get it checked! Talk to your doctor. (And see the chapter on high blood pressure on page 270.)

Additional Measures to Take to Heart

Beyond quitting smoking, limiting the cholesterol in your diet, and controlling high blood pressure, there are several additional factors, also well within your control, that will determine your risk of heart disease. A number of studies over the years have linked heart disease to a sedentary lifestyle, being overweight, leading a stressful life, and having diabetes.

Exercise Primes the Pump

Studies indicate that people who don't exercise have a greater risk of heart disease than those who are active. In one study of over 3,000 male railroad workers, researchers found that sedentary men were 30 to 40 percent more likely to die of coronary heart disease (or some other disease) than were active men.

If you can't see yourself running steps with Rocky and dripping sweat at 6:00A.M., take heart—you don't have to. The railroad study and others show that moderate activity such as brisk walking offers as much heart protection as strenuous huffing and puffing.

Take It Easy

Just because you're a success-driven, 12-hour-a-day, Type-A workaholic doesn't necessarily mean you're headed for a heart attack. What can put you at serious risk, however, is the hostility and distrustfulness that often go with Type-A behavior, according to Redford Williams, M.D., professor of psychiatry at Duke University School of

Medicine and author of *The Trusting Heart*.

Want to avoid heart disease? Dr. Williams recommends that you monitor your cynical thoughts and try to control them, relax more, learn to laugh at yourself, and practice trust and forgiveness as often as you can.

Down with Diabetes, Down with Extra Pounds

Diabetes, a condition in which the blood sugar level is abnormally high, can sharply increase your risk of a heart attack. That's because, as a large number of studies have shown, the person with excess sugar in the blood is much more likely to develop plaque in the arteries. If you have diabetes, work closely with your doctor to bring it under control and pay particular attention to controlling the other risk factors for heart disease discussed throughout this chapter.

Carrying around too many pounds is unquestionably a contributing factor in heart disease. Being overweight adds strain to your heart and increases your risk of coronary heart disease primarily because of its link to high blood pressure and blood cholesterol, and also because it can lead to diabetes.

Surviving a Heart Attack

Thanks to advances in modern medicine, your chances of surviving a heart attack are better than ever. Statistically, two of every three heart attack victims do survive. What separates the winners from the losers can be a matter of only seconds. That's why it's *critical* to seek medical attention as soon as you first suspect a heart attack.

The symptoms of heart attack vary, but the usual warning signs, according to the American Heart Association (AHA), are:

- Uncomfortable pressure, fullness, squeezing or pain in the center of the chest lasting for 2 minutes or more.
- Pain spreading to the shoulders, neck, jaw, arms, or back.
- Dizziness, fainting, sweating, nausea, or shortness of breath.

Not all of these signs have to be present for you to be having a heart attack. And in some cases, the symptoms go away and then come back.

How to Mend a Broken Heart

We've saved for last what may be the best news for people who have already suffered heart attacks. Studies are now showing that even if you've had a heart attack, you can probably lead a normal life—and a *long* one, too—with the right changes in the way you live. Those changes include the factors you've already read about and more.

First, consider exercise. You know it's good for *preventing* heart disease. What about *after* a heart attack? You'd have to be downright crazy to go out and exercise, right? Wrong. In a report published in *Circulation*, a professional journal, scientists concluded that rehabilitation programs that include 20 to 30 minutes of physical exercise three times a week significantly reduce the risk of dying from a second heart attack. Specifically, they say that if you've had a heart attack, undertaking an exercise program decreases your odds of succumbing to another attack by 20 percent over three years.

The researchers can't say for sure how exercise helps to mend broken hearts, but some conclusions are not hard to draw. "There's no evidence for increased risk with exercise; there's lots of evidence to the contrary. My advice is clear: Go ahead and exercise," says Gerald T. O'Connor, Ph.D., D.Sc., assistant professor of medicine at the Dartmouth-Hitchcock Medical Center in New Hampshire and one of the report's authors. Of course, you should only proceed under your physician's guidance.

In addition to exercise, you'd be wise to eat lots of fish. The prestigious British medical journal *Lancet* reports that people advised by their doctors to eat fish were 29 percent less likely to die for another two years after a heart attack. The best fish are those that contain lots of a substance called eicosapentaenoic acid, more commonly called EPA. These include mackerel, herring, sardines, salmon, and trout.

Aside from EPA, you've undoubtedly heard a lot about what aspirin can do for your heart. Is it true? Yes, aspirin is known to decrease the risk of a second heart attack, and more recently, a large study has shown that taking aspirin may reduce the risk of a first heart attack, too.

The study, done by researchers from Harvard Medical School and Brigham and Women's Hospital in Boston, showed that the risk of heart attack for those who took aspirin (325 milligrams of buffered aspirin every other day) was 47 percent lower than for those who did not.

Should you start popping aspirin tablets immediately? Not without consulting your doctor. Aspirin shouldn't be used by everyone, warns the AHA. And by no means should you count on it to protect you from heart disease. Aspirin works by making your blood less likely to clot, but it won't clear clogged arteries.

Love Your Heart

Unfortunately for some, fortunately for others, some of the risk factors of heart disease are far beyond our control. An older man with a history of heart disease in the family is much more likely to get heart disease than a younger woman with no family history.

But regardless of who you are, no one is immune to heart disease. That's why it's important to "listen" to your body and to be aware of heart disease's warning signs.

That warning is most often chest pain, a kind that generally comes with physical exertion or stress and is relieved when you sit down and relax. It's called angina, and it demands medical attention. If you're not sure whether your chest pain is angina or merely indigestion, play it safe and have it checked out. "It's my job as a cardiologist to tell the difference," says Dr. Watkins.

It's also a good idea, says Dr. Watkins, to check with your doctor if you're over 40 and embark on a vigorous exercise program, even if you've never had any warning signs.

With proper care, your ticker can be like one of those watches you see advertised on television—it'll keep on ticking.

Russell Wild

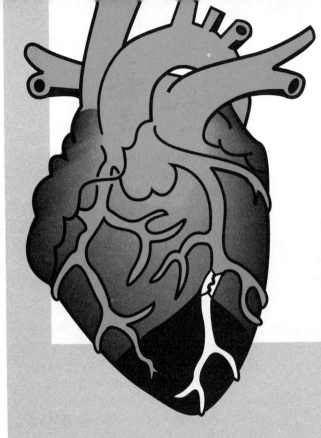

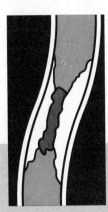

Left and below, Heart attacks are usually caused by coronary thrombosis, the formation of a blood clot in a narrowed artery that blocks the flow of blood to the heart.

The Anatomy of a Heart Attack

The very worst thing about heart disease is that it sometimes leads to a heart attack. More Americans die of heart attacks than anything else. But what exactly happens during an "attack"?

In doctor talk, a heart attack is called a myocardial infarction. It means that the supply of blood to a part of the heart muscle has been cut off. When the heart muscle is deprived of blood, the muscle cells suffer irreversible injury and die.

Depending on how much of the heart muscle has been affected, the heart attack victim suffers disability or even death. About two out of three heart attack victims do survive; they are often those who receive quick medical attention.

Heart attacks do not occur out of the blue. They are often the end result of atherosclerosis, a slow degenerative process that clogs the coronary arteries with fatty deposits and other debris.

In a way, a heart attack is not too different from an earthquake. In one case, slow changes underneath the earth's surface eventually result in a serious shock to things up above. In the other case, slow changes along the walls of the blood vessels eventually result in a serious shock to the heart.

HEART DISEASE

A Heart in Trouble

Just as the terms *arthritis* and *cancer* refer not to a single disease but to a group of diseases, so, too, does the term *cardiovascular disease*. A sick heart may be suffering from a congenital defect, that is, something a person is born with. Or heart disease may develop later in life. Similarly, some diseases of the heart affect the heart muscle, while others affect the heart valves or the blood vessels.

Heart attack symptoms vary, but the usual warning signs can include uncomfortable pressure, fullness, and squeezing pain in the center of the chest for two minutes; chest pain spreading to surrounding areas; dizziness; sweating; nausea; and fainting.

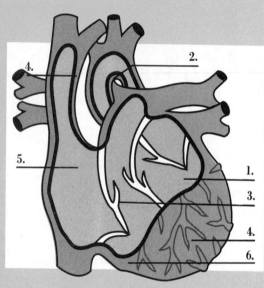

Pity the poor guy who has the heart you see above. This composite ticker has just about every form of ailment that a heart can get.

(1) Congenital defects. These aren't common, and doctors aren't sure why they occur, but some babies are born with heart problems. One of the two most common forms of defect is a hole in the wall between the heart's upper chambers.

(2) The other most common form of defect is an opening that allows blood to mix between the pulmonary artery and the aorta. Such an opening is normal before birth, but in some people it doesn't close the way it should. This defect is much more common in premature babies than in full-term babies.

(3) Diseases of the valves. Sometimes the valves in the heart, which help control the flow of blood, malfunction. This may happen because of a congenital defect or as the result of an infection. When the valves don't open and close properly, they can obstruct the forward flow of blood or cause it to leak backward.

(4) Atherosclerosis. Atherosclerosis refers to the filling of the arteries with deposits of plaque, which can narrow the coronary artery and lessen the flow of blood to the heart muscle.

(5) Arrhythmias. Everybody has a pacemaker—not a mechanical one, but a natural one. If the pacemaker isn't sending signals as it should, the rhythm of the heartbeat will be thrown off.

(6) Congestive heart failure. This condition occurs because of damage to the heart muscle. The damaged muscles keep the heart from working as efficiently as it should.

Your Pulse and Your Heart

No complicated medical tests are needed to measure your heartbeat. You can do it yourself, anytime you like, by taking a reading of your pulse. The pulse is a regular expansion of the artery that can be felt with the finger. It can be used to measure the speed, strength, and regularity of the heartbeat. Normally, your pulse rate will be between 50 and 100 beats per minute and vary according to your level of activity and stress.

Below, A day in the life of Jane Doe, as measured by her pulse rate. Notice that her pulse rate jumps as a result of either healthy exercise (such as her racquetball game) or unhealthy stress (such as rush-hour traffic). As Jane relaxes, so does her pulse. Whenever the pulse rate jumps, it indicates increased demand on her heart.

How to Take Your Pulse

The drawing below illustrates the best place on your wrist to feel for your pulse. Place the first three fingers of your right hand on the inside of your left wrist, slightly below the base of the thumb, and press gently. With a watch at your side, count the number of beats for 20 seconds, then multiply by three for the rate per minute.

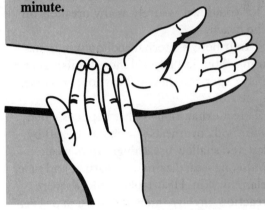

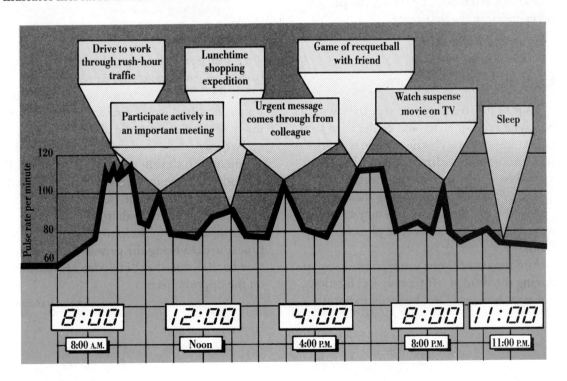

Drive to work through rush-hour traffic

Lunchtime shopping expedition

Game of recquetball with friend

Participate actively in an important meeting

Urgent message comes through from colleague

Watch suspense movie on TV

Sleep

Pulse rate per minute

120
100
80
60

8:00 | 12:00 | 4:00 | 8:00 | 11:00

8:00 A.M. | Noon | 4:00 P.M. | 8:00 P.M. | 11:00 P.M.

Heat Exhaustion/ Heatstroke

Go ahead. Have your fun in the sun. Just remember that heat waves can knock you down as surely as any breakers on the beach.

Your body's internal cooling system has its limits. Step just beyond those limits, and you may experience heat exhaustion, or worse, heatstroke.

Heat exhaustion—what happens when your body overheats—is characterized by fast and shallow breathing; rapid, weak pulse; nausea; dizziness; sweating; and pale, clammy skin. Heatstroke, a more severe reaction, involves mental confusion or even loss of consciousness.

You can avoid both by taking the proper precautions in the first place.

Cool It

Your body's temperature regulator works best when the air is dry and cooler than your body temperature. As the outside temperature and humidity climb, you need to take special care to keep from overheating.

Try to avoid exertion during the hottest part of the day. If you must be active, wear a wide-brimmed hat and drink plenty of fluids.

And remember, your sunny vacation escape during the dead of winter may feel fabulous, but your body may not be ready to handle strenuous outdoor exercise as soon as you alight from the airplane. Experts say your body needs at least two weeks to adjust to a hotter climate. All the more reason to relax poolside with a cool drink.

If the queasy, dizzy sensations of heat exhaustion do overtake you, follow this prescription for quick relief.

- Get out of the sun immediately.
- Find a cool place to rest.
- Wrap yourself in cool, wet towels.
- Sip a cold drink.

Your body should return to normal fairly quickly.

Strike Back at Heatstroke

Unlike heat exhaustion, heatstroke constitutes a real medical emergency. Without prompt treatment, a person can die. It's not unusual, either. Every year 5,000 Americans, many of them elderly, die of heatstroke.

Two important warning signs to look for are mental confusion and lack of sweating. If a person is acting inappropriately belligerent or strangely and has hot, flushed *dry* skin, get medical help immediately.

While waiting for help to arrive, start procedures to bring the person's temperature back down. (See "Help for Heatstroke" on the opposite page.)

Deborah Grandinetti

238

Help for Heatstroke

You are with a person suffering from heatstroke, and you've called for emergency medical help. While you are waiting, move the person to the coolest possible place. Have him lie in a tub of cold water, wrap him in a wet sheet, or sponge him with cool water and fan him. If his temperature rises, wet the sheet again or reapply the sponge. If the person loses consciousness, place him in the recovery position.

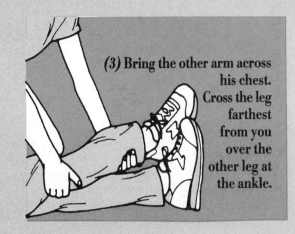

(3) Bring the other arm across his chest. Cross the leg farthest from you over the other leg at the ankle.

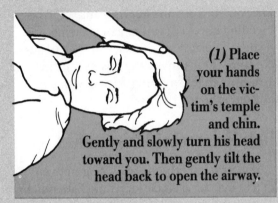

(1) Place your hands on the victim's temple and chin. Gently and slowly turn his head toward you. Then gently tilt the head back to open the airway.

(4) Support the head. With your other hand, grasp the victim's clothing at the hip and pull him toward you.

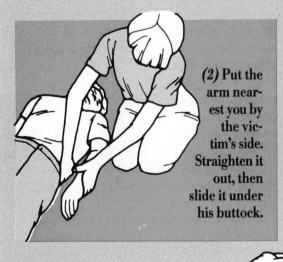

(2) Put the arm nearest you by the victim's side. Straighten it out, then slide it under his buttock.

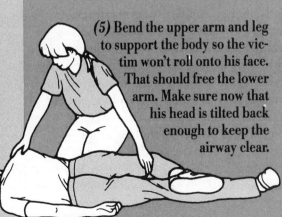

(5) Bend the upper arm and leg to support the body so the victim won't roll onto his face. That should free the lower arm. Make sure now that his head is tilted back enough to keep the airway clear.

HEMORRHOIDS

Your grandmother called them piles. You probably call them painful . . . if you bother to call them anything at all.

The fact of the matter is that 70 to 80 percent of us are walking around with hemorrhoids, and most us don't even know it. It's only when hemorrhoids act up—by itching, bleeding, or protruding—that people realize they have them.

Often, people with hemorrhoids have no obvious symptoms, says Max M. Ali, M.D., director of the Hemorrhoid Clinics of America.

How can that be? Hemorrhoids come in two varieties: internal and external. Internal hemorrhoids, which are tucked inside the rectum, can sometimes be felt if they protrude when stool is passed. Even external hemorrhoids can be so small and unobtrusive that you can't tell they're there.

So, What's a Hemorrhoid?

Maligned as it is, the hemorrhoid is simply a mass of dilated blood vessels in swollen tissue inside or outside the rectum. Straining to have a bowel movement causes the delicate tissue near the anus to become engorged with blood. If the blood vessel ruptures, it can cause further swelling. Sometimes the hemorrhoid is simply a displacement of the anal canal lining.

"Most people don't suspect they have a problem until they see blood in the toilet or in their stool or experience pain when they have bowel movements," says Dr. Ali.

If you experience pain or bleeding, consult your doctor. Pain is often a sign of some other common anal problem, such as a fissure or abscess. Rectal bleeding can also be a sign of cancer of the rectum or anus, says Dr. Ali. "If you don't get the cause of bleeding checked, you're jeopardizing your health. This type of cancer, caught early, is curable." Don't make the mistake, he says, of assuming that "anything wrong with your bottom is hemorrhoids."

Halt Hemorrhoid Discomfort

If your hemorrhoids are acting up, you don't have to reach far for immediate relief.

An application of petroleum jelly to the area will protect it when hard stools pass, says Dr. Ali. Or you can use an over-the-counter hemorrhoid product of your choice, although none of them works any better than petroleum jelly, says Dr. Ali.

In the long term, however, you need to make some lifestyle changes that can both prevent hemorrhoids and speed healing of existing conditions.

You may well wonder how what you put into your mouth can have any impact on your anatomy at the far end of your digestive tract . . . but it does.

If you're the type who favors coffee and Danish for breakfast, who thinks veggies are fine (for rabbits), who thinks fruit is okay (as a soft drink flavor), you might as well make your peace with hemorrhoids. Your body needs lots of dietary fiber in order to transport waste through your digestive system efficiently. And if you don't get it, you pay a price.

Fiber from whole grains, beans, fresh fruits, and vegetables helps make stool softer, bulkier, and easier to pass. Drinking more liquids can also help prevent hemorrhoids. You'll probably need it to help keep all that fiber moving through your system.

Regular exercise is important, too. "A physical exercise program will help establish good bowel habits," says Dr. Ali. "You may have heard that some people get hemorrhoids from heavy straining and lifting, but for most people lack of exercise is more of a problem."

If your hemorrhoids don't respond to home treatment, see your physician. There are several outpatient procedures to remove hemorrhoids that can have you back to work in two or three days.

Deborah Grandinetti

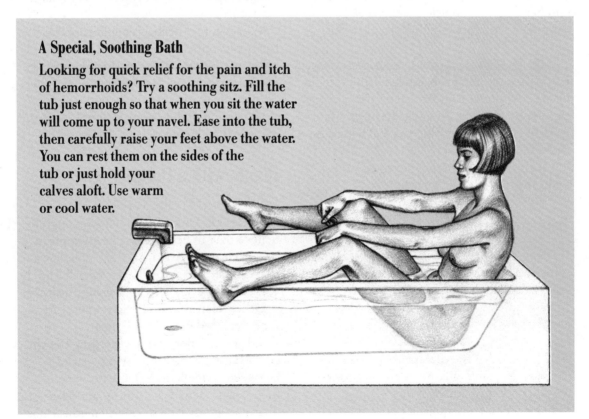

A Special, Soothing Bath

Looking for quick relief for the pain and itch of hemorrhoids? Try a soothing sitz. Fill the tub just enough so that when you sit the water will come up to your navel. Ease into the tub, then carefully raise your feet above the water. You can rest them on the sides of the tub or just hold your calves aloft. Use warm or cool water.

HERBS

So, you finally caught the bug that's been going around. You feel like one of the characters in those cold medicine commercials—achy, stuffy, sneezy, miserable.

Your next door neighbor stops in, offering to bring you something to help you feel better. You nod your head yes, but before you can say double-strength-time-released-cold-combat-formula-from-the-drugstore-please, she's gone and back in a snap, brewing you a pot of fresh eucalyptus tea, pouring witch hazel into a steaming bath, and handing you a bottle of echinacea capsules—"for a good night's sleep," as she puts it.

Though it all seems pretty suspect to you, pretty far-out, you go ahead and drink the tea, jump into the tub, and take a couple of capsules before bed. And to your pleasant surprise, the next morning you feel better. A *lot* better.

Maybe there's something to these faddish new remedies after all, you think.

Traditional Healing Returns

Using herbs for therapeutic purposes is actually anything but new. Herbal medicine enjoys a tradition that stretches back to ancient times. Egyptian scribes recorded the use of plants for medicinal purposes. A document written by a Greek physician in A.D. 78 describes the therapeutic properties of some 600 plants, a large number of which are still used medicinally today.

In fact, about one-quarter of commercial medications contain ingredients derived from plants. But it's not the pills that generate the most excitement among people who want to be healthier, it's the plants—healing plants that can, some claim, shorten a cold or lengthen a life.

America is undergoing an "herbal renaissance" as increasing numbers of people seek alternatives to modern medicine, says James Duke, Ph.D., author of the *CRC Handbook of Medicinal Herbs,* which details 365 herbs commonly available in almost every health food store.

What's more, herbal remedies are routinely prescribed by the 12,000 licensed homeopathic and naturopathic physicians who practice in the United States. (In other parts of the world, Dr. Duke notes, as much as 90 percent of the population relies mostly on herbal medicines.)

Plants with a Purpose

But do herbs really work?

Writes Dr. Duke: "I am folksy enough to believe that an herb a day, like an apple, a beet, a carrot, a citrus, and/or a coleslaw a day, can help keep the doctor away." And, he adds, maybe even help keep cancer away.

Other scientists and herbal experts are more reserved in their judgment.

"More misinformation regarding the efficacy of herbs is currently being placed before consumers than at any previous time," says Varro Tyler, Ph.D., professor of pharmacognosy (the science of medications

242

derived from natural sources) at Purdue University, author of *The New Honest Herbal*, and adviser on herbs to *Prevention* magazine.

Using herbs might be somewhat helpful, but doing so unwisely can be quite harmful, he says. One big danger is that of inaccurately diagnosing your illness.

"The person who self-diagnoses," says Dr. Duke, "has a fool for a doctor." Even if you properly identify your ailment, Dr. Tyler points out, it may be one that should be treated by a doctor, such as a heart problem or a tumor.

For any minor health problems, however, Dr. Tyler says he thinks herbs may be a fine treatment. "If you have a sore throat, chances are you're not going to immediately rush to the doctor. You might try a cup of herb tea first. I certainly have no problem in seeing people use herbs in a sensible fashion."

How to Select Herbs

But what exactly is sensible? How do you know where to buy your herbs? Which herbs are used for treating various symptoms? How much of each herb is appropriate?

First, Dr. Tyler advises buying your herbs from a reliable supplier because there are no laws or regulations governing the quality of herbs on the market. Larger companies, such as those that sell their products in health food stores, generally offer high-quality products.

Dr. Tyler especially cautions against picking herbs in the wild. Some herbs are deadly, and numerous cases of poisoning are reported each year, often the result of misidentification of herbs.

Another reason to avoid wild herbs is that they may not be as effective. "The amount of the active, therapeutic constituent in a particular herb can vary considerably," says Dr. Tyler. "It depends on where the plant was grown, how it was harvested and dried, how long it has been kept, and so on."

Caution: It's More Than Tea

Once you've selected and purchased the herb you want to use, be careful how you prepare it. Preparation method varies from herb to herb. And some methods of preparing herbs are less effective than others, Dr. Tyler points out.

For example, an herb's leaves may contain a potent, volatile oil that, when put in boiling water for tea, tends to evaporate, leaving you with very little of the therapeutic substance in the herb. Also, keep the dosage minimal: Just because a little bit may be healthful doesn't mean that double the amount is better. Large doses of some herbs can be quite dangerous.

Fortunately, the herbs on the following pages were chosen for their safety and effectiveness.

One final note of caution: Before taking any herbal remedy, give your doctor a call and get his approval. That way, you'll have the best of medical care and self-care.

Deborah Grandinetti

AN ENCYCLOPEDIA OF SAFE HEALING HERBS

The Ins and Outs of Herbal Tonics

Overwhelmed at the prospect of preparing and using herbs yourself? When? How much? Of which? Prepared how? For what? How often? . . . *Whoa!*

Think about potatoes. You can boil, bake, fry, deep-fry, or steam. You can slice, grate, chop, puree, quarter, cut plain or fancy, mash, or leave whole. You can enjoy them as a separate dish or add them to compatible foods. Folklore says you can use a slice of potato to soothe your eyes or soften a wart.

Herbs are no more intimidating than potatoes. They can be consumed or applied externally. You can use whole herbs or parts. You can crush, bruise, pound, break, chop, boil, simmer, or steep them. You can use a single herb or combine them. Here are a few traditional ways to enjoy nature's bounty.

Making the Tea

Thanks to the growing interest in health, herbal teas have become supermarket staples. To enjoy a *real* cup of tea, however, make it yourself.

Start with the right teapot. Ideally, it should be made of a "thick-walled ceramic material," explains Varro Tyler, Ph.D., Purdue University pharmacognosist and author of *The New Honest Herbal.* "The problem with a glass container is that the walls are too thin, and heat escapes. I'd advise against using any metallic container because an herb might react with the metal to produce a taste."

For superb tea, bring pure bottled water to a boil in a nonmetallic container. Pour it into your teapot and let it sit covered for 3 minutes to warm the pot. Pour the water back into the original container.

Toss an ounce (a handful) of dried herbs into the warm pot and pour in the boiling water. Use 1 pint of water for each ounce of herbs. Let it steep for 3 to 5 minutes.

To the tea lover, a teapot is rather like a cat: It enhances solitude, revives spirits, enriches the ordinary. The ideal teapot conforms to the song's description, ". . . short and stout," and is made of ceramic material or china.

If you add more herbs and steep the tea longer, you have an infusion. Infusions are used to extract more of the medicinal properties from the herbs.

And there is a third way — decoction — to prepare an herbal liquid. "You use the decoction method when you need to extract active ingredients and flavors from roots, barks, or tough fruits," explains Mark Blumenthal, executive director of the American Botanical Council and publisher/editor of *HerbalGram*. "You bring the plant material to a boil and keep it at a low, rolling boil for 15 to 20 minutes. You decoct when you want to get every iota of healing power out of the herb."

In all three processes, when the beverage is ready, strain, and add honey if you wish.

Use a reliable herbal source, such as a respected medicinal herbal guide written by an authority, a naturopathic physician, or an herbalist to learn the proper herbal ingredients, preparation, and application.

You may also apply herbs externally to treat bruises, sprains, swollen, aching muscles, congestion, tension, respiratory infections, and bee stings. Three common methods of external application are a compress, a poultice, and a plaster.

A compress is a clean towel made of cotton, gauze, or linen that has been soaked in either an infusion or a decoction. Simply dip the clean cloth into the hot (not too hot!) liquid, wring it out, and place it on the injured skin area.

Think of a poultice as an upside-down, open-faced sandwich. The "fixings" of this open-faced sandwich are a mass of fresh, dried, or steeped herbs, or a paste of herbs

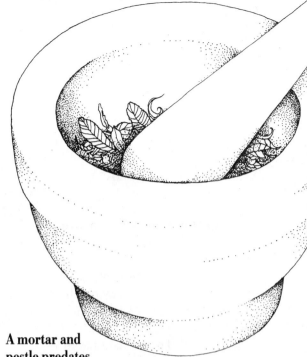

A mortar and pestle predates food processors yet excels in reducing small quantities of herbs to as fine a consistency as powder. There are even advantages to using these time-honored implements—once crushed, the herbs are easier to remove, and cleaning is a snap.

mixed with water, cider vinegar, flour, or oatmeal. Apply this herbal mixture directly to the skin. The "bread" of this sandwich is a warm cloth, towel, or bandage applied over the mixture to keep it in place. Poultices are frequently used to draw out pus.

A plaster is an herb sandwich with clean muslin serving as the "bread." Between it goes an herb "filling" of hot, stimulating herbs that have been bruised or made into a paste. Place the plaster directly on the aching or bruised area. For respiratory problems, use a plaster on the chest. The herbal mixture increases circulation and sweating, which herbalists say may help flush impurities out of the system.

245

HERBS

ALOE

This thick-leaved plant, a native of Africa, has long been used to heal and beautify the skin.

The herb's therapeutic ingredients are found in the clear, sticky gel that oozes out when you break open a leaf and squeeze it.

Many people keep a plant handy— particularly in the kitchen, where minor burns are common—and use the gel as a soothing salve. Some herbalists also claim the gel can reduce itching and use it to relieve poison ivy.

Scientists studying aloe have found that it breaks down dead tissue in a wound even as it helps regenerate new tissue, speeding the healing of burns. But it also helps repair skin damaged by cold; one study shows that it can greatly reduce the damage caused by frostbite.

Aloe also shows promise as a topical treatment for the pain of rheumatoid arthritis. A study at the Pennsylvania College of Podiatric Medicine found a special cream of aloe, vitamin C, and other ingredients reduced arthritis inflammation.

Experts say fresh aloe gel is much more potent than gel that has been stored and added to commercial preparations. So the best (and maybe the easiest) way to put this healing herb to work for you is to keep a pot of aloe on a sunny windowsill.

When you need it, break off a leaf, squeeze

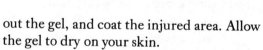

out the gel, and coat the injured area. Allow the gel to dry on your skin.

How often should you apply it? Once a day is probably enough. Researchers who studied the effects of aloe vera preparations on rheumatoid arthritis and burns in experimental animals got great results from applying the gel once each day over a period of weeks. The burn wounds were also covered with a bandage that was changed every day.

Go easy the first time you use it—some people can get a mild skin irritation. If you find that you are sensitive to aloe, you can continue to enjoy it as an attractive house plant—just don't apply it to your skin.

CASCARA SAGRADA

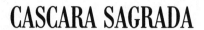

Spanish explorers on the Pacific Coast of North America must have been mightily relieved when they learned about the laxative properties of a certain kind of tree bark. They called it *cascara sagrada*—sacred bark. Still popular to this day, extracts of this herb have been used in various commercial laxative preparations, some of them available by prescription only.

The principal suppliers of cascara sagrada are concentrated in Oregon, Washington, and southern British Columbia. Cascara sagrada is derived by stripping the bark from the *Rhamnus purshianus* tree in the spring and summer, before the rainy season sets in, and leaving it to dry in the sun for at least a year. The inner surface is not exposed to the sun, which allows the herb to retain its yellow color.

The cured bark is then steeped in a tea or added to other ingredients. (On its own, cascara sagrada is bitter-tasting.) Herb experts say cascara sagrada can correct even the habitual constipation caused by misuse of other laxatives. If you want to try it, Nature's Remedy is one commercial product that contains cascara sagrada.

Humans are not the only ones to benefit from the sure action of this herb. Veterinarians often prescribe products containing cascara sagrada, especially for constipated dogs.

Some herbalists believe that cascara sagrada can restore normal tone to the colon. It was used in folk medicine in small amounts to treat gallstones and by nineteenth-century American doctors to treat liver ailments, according to Daniel B. Mowrey, Ph.D., author of *The Scientific Validation of Herbal Medicine*.

No matter what you use it for, just be aware that the herb is potent stuff when it's fresh. You are better off buying the herb than harvesting your own, unless you like long-term projects. Herbalists recommend aging fresh bark for at least a year before using it.

247

HERBS

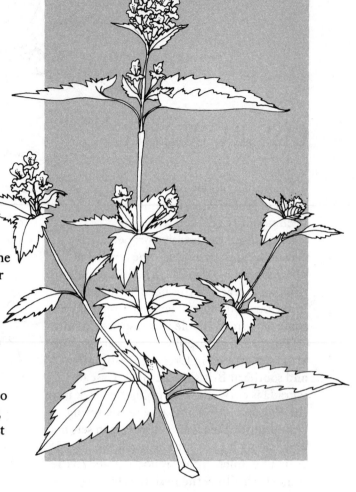

CATNIP

Herbalists say you're likely to find relaxation in a soothing, minty-tasting cup of catnip tea. But while you're unwinding, your cat will be anything but relaxed. The smell can drive cats wild. A component of the volatile oil inside the plant is responsible for both effects. That component—cis-trans-nepetalactone—has a chemical makeup very similar to sedatives in the herb valerian. (Obviously, it affects your brain and your cat's very differently.)

"There just may be some basis in fact for the cup of hot catnip tea taken at bedtime to get a good night's sleep," notes Varro Tyler, Ph.D., Purdue University pharmacognosist and author of *The New Honest Herbal.*

To make this pleasant-tasting tea for yourself, simply pour boiling water over dried catnip and let it steep. You may want to cover the tea as it steeps because the flavorful oil in catnip is volatile. This beverage is especially nice if you have a sore throat in need of soothing. Herbalists claim that it will also help loosen phlegm if you have a cold. Some research shows that catnip has antibiotic properties, too.

There are some folks who even call catnip "Nature's Alka-Seltzer"—a natural antacid and stomach soother—although that accolade fits the entire mint family of plants, of which catnip is a member.

Drink a cup of catnip tea before meals to stimulate your appetite. Take it after dinner to rev up your digestion.

Through the years, catnip has been used to treat just about everything from colds to cancer. Native Americans used it to ease childhood colic. In some cultures, people chew the leaves to ease the pain of toothaches.

Others have used the whole plant to make a poultice. The poultice was then applied to relieve corns and reduce swelling.

But cats love catnip even more than people do. It isn't the taste of the herb but the smell that drives them wild. They love to roll in catnip, crushing the leaves so they release more of their fragrance.

248

CAYENNE

As a seasoning, cayenne is hot stuff. As a medicinal herb, it may be even hotter. You know cayenne as the ground red powder you use to pep up your chili, or as the long red pepper from which the powder is made. It's this pepper that puts the fire in Tabasco and Louisiana Hot Sauce.

But right after your taste buds register their three-alarm fire, components of this herb are blazing through your bloodstream. Animal studies suggest it may be helping to clear away cholesterol and stimulate circulation.

Animal studies in India found that cayenne helps avert a rise in dietary cholesterol when eaten along with food that contains cholesterol. That's enough to make you want to order your chili extra hot the next time you sit down to a Mexican meal of cheese enchiladas garnished with sour cream.

Other studies suggest that cayenne speeds the rate at which the body sweats off waste products. Because cayenne stimulates circulation, adding a tiny amount of it to other herbs dramatically increases the efficiency of those herbs, says Daniel B. Mowrey, Ph.D., author of *The Scientific Validation of Herbal Medicine*.

If you avoid using cayenne because you're afraid its fiery heat might do damage, you may want to reconsider. A study using miniature cameras suggests that eating meals spiced with cayenne doesn't damage internal tissue. However, those with duodenal ulcers or chronic bowel diseases should probably avoid cayenne just to be extra safe.

Herbalists have long used cayenne externally, as a rub and poultice to warm chilled skin and relieve painful joints. Although cayenne can cause an intense burning sensation when applied to the skin, it seldom results in blisters. Herbalists claim that this irritation is what stimulates blood flow to the area, which is useful when you have congestion or painful swelling from arthritis.

249

HERBS

CHAMOMILE

Chamomile is loved the world over. Here in America, it ranks among the five top-selling herbs. And no wonder—it's pretty as a flower, sweet as a tea, and tradition has it that the herb is packed with medicinal benefits.

There are two major kinds of chamomile—German and Roman. They're actually fairly similar in the way they work. The one big difference is that German chamomile may help put you to sleep, while its Roman cousin may mildly stimulate your digestion, notes Michael A. Weiner, Ph.D., author of *Weiner's Herbal: The Guide to Herb Medicine.*

The medicinal power of this useful herb comes from the volatile oils in the flowers.

Remember when you prepare chamomile at home that boiling destroys the oil, so boil water separately and then pour it over the flowers to steep. Use ½ ounce of flowers to a pint of water to make an infusion, tea, or even a hair rinse that creates blond highlights.

Roman chamomile is best known for its ability to help relieve an overly acid stomach, according to Dr. Weiner. He adds that the herb is useful for treating colic, gas, and gout.

The oil of the German chamomile flower is valued for its ability to relieve muscle spasms, stimulate digestion, and guard against ulcers, notes Dr. Weiner. Laboratory studies suggest that this oil can even relax the muscles of the intestine, making chamomile useful for treating mildly upset stomachs or cramps, he says.

Additionally, chamomile may help cut down on the inflammation that accompanies arthritis. Researchers who studied arthritis in experimental animals verified its anti-inflammatory effect.

If you have allergies to ragweed pollens, chamomile isn't risk-free. Some individuals have developed skin rashes or more serious allergic reactions.

ECHINACEA

This plant's purple cone of flowers is pretty enough, but there's more to echinacea than meets the eye. The healing properties of this American plant lie hidden underground—in the root. The roots contain properties that boost immunity and speed wound healing, according to scientists who have studied the herb.

Used topically, echinacea is an anesthetic, anti-inflammatory, and antiseptic, notes Daniel B. Mowrey, Ph.D., author of *The Scientific Validation of Herbal Medicine.* In laboratory studies, an ointment made from echinacea and vitamin E even helps put an end to recurrent vaginal yeast.

And echinacea has a reputation as a whiz when it comes to wounds. This action may be due to a substance in the herb—caffeic acid glycoside—that is known to aid wound healing, scientists say.

Taken internally, echinacea stimulates the immune system, helping to produce and transmit infection-fighting cells. A sore throat, a common cold, or an overall ill feeling may all be sent into quick retreat by echinacea, says Varro Tyler, Ph.D., Purdue University pharmacognosist and author of *The New Honest Herbal.* The herb may eventually prove useful in the fight against cancer. U.S. Department of Agriculture researchers have discovered that a constituent of echinacea has the ability to inhibit tumors, says Dr. Mowrey.

If you'd like to try echinacea, you'll find it available commercially in a liquid extract, tablets, and tea. You can also make a decoction or infusion from the fresh root. If you are using it to strengthen your immune system, herbalists advise that you take it periodically—a few weeks on, a few weeks off. Continuous use may actually stress certain components of your immune system, advises Dr. Mowrey.

Echinacea doesn't appear to be toxic in large doses. Be warned, however, that heavy use has been shown to induce temporary infertility in men.

EUCALYPTUS

The bracing scent of eucalyptus may be a breath of fresh air for anyone suffering from respiratory ills. Herbalists say inhaling steam laced with eucalyptus oil provides welcome relief from the annoying symptoms of colds, flu, bronchitis, laryngitis, rheumatism, and similar problems.

If you've ever tried to fight a cold with one of the various nasal inhalers available at your drugstore, chances are that you've already experienced the healing vapors of eucalyptus. Many of these products contain eucalyptus, as do a number of lozenges, liquid medicines, and rubs, all of them formulated to help clear disturbing deposits of mucus from your nose, throat, and lungs.

The magic ingredient behind this herb's medicinal properties is a potent substance called cineole oil, or eucalyptol, which is contained in large quantities in the fresh leaves of the eucalyptus tree. Colorless or pale yellow, aromatic eucalyptus oil has a somewhat camphorlike odor and a pungent, spicy cool taste.

The oil is often used as an antiseptic and to induce sweating, notes Varro Tyler, Ph.D., Purdue University pharmacognosist and author of *The New Honest Herbal*. It is also used as an ingredient in commercial cold-relief products such as Vicks VapoRub.

Eucalyptus contains antibiotic properties, too. Because of its germ-fighting abilities, it's a popular choice among herbalists for treating skin problems such as abscesses. The leaves can be applied to the skin in a poultice. You can also apply a diluted form of the oil directly as an antiseptic, herbalists say. To make your own, add up to 2 teaspoons of eucalyptus oil to a pint of vegetable oil, water, or rubbing alcohol.

Herbalists say that an infusion of eucalyptus may be helpful for respiratory problems. They recommend either drinking the infusion or simply adding it to a vaporizer. To make an infusion, steep a handful of fresh or dried leaves in a quart of boiling water for 20 minutes.

FENNEL

If you like licorice, you'll love fennel, a Mediterranean herb with a subtle licorice flavor. Its cool, refreshing taste combined with its powers as a digestive aid make fennel just the right food to serve at the finale of a heavy meal. Traditional Italian-American families still observe the ancient custom of closing a meal with crunchy, celerylike stalks of fennel.

While the stalks are delicious, the dried, ripe fruits are the portion of the plant most commonly used in healing. The fruits are so tiny, they're commonly referred to as seeds. These "seeds" contain a concentrated amount of a powerful oil that has been shown to relieve muscle spasms in laboratory animals. This antispasmodic property is probably what makes fennel such an effective remedy for flatulence, say herbal experts.

Fennel was traditionally used as a dieter's herb, too. People in medieval times chewed the seeds to suppress their appetite. Scientists have found that fennel doesn't directly affect weight. However, its stomach-soothing properties can be a big help when the body is adjusting to dietary changes. Fennel seed helps maintain the tone of the stomach muscles and fight infection in the gastrointestinal tract, according to herbalist Daniel B. Mowrey, Ph.D., author of *The Scientific Validation of Herbal Medicine.* Perhaps that's why you'll find fennel in weight-loss products.

Traditional herbalists have long used tea made from fennel to prevent infant colic. This use of the herb now has some support from scientific studies done in Europe.

The best way to prepare fennel beverages is as a tea or decoction made from the dried seeds that are at least one year old, according to Michael A. Weiner, Ph.D., author of *Weiner's Herbal: The Guide to Herb Medicine.* Seeds are readily available on the spice shelf in supermarkets. Add ½ ounce of the seeds to a pint of water and boil slowly, covered, for a half hour. Keep the cover on and let the brew cool. Drink the decoction cold, 1 teaspoon at a time, up to 2 cups a day.

253

HERBS

GARLIC

Once upon a time, people wore garlic as an amulet against evil. Demons, witches, and vampires were apparently no match for the "stinking rose." These days, garlic is respected by some scientists for a very different sort of "magic"—its possible protective power against some types of disease. Modern research shows that garlic may help lower blood pressure and cholesterol levels, combat infection, and even stimulate the immune system. Not bad for a little brown bulb.

The first benefit you get when you chew on a clove of garlic is nutrition. Garlic contains thiamine and trace minerals such as calcium, magnesium, iron, potassium, phosphorus, and zinc.

The next benefit you'll get is a natural and potent anti-infection agent. Whole garlic bulbs contain an odorless substance called alliin which, when ground or chewed, turns into allicin. This latter substance carries the strong odor most of us associate with garlic, as well as the healing powers of the herb. Allicin inhibits or totally destroys many types of bacteria and fungi, including the microorganisms most likely to cause vaginal yeast infections, says Daniel B. Mowrey, Ph.D., author of *The Scientific Validation of Herbal Medicine.* Two studies found that garlic even offers protection against the influenza virus.

It should come as little surprise that garlic can also *stimulate* your immune system. In one study, people who ate two to three heads of garlic a day for three weeks showed significantly more activity in special white blood cells that fight tumors. When these white blood cells were placed in a laboratory dish with cancerous cells, the garlic-eaters' cells knocked off more than twice as many tumor cells as white blood cells taken from people who did not eat garlic.

When using garlic for medicinal purposes, remember that its odiferous constituents are its most active parts. Eat it fresh or freeze-dried for best results.

254

GINGER

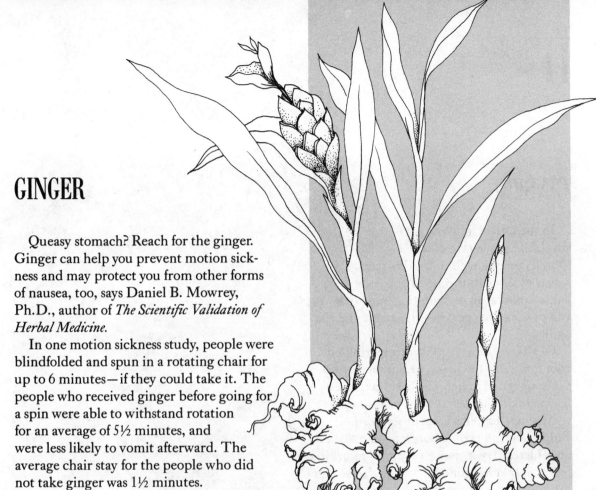

Queasy stomach? Reach for the ginger. Ginger can help you prevent motion sickness and may protect you from other forms of nausea, too, says Daniel B. Mowrey, Ph.D., author of *The Scientific Validation of Herbal Medicine*.

In one motion sickness study, people were blindfolded and spun in a rotating chair for up to 6 minutes—if they could take it. The people who received ginger before going for a spin were able to withstand rotation for an average of 5½ minutes, and were less likely to vomit afterward. The average chair stay for the people who did not take ginger was 1½ minutes.

If you'd like to see how well ginger works for you, take two to four capsules just before you travel, recommends Dr. Mowrey. Then take two more each hour or so. If your stomach begins to feel even mildly upset, take the ginger even if the hour is not up yet. You may find you need less and less as you get used to the sensations of travel.

Ginger also can aid your digestion by stimulating salivation and gastric secretions, reducing gas, and inhibiting muscle spasms, according to Hiroshi Hikino of the Pharmaceutical Institute of Tohoku University in Japan. There is even some evidence that it can prevent the rise in blood cholesterol levels that accompanies cholesterol-rich meals, notes Dr. Mowrey.

Ginger is stimulating to the heart, helping to regulate its function. Studies show a component of ginger has a balancing effect, lowering high blood pressure and raising low blood pressure, according to Hikino, coauthor of *Economic and Medicinal Plant Research*.

To take advantage of ginger's mild stimulant properties, make a tea by pouring a pint of boiling water over an ounce of grated root and letting it steep for up to 20 minutes, suggests Michael A. Weiner, Ph.D., author of *Weiner's Herbal: The Guide to Herb Medicine*. You'll find the tea invigorating on a cold winter day and useful when you're trying to sweat out a cold, he notes.

255

GINSENG

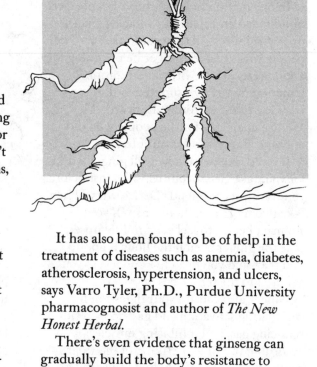

In the Orient, ginseng is so prized it has sometimes cost *more* than its weight in gold. Used to treat scores of ailments through the ages, it is valued most as an invigorating tonic that can preserve physical health and mental agility.

Of all the claims made for this wrinkled root, probably the most curious one is this: Ginseng is said to help the brain retrieve a learned skill that hasn't been practiced for some time. The effect was observed in Bulgarian studies on laboratory animals and on athletes. Try it yourself if you're returning to a skill that has gone rusty from disuse. For example, if you're a winter skier who doesn't get much chance to practice between seasons, you may want to see for yourself if ginseng root really can improve your performance that first day back on the slopes.

Ginseng's effect on the brain has been noted in many studies. Some studies suggest that it can improve memory and learning and increase mental alertness in the aged. It has also been shown to increase concentration and hand coordination.

Ginseng seems to also exert a protective effect on the body's adrenocortical system—the system that orchestrates the chemistry of stress. It acts as a kind of shock absorber, allowing the body to bounce back more quickly than it might without the ginseng, notes Daniel B. Mowrey, Ph.D., author of *The Scientific Validation of Herbal Medicine.*

It has also been found to be of help in the treatment of diseases such as anemia, diabetes, atherosclerosis, hypertension, and ulcers, says Varro Tyler, Ph.D., Purdue University pharmacognosist and author of *The New Honest Herbal.*

There's even evidence that ginseng can gradually build the body's resistance to fatigue, notes Dr. Mowrey.

Some athletes like Siberian ginseng for its ability to increase endurance, a claim that is backed up by studies on animals and Russian telegraph operators. In Russia, ginseng is part of the Olympic training diet.

HOPS

Late, late at night, you lie awake, restless, certain the sandman has abandoned you forever. You're too wound up to sleep, but not too exhausted to worry about how you'll feel the next day with the sleep deficit you're racking up.

Maybe hops can help.

Hops are the conelike fruits that have been used in brewing beer for thousands of years. They contain a form of alcohol that contributes to the sedative powers of this herb.

Fresh hops contain little of this alcohol. But allow hops to dry at room temperature, and the concentration of this active ingredient increases, reaching its peak in about two years. Hops tea, freshly prepared from the dried herb, has been shown to have a significant and active component of this alcohol.

According to herbalists, you can try hops as a sleep aid in one of two ways: imbibe it or lie on it.

An herb pillow, stuffed solely with hops, is an age-old remedy for insomnia. Probably the most famous head to lie on a hops pillow was that of King George III. To make a pillow for yourself, pack the herbs into a natural fiber casing. Choose a slightly porous material, so the scent can waft through.

The other way to use hops to help induce sleep is to brew an infusion. Steep ½ ounce of the dried fruit in a pint of boiling water. The traditional dose is 4 ounces of the infusion.

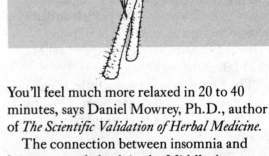

You'll feel much more relaxed in 20 to 40 minutes, says Daniel Mowrey, Ph.D., author of *The Scientific Validation of Herbal Medicine*.

The connection between insomnia and hops was made back in the Middle Ages, when it was observed that laborers who toiled in fields of hops tired very easily. Apparently this was due to the accidental transfer of the hops' resin from the laborers' hands to their mouths.

Be cautious about picking or handling fresh hops if you are prone to allergies. As many as 1 out of 30 workers picking hops may suffer dermatitis on their hands, face, and legs.

257

HORSERADISH

Mention the word horseradish and most people think of roast beef and delicatessen fare. Yet this pungent herb was popular as a healing agent long before it caught on at the dinner table.

Horseradish is a member of the mustard family. The most useful part of this flowering plant is its tapered white root. The chief active ingredient in the root is a substance most commonly known as mustard oil.

Herbalists use the root externally by grating or chopping it and mixing it with water to form a paste. The paste is added to a cloth compress to make a topical pain reliever for neuralgia, stiffness, and aches at the back of the neck.

The compress may sting a little. Keep it on until you feel it begin to burn. The heat will bring blood to the area and may hasten healing.

Herbalists say that horseradish has healing properties when taken internally. A syrup made of grated horseradish, honey, and water is one of the standard remedies for hoarseness. Just be careful not to overdo it. In sensitive individuals, too much can cause dizziness, pharmacology experts say.

Herbalists also have long maintained that horseradish is a potent diuretic—one of the most effective herbs for treating water retention. It has a history as a treatment for kidney conditions that cause the body to retain lots of water. In some traditional recipes, the horseradish is mixed with bruised mustard seed and water to further enhance its power as a diuretic.

There are plenty of other reasons to enjoy horseradish. The root contains impressive amounts of vitamin C. Roots kept in cool storage retain that vitamin C.

Perhaps one of the most enjoyable ways to use horseradish is to slather some on your roast beef sandwich or serve it as an accompaniment to fish. If you prefer a milder condiment, add some vinegar.

PARSLEY

Bet you thought parsley was just a garnish—something restaurant chefs use to add a touch of color to that fish entree.

Of course, you could leave the parsley on the plate as you usually do. But you'd be missing out on potassium, vitamin A, and more vitamin C ounce for ounce than an orange. The leaves of this flowering and fruit-bearing plant contain up to 25 percent protein. It is also rich in calcium and iron.

You can also count on the high chlorophyll content of parsley to help freshen your breath, so it won't go around announcing what you had for dinner. "Fish-breath" never has been, and never will be, a compliment. You've probably never heard anyone called "parsley-breath," though, have you?

Similarly, parsley can sweeten your bath. To help you relax and feel superclean, add an infusion when you fill up the tub. Or look for toiletries that contain parsley extracts.

As a medicinal herb, parsley functions primarily as a diuretic to promote urination. It contains some laxative properties, as well. Men may find that a cup of parsley tea, made from the roots and leaves of some fresh parsley, may make urination less painful if the prostate gland is enlarged, according to Daniel B. Mowrey, Ph.D., author of *The Scientific Validation of Herbal Medicine*. Of course, this is a condition that should be treated by a doctor.

Fresh parsley is also said to help with menstrual problems, notes Dr. Mowrey. Try adding parsley to your meals to alleviate discomfort on those problem days.

There is some evidence to suggest that parsley is also a mild antibiotic, notes Dr. Mowrey. Couple that with its vitamin C content, and it makes sense to toss the green leaves and root into the chicken soup you're brewing for that special someone with a cold.

Pregnant women should be extra careful to limit their intake and stay away from parsley oil altogether.

259

HERBS

PEPPERMINT

That anchovy and sausage pizza, side order of fries, and double-chocolate milk shake were a hit with your taste buds. But now your poor digestive system just can't stomach the combination. Is there anything you can do besides sit there and clutch your innards?

Moments like these were made for peppermint tea. At least, that's what herbalists would recommend, and according to researchers, they may be right.

Peppermint is probably the best-known natural remedy for stomach complaints, says Daniel B. Mowrey, Ph.D., author of *The Scientific Validation of Herbal Medicine*. People have relied on it since the hybrid plant first appeared late in the seventeenth century.

Peppermint has been shown to relieve indigestion, colic, and gas. It can also help an overacid stomach and alleviate nausea, says Dr. Mowrey.

The herb's digestive action is due primarily to the powerful essential oils contained in its leaves and flowering tops. Peppermint oil contains components that stimulate the flow of digestive juices and promote better digestion overall, says Varro Tyler, Ph.D., Purdue University pharmacognosist and author of *The New Honest Herbal*.

The oil in peppermint can even awaken your appetite. At first it relaxes the muscular activity responsible for hunger pangs. But once that muscular activity resumes, it is stronger than ever.

If that weren't enough, peppermint oil may help you fight disease. Studies show that it can inhibit the action of 30 different "bugs," including the ones responsible for Asian flu, sinusitis, cold sores, and mumps, notes Dr. Mowrey.

Peppermint tea is considered nontoxic, although some people may find themselves allergic to it. The tea should not be given to young children, according to Dr. Tyler. And make sure you never take peppermint oil straight. As little as 0.2 ounce can cause drowsiness and vomiting.

PSYLLIUM

It seems you just can't beat psyllium seed for fiber. Doctors say that taking some powdered seed with water can relieve constipation, help you stick to your diet by making you feel full, and may help keep your cholesterol count in the healthy zone.

Americans have relied upon this herb as a laxative since the 1930s. Today, psyllium seed is available in a number of commercial preparations, such as Metamucil, and in some high-fiber cereals.

The seeds work their magic by means of their unique ability to swell far beyond their original size. One gram of seed, placed in water, will swell 8 to 14 times in volume. It's actually the husks that absorb the water. They retain this nifty property even when they're ground up.

Inside the body, the soaked seeds soothe the mucous membranes as they expand, transforming themselves into a bulk laxative, according to David G. Spoerke, Jr., author of *Herbal Medications*. This soothing effect on the entire gastrointestinal system appears to lead to smoother movement of food substances along surfaces that might be inflamed.

Remember, however, that you have to take psyllium with plenty of water to get the full benefit. An 8-ounce glass of water per teaspoon of the powdered herb is just about right.

In one Italian study, dieters who took psyllium seeds in water before meals twice a day lost more weight than those who simply followed the diet.

Psyllium does more than help you lose weight, however. Researchers in the Soviet Union and Italy found that psyllium, taken before meals, helps to decrease the bad kind of cholesterol while proportionately raising the good kind. Scientists say that it's possible that the cholesterol status changed because the individuals studied ate less fatty foods.

Generally speaking, psyllium is very safe. If you have a bowel obstruction or disease, however, you need to ask your doctor before you use it.

ROSE

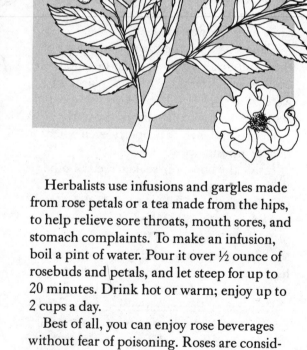

Roses are always therapeutic. Just think back to the last time you received some.

How did you feel?

Great, right?

Case closed.

All kidding aside, roses have been used medicinally for centuries. Fresh rose hips, the fruit of the plant, are highly nutritious. Ounce for ounce, rose hips contain more vitamin C than oranges. They also boast an ample supply of vitamin A, which has been found to help boost immunity.

Rose hips also contain organic acids and pectin, which make them a mild laxative and diuretic, helping to treat water retention, herbalists say.

Be aware that you may not get all these benefits from the rose hips you buy dried or in tea blends. The actual vitamin content varies depending upon which type of rose plant is used, the climate and soil in which it was grown, where and how it was harvested, and how it was dried.

You're probably better off harvesting your own hips and buds from roses grown at home without pesticides.

You can use the rose hips to make a vitamin-rich tea, an infusion, or a soup base.

You might want to collect the petals too. Rose petals are valuable for their ability to shrink inflamed mucous membranes, herbalists say.

Herbalists use infusions and gargles made from rose petals or a tea made from the hips, to help relieve sore throats, mouth sores, and stomach complaints. To make an infusion, boil a pint of water. Pour it over ½ ounce of rosebuds and petals, and let steep for up to 20 minutes. Drink hot or warm; enjoy up to 2 cups a day.

Best of all, you can enjoy rose beverages without fear of poisoning. Roses are considered safe.

If you go overboard, however, and consume too many rose hips or petals, you could end up with diarrhea.

262

ROSEMARY

You're probably familiar with rosemary's many talents as a seasoning. But did you know it contains painkillers?

Even the aromatic oil that gives rosemary its characteristic woodsy smell is said to be beneficial to nerves. It is credited with the ability to calm irritated nerves and reduce anxiety, according to Daniel B. Mowrey, Ph.D., author of *The Scientific Validation of Herbal Medicine*.

If you want to give it a try, there are plenty of ways to enjoy this herb. Indulge yourself in fresh, hot-from-the-oven rosemary herb bread and let the carbohydrates contribute their calming influence, too. Or toss a handful of fresh rosemary on your salad.

As a medicinal herb, rosemary has been used for everything from soothing headaches to treating malaria. But few of those claims have been seriously tested.

However, Italian researchers have found it to contain mild painkillers. And the Chinese have known about the herb's painkillers for a long time—they use rosemary to treat headaches and stomach pain.

Other studies show that rosemary's essential oil contains an antibacterial agent and a chemical (rosmaricine) that stimulates the smooth muscles of the body, notes Dr. Mowrey.

One safe and easy way to use rosemary as a therapeutic aid is to add a few drops of rosemary essential oil to your morning bath.

Don't take a rosemary bath at night, however, or you may feel too alert.

You can also add 6 drops of the essential oil to 2 ounces of a light oil such as almond oil to create an invigorating massage oil. Rosemary essential oil is readily available in many health food stores.

Rosemary is fine to eat as a spice, but if you want to use the oil, use it externally only. There are no documented cases of serious poisoning with rosemary, but the oil is classified as an irritant. In large quantities, rosemary oil is known to irritate the stomach, intestines, and kidneys.

SAGE

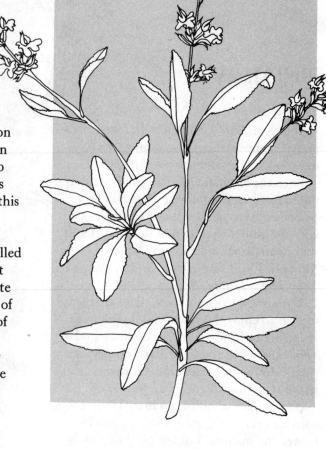

Perspiring heavily? If you sip an infusion of sage leaves, you may experience relief in about 2 hours, according to scientists who have studied this flowering herb. (There's even a German drug made from sage for this very purpose.)

Just be sure that you use sage only occasionally. Sage contains a potent oil called thujone. There is evidence to suggest that long-term intake of thujone can contribute to physical deterioration. Large amounts of thujone can induce convulsions and loss of consciousness.

Cooking with sage apparently is a safer alternative. The heat burns off most of the thujone.

You're also safe using sage preparations externally or as a gargle.

Studies have shown that sage contains chemicals that are astringent. Applied externally, it stimulates blood flow to the area where it's used, says Varro Tyler, Ph.D., Purdue University pharmacognosist and author of *The New Honest Herbal.* These qualities contribute to the value of a sage infusion as a gargle for tonsillitis, bleeding gums, and other inflammatory conditions of the mouth and throat.

The Native Americans also knew how to use sage externally. Infusions were used for baths, rubdowns, and topical applications to sores. They used fresh sage to keep their teeth clean.

Other cultures have used sage decoctions to help relieve toothaches.

Lotions made from sage have been used as hair rinses and scalp tonics, in the hope they'd stimulate hair growth. There's no proof these lotions work, however.

You can use sage oil with good results as part of therapeutic massage. Aromatherapists use sage oil to counter fatigue, nervousness, bronchitis, and menstrual difficulties.

If you'd like to try therapeutic massage, add 6 drops of the essential oil to 2 ounces of a lighter oil such as almond oil. Don't apply the essential oil directly to the skin.

THYME

Thyme is a seasoning. It seems though, that the spice is also a seasoned and versatile healer. Herbal experts maintain that thyme may soothe your tummy, relieve toothache, and treat menstrual problems.

Thyme is also nutritious. Ounce for ounce, it contains 100 times as much chromium and 400 times as much manganese as meat.

Every part of the thyme plant is useful as a medicinal herb, although the leaves and flowers are much more important than the stems.

There are several ways to use the entire herb. If you want to treat indigestion, make an infusion by adding ½ ounce of thyme to a pint of boiling water, says Michael A. Weiner, Ph.D., author of *Weiner's Herbal: The Guide to Herb Medicine*. Steep it for 15 to 20 minutes. Enjoy it warm or cool. Drink up to 2 cups a day.

Thymol, the essential oil in thyme, has been found to help relax the smooth muscles of the stomach and to release gas from the stomach, notes Dr. Weiner.

A tea made of 1 teaspoon of thyme leaves steeped in 1 cup of boiling water may be useful as a bronchodilator. Human and animal studies have shown that thyme acts as an expectorant and bronchodilator and as an antiseptic and helps clear mucus from the respiratory system, notes Dr. Weiner.

You can also try the tea to calm a cough, herbalists say. Thyme is used in a number of commercial cough and bronchitis medications.

You can also make a poultice by mashing the leaves into a paste and applying it to the skin. Be aware, however, that thyme can irritate sensitive skin. Test a small area first.

Historically, thyme poultices have been used for treating inflammation, sores, burns, eczema, and psoriasis.

Do not take thyme oil internally. It can cause dizziness, nausea, vomiting, and muscle weakness.

VALERIAN

You've heard of Valium. It's a tranquilizer available by prescription only. But chances are you've never heard of valerian, a flowering plant that herbalists claim is, in some respects, the better tranquilizer by far. It's better because clinical studies show that properly prepared valerian has fewer side effects than synthetic tranquilizers. Studies also show that valerian won't aggravate the depressant action of alcohol the way synthetic tranquilizers do, according to Varro Tyler, Ph.D., Purdue University pharmacognosist and author of *The New Honest Herbal.*

The root is the medicinally useful part of the plant. Despite its characteristic, disagreeable odor, valerian root is a valued and often-studied herb. It has been used to soothe jangled nerves and conquer sleeplessness for more than a thousand years.

Recent studies have confirmed what ancient herbalists suspected. In one study, men who drank a glass of water containing an extract of valerian root showed the recognizable changes in brain wave activity that occur after taking tranquilizers.

There is some talk that valerian is more of an "equalizer" than a sedative. Certain studies suggest it soothes the agitated but stimulates people suffering from fatigue.

You can experience the calming effect of valerian at home. Use a fresh valerian root (if you can find it); the fresher the better. (Old,

improperly stored valerian root won't do much for you because certain of the active ingredients evaporate as the root dries.)

Make an infusion using 1 teaspoon of grated root in 1 pint of water. The resulting brew will taste bitter. Take no more than a cup in any single day.

If you have trouble sleeping, try drinking your allotted cup just before bedtime. Valerian has been found useful as a treatment for insomnia, especially when anxiety, exhaustion, or headaches are at fault, according to Daniel B. Mowrey, Ph.D., author of *The Scientific Validation of Herbal Medicine.*

WITCH HAZEL

Forget for a moment about the kind of witch hazel you can buy bottled at your local pharmacy or supermarket. Let's focus instead on its source, a small, hardy, winter-blooming tree that grows best in moist woods and along rocky streams. You won't have any problem identifying the tree because it will be ablaze with threadlike yellow flowers long after autumn winds have bared the neighboring trees.

The medicinal part of this tree is found in its leaves, bark, and twigs. These—and the dried herb derived from them—contain tannic acid. Herbalists think the tannic acid gives unadulterated witch hazel its ability to affect the veins of the body and help stem bleeding.

Witch hazel water can be used as a topical skin-soother; its refreshing scent will offer a quick pick-me-up when your spirits are flagging. But you'll find more uses for the ground-up leaves and/or bark.

Because of witch hazel's ability to affect the veins, you may find a witch hazel poultice helpful for stopping a nosebleed or bleeding from cuts and scratches, according to Daniel B. Mowrey, Ph.D., author of *The Scientific Validation of Herbal Medicine.*

To soothe inflammation, add 1 teaspoon of the granulated leaves and/or bark to a cup of boiling water, according to Michael A. Weiner, Ph.D., author of *Weiner's Herbal: The Guide to Herb Medicine.* Then let the liquid cool and apply to the problem area. You can also moisten a compress with this witch hazel recipe and use on insect bites, minor skin irritations, bruises, and sprains. Headaches and inflamed eyes may also benefit from a witch hazel compress, herbalists say.

To treat vaginal yeast infection, try adding an infusion from the leaves to a sitz bath, says Dr. Mowrey.

You can also mix a liquid extract of witch hazel with petroleum jelly and apply it directly to hemorrhoids. In fact, you'll find witch hazel in several commercial hemorrhoid preparations, notes Dr. Mowrey.

HICCUPS

The all-time "King of the Hiccups" title has to go to farmer Charles Osborne of Iowa, father of eight.

His hiccups started in 1922 as he was slaughtering a hog and have persisted all these years, even through a second marriage. According to the record books, Osborne has hiccuped more than 430 million times.

If you're like most people, even a few *minutes* of hiccuping are unbearable. Fortunately for most of us, episodes don't last long.

A hiccup is an involuntary contraction of the diaphragm, the dome-shaped muscle that rests beneath your lungs. If you irritate the nerves that govern the movement of this muscle, you're likely to bring on hiccups.

Unfortunately, it's all too easy to irritate these nerves—everything from food to stress can set them off.

Usually the diaphragm calms down fairly soon on its own, and hiccups disappear. (Hiccups that persist for more than a day or two should be reported to your doctor.)

What do you do in the meantime? Modern medicine has yet to come up with a definitive cure. The remedies that do exist are from Grandma's textbook.

"They're free, not dangerous, and sometimes work," says Kansas City physician John Renner, M.D. He suggests "taking a few sips of water, a few sips of pineapple juice, or a pinch of sugar."

Three Homey Ways to (Maybe) Halt the Hic

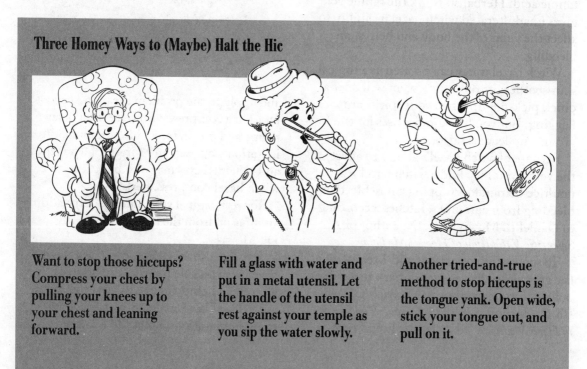

Want to stop those hiccups? Compress your chest by pulling your knees up to your chest and leaning forward.

Fill a glass with water and put in a metal utensil. Let the handle of the utensil rest against your temple as you sip the water slowly.

Another tried-and-true method to stop hiccups is the tongue yank. Open wide, stick your tongue out, and pull on it.

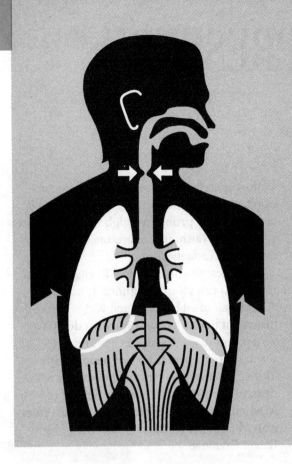

How a Hiccup Hics

Hic-CUP! That sound is your nerves' way of saying "I'm irritated."

The nerves responsible for producing the annoying reflex extend in a network that includes the cervical nerves in your neck and those deep down in your abdomen.

Normally, as your lungs take in air, your diaphragm functions smoothly, allowing the column of air to pass unimpeded through the voice box.

But when your diaphragm spazzes out, the vocal cords and voice box snap shut. That column of air, now denied entrance to the voice box, is what causes the telltale noise.

You can also try rubbing a cotton swab on the roof of your mouth where the palate changes from hard to soft. This technique can short-circuit the nerve that's causing the diaphragm to spasm.

Or, for something more exotic, you can soak a lemon wedge in bitters and suck on it, rind and all. Just remember to brace yourself for a superpucker.

"It takes your breath away," says Jay Herman, M.D., medical director of the Penn-Jersey region of the American Red Cross. "Can you imagine biting into a lemon you've made even more bitter?"

It was Dr. Herman who helped popularize this lemon-and-bitters cure for hiccups, when he sent a tongue-in-cheek letter to the *New England Journal of Medicine*. He says he was having dinner with his bartender friend

David Nolan, when Nolan asked the restaurant bartender for the standard hiccups cure. Dr. Herman was intrigued that the bartender knew exactly what Nolan meant.

"It's part of the lore bartenders hand down. I was impressed with it because it works," says Dr. Herman. "I'm talking about temporary cases, of course." He says he tried it on 20 friends, and it worked 19 out of 20 times.

Why does it work? Dr. Herman's not sure, but he suspects that the concoction creates "noxious stimuli" that compete with the nerve impulses causing the diaphragm spasm.

Will any brand of bitters work? "Probably," says Dr. Herman. "But I haven't tried it yet with Grenadine."

Deborah Grandinetti

269

HIGH BLOOD PRESSURE

If Stephen King ever runs out of ideas for horror thrillers, we have one for him. It's a story about a killer that quietly stalks its victims, often for years, then strikes without warning. Its name is high blood pressure.

This story does not have to climax in bone-chilling horror, however. There's even a good chance for a happy ending. For while it's true that high blood pressure is nasty, the heroes of this tale, the high blood pressure police, are mighty resourceful. They have an arsenal of weapons that can stop the killer, including weight control, dietary modifications, exercise, medications, and more.

Profile of a Killer

Blood pressure refers to the amount of force with which your blood pushes against the artery walls. Without any pressure, your blood would just sit around in your blood vessels, like water in a turned-off hose. With high blood pressure, also known as hypertension, your blood is being pushed too hard against the arteries.

If you twisted shut the nozzle on a hose while the faucet at the other end was still turned on, the hose would start to bulge. If it were too weak, it might pop. Similarly, high blood pressure, if unchecked, can lead to serious damage in your body.

More than 60 million Americans, or about a quarter of the population, have high blood pressure. Even though the cause of most of these cases isn't known, the disease is easily detected and usually controllable.

Unfortunately, many people who have it don't even know it. That's because, until it causes serious problems, high blood pressure can't be felt (although sometimes it causes morning headaches).

Just because you can't feel it, that doesn't mean you can afford to ignore it, however. About half of all heart attack victims have a history of high blood pressure, as do 80 to 90 percent of all stroke victims and a similarly high percentage of people with kidney disease, says Aram Chobanian, M.D., dean of the Boston University School of Medicine and former chairman of the American Heart Association's Council on High Blood Pressure.

Stopping the Killer Cold

How do you find out if you're on the high blood pressure list? Go to your doctor and ask to have your blood pressure checked. It's fast. It's simple. It's painless. Every adult should have a blood pressure check at least once every two to three years. (People who already have hypertension need to be monitored more often.)

You will get a reading consisting of two numbers. The first number is the systolic pressure, and the other is the diastolic pressure.

The systolic reading represents the pressure of your blood as it is pumped from the heart, while the diastolic number refers to the pressure of your blood while the heart is at rest, between beats.

If you have a mild case of high blood pressure—a systolic (top) reading of 140 to 160, with a diastolic (bottom) reading of 90 to 100—lifestyle changes alone may be enough to bring your problem to an end, says Dr. Chobanian. The very same lifestyle measures may also prevent high blood pressure in the first place.

Just remember: High blood pressure is serious stuff, so if you have it, you should be under a doctor's supervision.

A Weighty Matter

What's the most important thing you can do, beside remembering to take your medication, to keep your blood pressure in line? It's hard to say for sure, but "if there's one thing that often works, it's weight reduction," says Marvin Moser, M.D., a clinical professor of medicine at Yale University School of Medicine, senior medical consultant to the National High Blood Pressure Education Program of the National Heart, Lung, and Blood Institute, and author of *Lower Your Blood Pressure and Live Longer.*

Losing weight—if you are 20 percent or more overweight—has a definite impact. In many instances, overweight people might lose one point off both their systolic and diastolic blood pressure for every 2 pounds they drop. Approximately a quarter of overweight people who have mild hypertension might reduce their blood pressure to normal levels by losing 10 to 15 pounds and keeping it off, says Dr. Moser.

Don't be discouraged if you're very overweight and you can't seem to get your weight down to normal levels. Studies show that losing even a bit can result in some lowering of blood pressure.

Dr. Moser urges those trying to lose weight not to be taken in by fad diets. Rather, he suggests a long-term strategy of regular exercise and smarter eating. One way to eat smart when you're trying to shed pounds is to cut your usual portions in half and to cut down on fat. This may bring double benefits. The evidence is far from conclusive, but some research suggests that intake of saturated fats (prevalent in red meat and many dairy products) may be linked to slight rises in blood pressure. And polyunsaturated fats (found in vegetable products such as safflower and corn oils) and monounsaturated fats (predominant in olive oil and a few other foods) may lower it, at least to some degree.

Experts advocate lowering your intake of all fats to less than 30 percent of total calories and keeping saturated fats to a minimum. No more than one-third of the fats you eat should be saturated. A tasty low-fat meal might include a portion of broiled fish or poultry, boiled or steamed vegetables, bread, and a dessert of low-fat yogurt or fruit ice.

The Sodium Connection

Excess sodium (the main component of salt) causes sodium-sensitive people to retain more fluid, which can raise blood pressure.

HIGH BLOOD PRESSURE

There's no easy way to determine who's sodium sensitive. But most of us consume far too much salt and could stand to cut back. So experts say reduce your total daily sodium intake to 1,500 to 2,000 milligrams—the amount you'd find in about 1 teaspoon of salt.

"If after two to three months on a salt-restricted diet you see no change in blood pressure, you're obviously not salt sensitive," says Dr. Moser. About 15 to 20 percent of all people with mild hypertension will find that restricting their salt intake is enough to pull their blood pressure down to normal levels.

The best way to cut down on salt might be to ease off on fast foods. They are typically loaded with sodium (and fat). A fast food hamburger has 950 milligrams of sodium. That same size burger with cheese has 1,164 milligrams of sodium, which by itself almost equals the recommended amount for people on sodium-restricted diets.

Cured meats, such as bacon, hot dogs, and sausage, are also quite high in sodium and fat. So are many (but not all) canned soups, some brands of canned tuna, prepared pancakes, some TV dinners, and regular soy sauce. Become a label reader when you shop.

The Antihypertension Diet

Besides eating less salt and perhaps eating fewer calories, what else constitutes the antihypertension diet? You might start by eating a baked potato.

A baked potato with no added salt has a powerful "K Factor," says potassium expert George Webb, Ph.D., associate professor of physiology and biophysics at the University of Vermont College of Medicine. It has 130 times more potassium than sodium. Lack of potassium has been associated with an increase in blood pressure. And some researchers feel that the key to keeping blood pressure down is to maintain a 2:1 or 3:1 ratio of potassium to sodium in your diet. In general, fresh fruits and vegetables have far more potassium than sodium. Top choices: beans, rice, fresh fruits, and grains.

Two other nutrients that may possibly help keep blood pressure in line are calcium and magnesium. One Belgian study involving over 8,000 people found that men who get lots of calcium (abundant in dairy products, collard greens, sardines, and kale) in their diet might expect lower diastolic blood pressure. And women who get lots of magnesium (abundant in soybeans, avocado, cashews, and almonds) might similarly expect lower systolic blood pressure.

A Word about Fish

Aside from these minerals, you might want to include some fish in your diet. Preliminary studies have suggested an association between eating fish or fish oil and lower blood pressure. Researchers theorize that it's the omega-3 fatty acids in ocean fish (such as mackerel, tuna, and salmon) that could somehow be counteracting hypertension. The experts' recommendation: Dine on fish at least two or three times a week.

And what do you wash all this great food down with? Think twice before you reach for the hard stuff. It's long been known that regular heavy drinking (more than three or four drinks a day) can lead to high blood pressure. On the other hand, "an occasional drink isn't likely to hurt anyone," says Dr. Moser. He notes, however, that alcohol has lots of calories—something to keep in mind if you're looking to lose weight. Not only that, but alcohol may not mix well with some hypertension medications; ask your doctor.

And what about coffee? Years ago caffeine was suspected as a major cause of high blood pressure. There is still a lot of debate; the latest evidence seems to show that switching to decaf has just a minimal effect on your blood pressure.

Go for a Walk

Research shows that regular aerobic exercise (brisk walking, cycling, swimming, and the like) may lower blood pressure four or five points. How much exercise does it take? Most of the studies had people working out for 30 to 60 minutes, three times a week. (You have to work up to this level slowly, though, and with your doctor's blessing.) Try to choose an activity that you find fun and relaxing. You do not have to run or jog to derive these benefits from exercise.

Destress Yourself

Taking the stress out of your life just may help knock a few points off your blood pressure reading.

"Anything that holds your attention so you're looking and listening, but not thinking and worrying, reduces blood pressure temporarily," says Aaron Katcher, M.D., associate professor of psychiatry at the University of Pennsylvania. "And this reduction could be from watching a fireplace, taking a walk in the park, going bird-watching, or watching fish in an aquarium." Dr. Katcher believes that doing any of these things for 15 minutes, twice a day, may be an effective treatment for some people with mild hypertension.

Fish and birds aren't the only members of the animal kingdom that can help reduce your blood pressure. Dogs and cats can, too. In fact, any animal that's soft and cuddly can help take the pressure off. Some researchers suspect that interacting with a pet may lower blood pressure, at least temporarily. "The minute you start talking to and petting your dog, your blood pressure goes down and stays down during the interaction," says Aline Halstead Kidd, Ph.D., professor in psychology at Mills College in Oakland, California. "Human-to-human interactions make certain demands. A pet allows you to interact with another living being that makes no demands and loves you without regard to anything."

Progressive muscle relaxation is also a proven technique for relieving stress. Sit or lie in a comfortable position. Start by clenching your fists for 3 or 4 seconds, concentrating on how the tension feels, then relax your hand muscles, letting go of the tension. Try this tensing/relaxing sequence for all major muscles—those in your neck, shoulders, back, arms, abdomen, buttocks, thighs, calves, and feet—for 10 minutes, twice a day. Ideally, you'll soon learn to relax these muscles without tensing them first.

HIGH BLOOD PRESSURE

A Word about Medications

All these lifestyle changes may still not be enough to get your blood pressure into a normal range. If that's the case, you'll need medication. Some drugs get rid of excess fluid and sodium, others open up narrowed blood vessels, and still others prevent blood vessels from constricting.

You and your doctor may need to experiment for a while to find the appropriate medication to bring down your blood pressure without side effects. "There are seven or eight classes of drugs, and over 100 individual drugs, so many options are available," says Dr. Chobanian.

Two particular medications worth mentioning are birth control and diet pills. Oral contraceptives raise blood pressure slightly in many women and are estimated to cause high blood pressure in about 5 percent. So if you use oral contraceptives, ask your doctor about a preparation with low estrogen/progestogen content. Low-dose formulas are less likely to have a pressure-raising effect.

And many diet pills, both prescription and over the counter, contain a substance that's a mouthful—phenylpropanolamine (PPA). PPA is believed to depress the part of the brain that controls appetite. But in some people it can also raise blood pressure, among other possible side effects.

A Lifelong Commitment

Say you've successfully reduced your blood pressure to a normal reading. Can you now rush back to potato chips and beer each night? Sorry, but no. "If you've got your high blood pressure under control, that doesn't

274

Diastolic and Systolic Pressure

Your blood pressure is the force of blood pushing against the blood vessel walls. When you get a measure of your blood pressure, it comes as two numbers, such as 120/75. What do they mean?

The higher number is your systolic pressure. It's generated by the contraction of the heart. The lower number is your diastolic pressure. It is the pressure in the arteries while the heart is resting between beats.

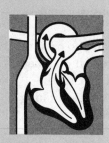

As blood surges out of your heart into the arteries, it attains its maximum, or systolic pressure. You need to be concerned when this number goes above 140.

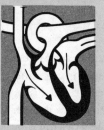

The heart fills with blood and rests between beats. The pressure in the arteries is now at its lowest, or diastolic pressure. Your diastolic pressure should be lower than 90.

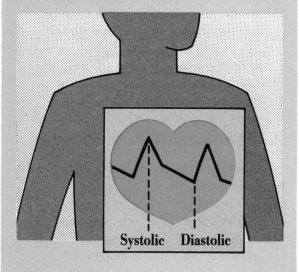

Systolic   Diastolic

How To Take Your Blood Pressure

If you want to monitor your blood pressure at home you'll need a stethoscope and cuff. Here's the proper procedure.

(1) Apply the cuff so the bottom edge is just above the elbow.

(2) Apply the stethoscope at the bend of the arm, just over the artery.

(3) Inflate the cuff until you can no longer hear your pulse.

(4) Release the air until you just begin to hear the pulse tapping once again.

(5) Look at the gauge for your systolic reading at exactly the point when you hear the pulse.

(6) Continue deflating the cuff. Look at the gauge for your diastolic reading at the point when the tapping sound stops.

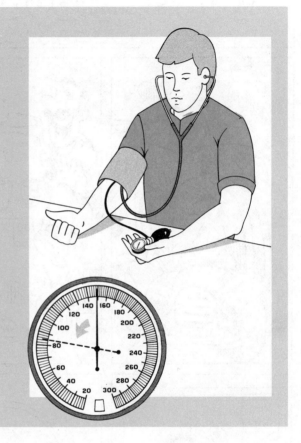

mean you've 'cured' it," says Dr. Chobanian. "You have to assume that once you're susceptible, you're always susceptible." That means a lifelong commitment.

Blood pressure experts say that you're more likely to stick with an antihypertensive regimen if you enlist the whole family in the effort. Some suggestions: Do exercises that other family members can enjoy with you, like walking and bicycling. Don't keep food in the house that one person can eat but another cannot.

Finally, keep in mind that high blood pressure is one of a package of what doctors call "risk factors" that can lead to a number of diseases, the most common of which is heart disease. It's especially important if you have high blood pressure to keep these other risk factors under control, says Dr. Chobanian. That means don't smoke, watch your cholesterol level, exercise regularly, and get a checkup for diabetes.

Russell Wild

HIGH BLOOD PRESSURE

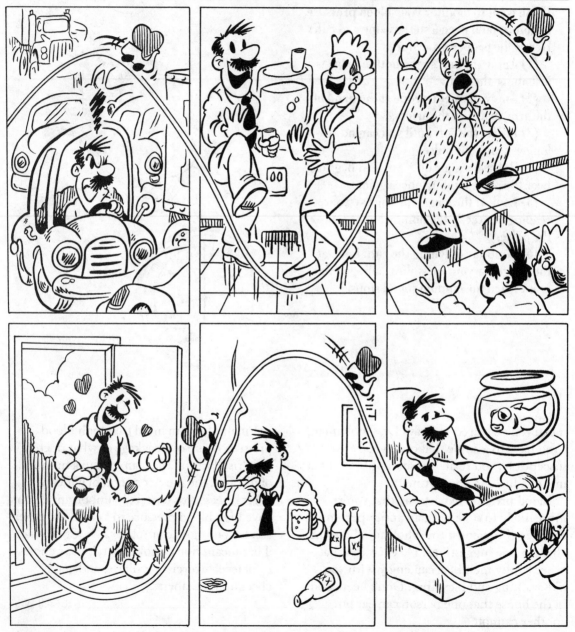

HYPERVENTILATION

In a typical minute, you inhale 4 to 5 quarts of air. But let something push your panic button, and you could suck in almost twice that amount. Now you're hyperventilating.

Hyperventilating leads to a loss of carbon dioxide from the blood, says John Clarke, M.D., a Harvard-trained cardiologist whose research focuses on the relationship between breath, cardiovascular functioning, and psychological states.

Dizziness often accompanies hyperventilation. Numbness in the fingers and toes, chest pain, pounding heart, and muscle cramps are also common symptoms.

Hyperventilation is a common body response to stress, experts say. In fact, you may find yourself taking in a little more air than normal whenever you do something that really requires you to be alert. Some studies show that respiration picks up in people asked to perform mental calculations even in a relaxed setting, says Dr. Clarke. This natural body mechanism may find its extreme response in hyperventilation.

To quickly end an attack, use the paper bag technique (see illustration at right). Try to breathe from your diaphragm. You'll know you're doing it right if your belly swells as you inhale and falls as you exhale. If you need to learn how to breathe from your diaphragm, lie face down on the floor and cross your arms in front of you under your head. Now rest your forehead on your arms and try to keep your face down. This position keeps your chest from moving, thus forcing you to breathe correctly. Observe the pressure of your stomach against the floor each time you inhale. Once you get the hang of that, roll onto your back and place a book on your stomach. Each time you inhale, try to raise the book.

Continue until you can do this without the book. Then practice until diaphragmatic breathing becomes second nature. If you learn this breathing technique, you may find that you don't have to resort to the paper bag. Practicing for 5 to 10 minutes at a time, several times a day, can go a long way toward helping you remain relaxed, says Dr. Clarke. And when you're calm, you're less likely to hyperventilate.

Deborah Grandinetti

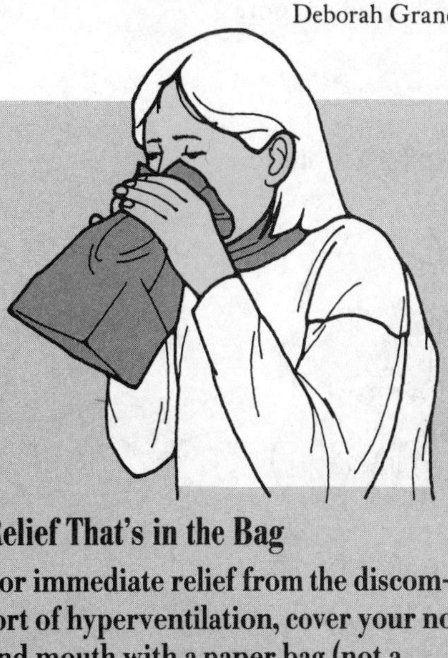

Relief That's in the Bag

For immediate relief from the discomfort of hyperventilation, cover your nose and mouth with a paper bag (not a plastic one) and breathe normally for 3 to 5 minutes. This helps restore carbon dioxide to your lungs and blood.

INGROWN HAIRS

Imagine a tiny army standing on your face. Each soldier holds a spear with a flexible shaft. Each day you slaughter them all. But this army has a *lot* of reserves. And sooner or later, one—just one—of those spears bends.

"An ingrown hair is nothing more than a hair that curls in on itself and grows back into your skin," says dermatologist Leonard Grayson, M.D., clinical associate professor of allergy and dermatology at Southern Illinois University Medical School in Quincy.

Men are usually the victims, and necks and chins are usually the sites. Those with straight hair are relatively immune; the curly-haired are not.

Trying to get the closest possible shave is the biggest cause of ingrown hairs. The best way to prevent them is "to grow a beard. Ingrown hairs only happen when the hairs are very short," according to Tom Meek, Jr., M.D., a dermatologist and assistant clinical professor of dermatology at Louisiana State University School of Medicine in New Orleans.

But if beards aren't your bag, "shave with the grain of your beard, not against it," says Dr. Grayson.

To get rid of an ingrown hair, "apply an antiseptic, like alcohol, first," says Dr. Grayson. "Then, with a fine tweezer, the kind that you use to remove slivers, pluck out the hair."

Don Barone

A Closer, Easier Shave

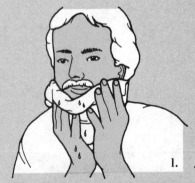

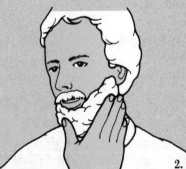

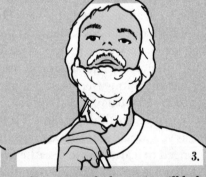

1. Wet whiskers are easier to cut than dry whiskers. Thoroughly soak your beard for at least 5 minutes before you shave. Better yet, shave after your shower.

2. Shaving cream helps your whiskers absorb water, which makes them easier to cut. Lather up and leave it on for a little while before you shave.

3. Shaving with the grain will help. On the sides of your neck, shave down and toward the center. In the middle of your neck, shave straight down.

INSOMNIA

You'll try anything. You flip the pillow over to the cold side, thinking that might help you sleep. You lie on your back. Turn over on your side. Your other side. Your stomach. Nothing works.

Fluffy pillows. One pillow. Two pillows. Your partner's pillow. No pillow. And still no sleep. As you lie there night after night suffering with insomnia, it may comfort you to know that you're not alone. Much of America is awake with you.

Wide Awake Coast to Coast

"Approximately a third of the population of the United States has trouble sleeping," says Michael Stevenson, Ph.D., clinical director of the North Valley Sleep Disorders Center in Mission Hills, California. "At some point in their lives, half of those people, about 15 percent of the country, will have chronic insomnia that lasts for months," he says.

It's a wonder all that rustling around at night doesn't keep more people awake.

Insomnia can occur at any age, even in childhood, but it tends to happen more often as you get older. "By the time people reach their sixties, about 80 percent of them will have at least some insomnia during the year," says Dr. Stevenson.

Take heart. You're about to learn how to drift off to the land of Nod effortlessly—to fall asleep faster and sleep more soundly than you have in years.

Technically, insomnia is classified as the inability to fall asleep or maintain sleep, but there is good news here. Research in sleep disorder laboratories shows that most insomniacs actually *do* sleep. "They may not be sleeping very well, but they are getting quite a bit more sleep than they think they are," according to Dr. Stevenson.

We all have individual sleep quotas. The range of sleep requirements is from 6 to 9 hours a night for most of us. (Doctors say we should get at least 5 hours and no more than 10 to be the healthiest.) Your sleep quota is genetically determined and remains the same throughout your adult life. It's possible to lengthen or shorten your sleep time, but only by an hour or so.

So how much sleep do you need? Enough to feel rested, alert, and able to stay active all day. If you find yourself frequently feeling irritable, nodding off while listening to a lecture that you need to pay attention to, or drinking more coffee than usual to get perking in the morning, you may not be meeting your sleep requirement.

The Fine Art of Sleeping

To sleep tight, you have to learn to sleep right. Use your bedroom only for sleeping and sex. "Plan all your evening activities so that you wind down slowly toward sleep. Don't work right up to the time you go to sleep. Relax. Take a warm bath," says Dr. Stevenson. "Sit and soak for a while. A warm bath will elevate your body temperature and help make you sleepy."

INSOMNIA

Develop a routine. "Establish and keep a regular bedtime and arising time," says Robert Golden, M.D., associate professor of psychiatry, University of North Carolina School of Medicine. "Try to wake up and get out of bed the same time every morning, even on holidays and weekends."

And while you're at it, "don't take naps during the day. A long nap following a night of insomnia may disturb the next night's sleep," says Dr. Golden.

Instead of napping, try taking a brisk walk around the block each day to fight the drowsies. In fact, engaging in regular exercise is another good way to ensure a night's sound sleep. Studies have shown that regular afternoon exercise increases sleep's deeper stages.

The key word is *regular.* If you try to cram all your exercise into the weekend, you'll wind up with aches and pains that will keep you up all night. So don't overdo it.

Do's and Don'ts for Dozing

In addition to regular exercise, make it a practice to watch what you eat and drink before bedtime. "Hunger may disturb sleep, as may caffeine, alcohol, and tobacco," says Dr. Golden. "A light snack or glass of warm milk may promote sleep, but avoid heavy or spicy foods."

Dr. Golden also advises against the routine use of sleeping pills. "While they can be effective when used as part of a coordinated treatment plan for certain types of insomnia, chronic use is ineffective at best and can be detrimental to sound sleep," he says.

If after all of this you still can't get to sleep, "don't lie in bed awake," says Dr. Stevenson. "If you can't fall asleep within 20 minutes, leave the bedroom. Go out into another room, such as your living room, and stay there until you feel sleepy, then go back to bed."

The Too-Early Bird

If you have a problem with waking up too early and not being able to go back to sleep, don't just lie there looking at your alarm clock. Get out of bed until you are sleepy again.

"Watching your alarm clock frequently creates insomnia, as it makes you feel anxious about not falling asleep. It's okay to have an alarm clock, but put it where you will hear the alarm without being able to see the clock dial," says Dr. Stevenson.

There are times when you need to see your doctor about insomnia. "If you find it impairs your ability to function during the daytime, if it affects your work, or you find yourself too tired or sleepy to get through the day, then you need to see a doctor," says Edward Stepanski, Ph.D., director of the Insomnia Clinic at Henry Ford Hospital's Sleep Disorders Center in Detroit. "Also, see your doctor if insomnia lasts for more than a month or so."

Don Barone

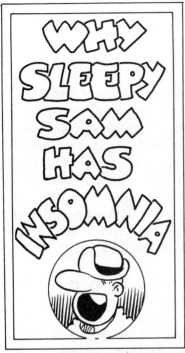

WHY SLEEPY SAM HAS INSOMNIA

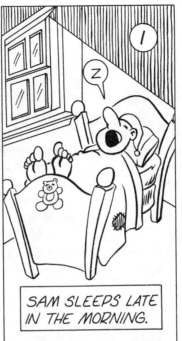

1

SAM SLEEPS LATE IN THE MORNING.

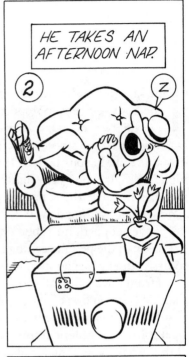

HE TAKES AN AFTERNOON NAP.

2

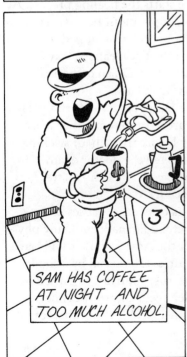

3

SAM HAS COFFEE AT NIGHT AND TOO MUCH ALCOHOL.

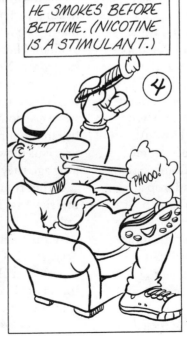

HE SMOKES BEFORE BEDTIME. (NICOTINE IS A STIMULANT.)

4

PHOOO!

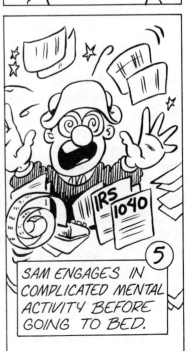

IRS 1040

5

SAM ENGAGES IN COMPLICATED MENTAL ACTIVITY BEFORE GOING TO BED.

281

KNEE PROBLEMS

The knee is the Rodney Dangerfield of the body—it gets no respect.

Do you respect yours? How are you treating the largest, most vulnerable, most unstable joint in your body? Do you wear high heels? Are you overweight? Do your feet turn in? Out? If you participate in sports, what training do you do? Have your knees ever popped, hurt, buckled?

Over half the people seeking help from sportsmedicine specialists are looking for relief from knee pain. All sports tax the knee. While you don't have to be an athlete to suffer knee pain, you can learn how to treat it from an athletic trainer who deals with knee pains as a matter of course.

"The basic rule of thumb is if it doesn't feel that severe, if you are able to walk on it, you don't have to see anybody that day," says Mark Howard, athletic trainer and orthopedic technician who spent 12 years with the San Diego Chargers.

And what does he recommend for temporary relief of knee pain? "You can't go wrong with the RICE treatment," says Howard.

RICE is the acronym for the best home care for a knee injury: Rest, Ice, Compression, Elevation. *Rest* means go easy and stop all activities that tax the knee. Don't scrub floors on your knees. Skip the aerobics class. *Ice* should be applied as soon after the injury as possible. Wrap it in a bath towel so it doesn't freeze the skin. Leave it on for 20 minutes. A few hours later, put ice on it again. Repeat this procedure for up to two days. *Compression* means wrapping the ice

package in an elastic bandage or anything that'll keep it snugly pressed against the injury. *Elevation* means keeping your knee higher than your heart—or "toes over nose."

"Even if something severe exists that would need medical treatment, the RICE procedure helps keep the swelling and discomfort down until the knee can be taken care of," states Bob Sauers, an athletic trainer with Sports Medicine Lehigh Valley in Pennsylvania.

The immediate thing is to get the weight off it. If your knee pain is the result of a minor injury, follow the ice treatment with a little soothing heat. "After about 48 hours, Mother Nature starts the healing process. At about this time, apply moist heat with a heating pad or a hot towel wrapped in a plastic bag from the dry cleaners," says William Hamilton, M.D., an orthopedic surgeon in New York City.

If swelling or pain persists after three days, seek medical care. Try to remember what you were doing before the pain or swelling began. Be sure to tell the doctor of any previous blows to your knee, no matter how long ago they occurred.

Either trauma or overuse causes knee injuries, says Peter Marshall, company physical therapist for the American Ballet Theatre. "Traumatic injuries are caused by a single occurrence. Overuse injuries are caused by repeated smaller events, known as microtraumas." If a knee problem persists, see your doctor.

Bejou Merry

The Joint That Can Bring You to Your Knees

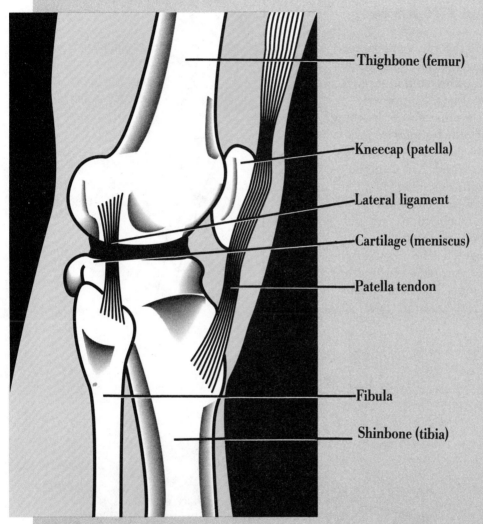

Thighbone (femur)

Kneecap (patella)

Lateral ligament

Cartilage (meniscus)

Patella tendon

Fibula

Shinbone (tibia)

The knee is a complex of bones, ligaments, cartilage, and muscles. It's nature's engineering marvel, but it's not perfect. The bursa, little sacs that contain a small amount of lubricating fluid, can become irritated. This condition is called bursitis, or "housemaid's knee," because it's associated with prolonged kneeling. Runners, aerobic dancers, weight lifters, and people with feet that turn inward are susceptible to "runner's knee." This condition results from the deterioration of the cartilage on the underside of the kneecap over time. When the kneecap gets knocked off the track or groove along which it usually runs, you've "dislocated" your kneecap.

NEE PROBLEMS

Exercise for Pain-Free Knees

Have you ever had to forgo a golf game or a stroll on the beach because your knees were acting up? If the muscles that support your knees are weak, they can't properly support your weight-bearing, shock-absorbing joints. Strengthening the leg muscles and keeping them flexible are knee-care musts.

Heisman Trophy winner Earl Campbell credits his trainer with convincing him that the key to pain-free knees is flexibility and training. "The guys who used to work out with this one trainer on our team, none of them had a knee problem," he says. Inadequate warm up, overexertion, and a "macho" obsession with accomplishment may make you more susceptible to knee injuries.

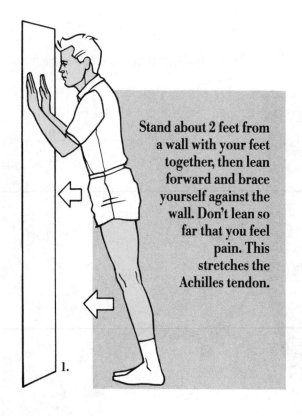

Stand about 2 feet from a wall with your feet together, then lean forward and brace yourself against the wall. Don't lean so far that you feel pain. This stretches the Achilles tendon.

1.

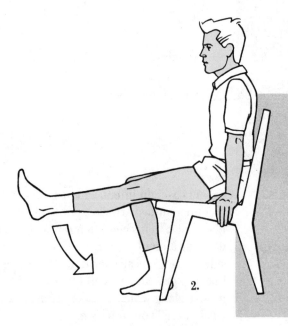

With your back erect, sit in a chair. Extend one leg. Hold it out for 5 seconds. Lower it slowly. Do this with your other leg. This strengthens the knee and helps improve knee flexibility.

2.

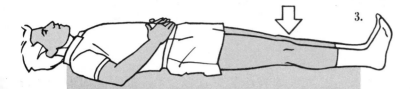

3.

Lie on your back and push your knees toward the floor. Hold for 5 seconds. Then relax your leg muscles. It might not feel strenuous, but this exercise strengthens the quadriceps, important muscles that support the knee.

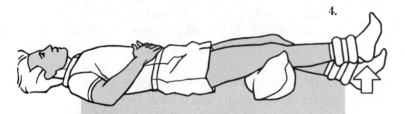

4.

Problems with kneecap pain? Lie on your back with a pillow under your knees. Straighten a leg and hold it raised for 5 seconds, then lower it slowly. Repeat ten times on each leg.

Lie on your right side with your right leg bent and your left arm supporting you. Lift the left leg, keeping it straight. Hold it raised for 5 seconds before slowly lowering it. Repeat ten times, then switch legs. For an extra challenge, add ankle weights.

5.

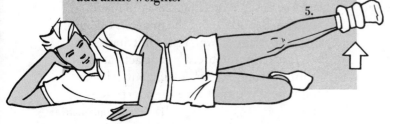

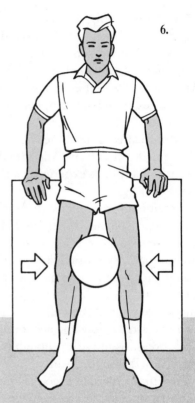

6.

If you can borrow your teenager's basketball for a few minutes, here's a new use for it. Place the ball (or any similar size ball, for that matter) between your legs above your kneecaps. Squeeze for 5 seconds. Repeat.

MENSTRUATION

Whoever dubbed menstruation "the curse" certainly had no feel for aesthetics. What a rich and complex symphony the entire menstrual cycle is. What a precise orchestration of glands, hormones, muscles, brain, nerves, and emotions.

Month after month, the symphony plays the same familiar tune. And month after month, many of us experience a few sour notes.

Hormones are responsible for much of the discomfort you may experience. (During your menstrual cycle, hormone levels fluctuate, preparing your body for pregnancy. If you do not become pregnant, you get your period and the cycle begins again.) Hormones help signal the milk secretion cells of your breasts to grow and accumulate fluid. If your breast tissues swell enough to stretch nerve fibers, you feel pain.

You may experience food cravings at the same time. Scientists have shown that as estrogen falls and progesterone rises, your metabolism gets revved up—and so does your appetite. What this means for you, according to independent researcher Paul Webb, M.D., of Ohio, is that you may burn as many as 200 calories more per day during the last two weeks of your cycle than you did when the cycle began. But Two-Zero-Zero isn't a license to kill your appetite. If you do give in to the munchies, don't eat the whole bag of chips.

Your moods may shift, too, triggered by the dance of adrenaline in your body. A Swedish study shows that adrenaline, a stress-response hormone, rises most sharply during the third week of your cycle. Not surprisingly, test subjects reported darker moods during the latter half of the cycle.

During your period and right before it, you're also subject to cramping, thanks to prostaglandins, hormones your uterus produces to help it contract and expel menstrual fluid. If the ratio of prostaglandins is off, your muscles may tighten more often and more intensely than they need to. Those contractions cut off blood supply to the muscles. Result? You cramp.

That's what's going on in your body. But you don't have to suffer in silence. There's a lot you can do to ease through your monthly menstrual discomforts.

The Dietary Solution

Diet is the easiest area to manipulate. You want to follow a diet low in fats and rich in whole grains, beans, and vegetables. A study at the National Cancer Institute of the National Institutes of Health found that women who switch to a low-fat diet retain less water during both their premenstrual week and their period. You also want to make sure you're getting plenty of niacin, vitamins B_6 and C, and the minerals calcium, zinc, and magnesium. These nutrients regulate prolactin, the breast-tissue activator.

Studies suggest that cutting out caffeine might help you beat breast tenderness.

Deborah Grandinetti

286

THE RIGHT MOVES CAN SOOTHE CRAMPS

Menstrual cramps and premenstrual discomfort don't have to put a crimp in your day. To ease discomfort fast, forsake the couch and grab your exercise mat. The right moves can help you relax the tense muscles that hurt.

Just be sure to go easy on yourself when you're working to relieve cramping that's already in progress. The key word here is *relax*. A relaxed muscle will cause less discomfort than a muscle that's clenched. Even anxiety about getting your period can cause you to tense up, and tension can only make the pain worse.

To relieve cramps, you have to get the tightened muscles of the uterus and nearby areas to unclench. (If you're suffering from premenstrual discomfort, try the exercises here and on pages 288 and 289. The exercises on pages 290 to 293 are designed to help relieve menstrual cramps.) Remember to breathe slowly and deeply. Listen to your body. If any of these exercises make you feel uncomfortable, go on to the next exercise.

There is some evidence that a daily exercise routine may reduce the discomfort of menstrual cramps. This is not a new idea. During World War II, an aircraft factory that involved its female workers in an on-site exercise program found that absenteeism blamed on menstrual cramps dropped by 80 percent. A three-year study of 302 junior high school students who had not yet begun to menstruate found that those who exercised subsequently developed fewer menstrual problems than those who did not.

Stretch Away PMS

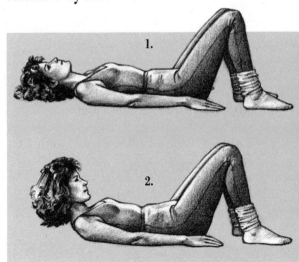

(1) Lie on your back with knees bent. Breathe in through your nose while you count to five. *(2)* Then as you exhale through your mouth to a count of five, tighten your stomach and slowly lift your head as high as you can. Hold this position as you breathe in and out, counting to five. On the next inhale, lower your head to the floor. Note: If you suffer from a stiff neck or headaches around the time of your period, don't do this one.

MENSTRUATION

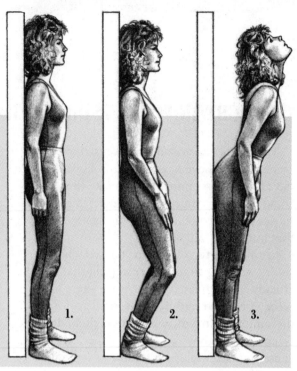

(1) Stand with your back and your heels touching a wall. *(2)* Tighten your buttocks and bend your knees until even the small of your back is flat against the wall. Now exhale for five counts while tightening your stomach muscles and tilting your pelvis and hips forward and up, all the while keeping your back flat against the wall. *(3)* Now inhale, straighten your legs, and arch your back so much that it feels like you are sitting on the wall. Repeat five times. Build to ten repetitions.

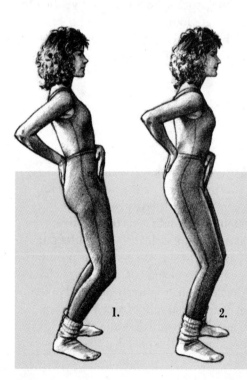

Once you develop a feeling for the exercise above, you can work the same muscle groups without using a wall for support. Here's how. *(1)* Place one hand on your lower back and the other on your stomach. *(2)* Now tilt your pelvis forward and backward, using your hands to guide the movement. This exercise will make your back more flexible and your stomach stronger.

If you have back ailments, consult your doctor before doing this exercise. It will really give your back a good stretch. *(1)* Stand with your back and your heels flush against the wall. *(2)* Bend your knees as far as necessary to eliminate the space between your lower back and the wall. Let your arms hang at your sides. Pull your stomach muscles in, keeping your pelvis muscles tucked under. Inch your body up the wall, keeping your back flush against the wall. Keep inching up until you no longer keep your back flat. Getting your calves to touch the wall without having your back arch may take months of work. *(3)* At your maximum stretch, extend your arms out in front of you. *(4)* Now slowly raise your arms overhead. Try to bring them all the way back as you keep your head, back, calves, and heels against the wall.

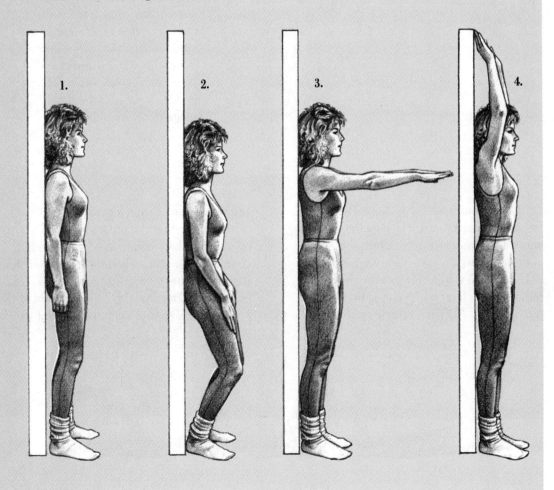

1.   2.   3.   4.

Menstruation

Unclench Those Cramps

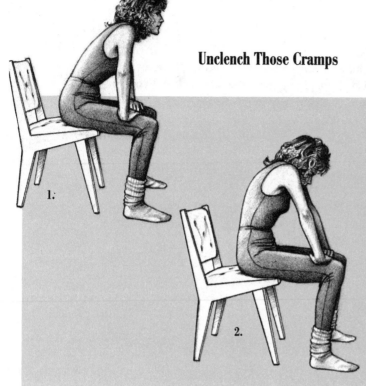

1.

2.

Sit halfway back on a chair and rest your feet on the floor, a chair's width apart. *(1)* Place your hands on your thighs, raise your shoulders, and lean forward a bit. Make sure that your back is straight. *(2)* Inhale through your nose. Then exhale forcefully through your mouth, emptying yourself of air. As you exhale, pull in your stomach muscles until your stomach is concave and your back arches like a cat's. Hold this position for a few seconds before you release.

(1) Lie on your back on the floor. Bend your knees and place your feet flat against the floor, about 1 foot away from your buttocks. Let your arms rest at your sides, palms down. *(2)* Now raise your knees to your chest and pull them in closer with your arms. Hold momentarily. *(3)* Then release your legs and slowly lower your feet to the floor. With your feet flat on the floor, inhale. *(4)* Then exhale slowly, contracting your abdominal muscles and lifting your hips slightly off the floor, making sure to keep your back pressed against the floor. Hold this position for five to ten counts. *(5)* Now slowly

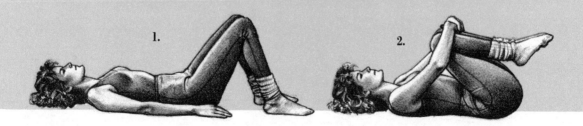

1.

2.

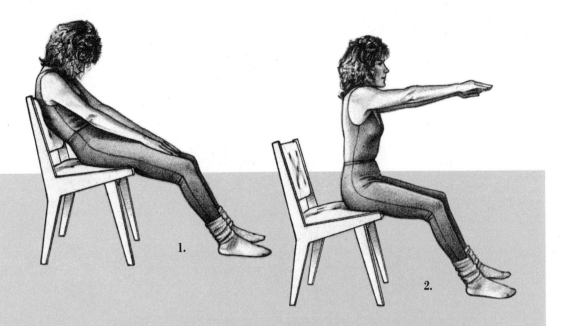

(1) Sit on the front half of the chair seat. Lean backward until your back touches the chair back. Stretch your legs in front of you, bending them slightly at the knees. Rest your arms on your lap. *(2)* Slowly breathe in and fill your lungs completely with air. Draw your arms up together as if you're about to dive. Exhale while you tighten your tummy and rise to a straight-back position. Hold for a count of three, then drop smoothly back into the starting position.

lower your hips back down to the floor. Focus on using the muscles of your thighs and stomach. Release and rest. Breathe deeply and allow your back to relax against the floor. Repeat the sequence if you feel the need.

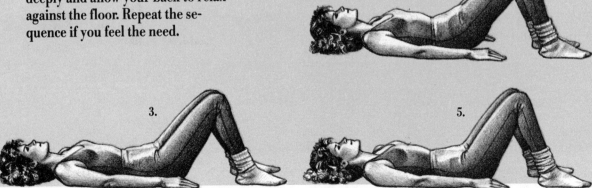

Menstruation

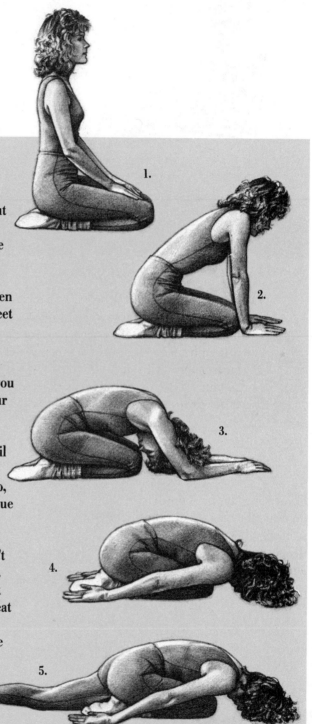

1.

This exercise is somewhat demanding, but it is worth the effort if you can manage it. The alternating stretches provide a gentle internal massage that can help to short-circuit pain from cramps. *(1)* Kneel on a carpeted floor or mat, knees together. Then sit back on your heels. The tops of your feet should rest against the floor. *(2)* Bend forward with your arms straight out and palms down, fingers facing forward. *(3)* Slide your palms out straight in front of you until your forehead touches the floor. Your rib cage should feel relaxed. Gently and slowly breathe in and out in this position. Close your eyes and hold the position until you feel very relaxed. *(4)* Now slide your arms back until your hands rest, palms up, alongside your feet. Let your chest continue to rest on your knees. *(5)* Now shift your body until the weight rests on your right leg. Extend your left leg behind you. Don't worry if your balance temporarily falters. Hold this stretch for a few moments. Tuck your right leg back in. Pause to rest. Repeat the leg stretches five times on each side, alternating the stretched position with the tucked. Remember to rest between sets.

2.

3.

4.

5.

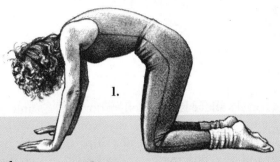

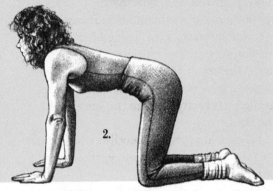

(1) Get down on all fours. Place your palms flat against the floor and make your back flat. Inhale slowly. Now exhale as you pull your stomach in and arch your back like a frightened cat. Lower your head and try to see your navel. Hold the position for five counts. (2) Release and breathe in slowly as you flatten your back and lift your head back up. Hold for five, rest, and then repeat the entire exercise.

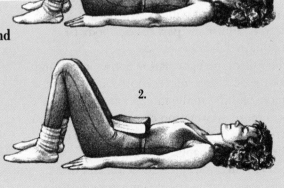

(1) Lie on your back with your knees bent and your feet resting flat on the floor. Practice bouncing your belly up and down as you take short, panting breaths. (2) Now put a large softcover book, such as a telephone directory, on your belly. When you inhale, push the book up and hold. Then exhale and let the book drop along with your stomach. Try to keep your stomach muscles tightened as you exhale.

293

MOTION SICKNESS

Part of travel's allure is that it offers novel sensations—the tilt of a plane, the gruff grumble of a train, the heave of a ship. Tilting, grumbling, heaving . . . the same sensations that set the mind astir can also stir up your stomach. Full-fledged motion sickness usually begins with dizziness and proceeds through nausea and vomiting. In the process, your skin turns pale and clammy as the blood retreats from the surface of the skin.

Women are more susceptible than men, and young people more susceptible than older people.

More-experienced travelers also seem to be more immune to it. Attitude seems to play a role, too. If you expect you'll get sick en route, you probably will.

Science can't say for sure why people get motion sickness. A leading theory is that motion sickness is the body's response to conflicting sensory information.

That's because your body is wired for balance. Your brain scans continuously for information that will reveal whether you need to adjust any part of your body to maintain balance.

Some of the information comes in through your eyes. Other information comes from nerve endings in the muscles and tendons. Still more information comes in from certain structures in the inner ear that report even the minutest change in position.

Typically, your eyes, muscles, and inner ears provide compatible information. But when you're reading in a car, for instance, and your eyes scan a page that remains stable while your body reacts to bumps in the road, the brain seems unable to reconcile the conflicting reports. And that may set in motion a process that results in nausea, says Michael W. Bungo, M.D., staff scientist and director of NASA's Space Biomedical Research Institute at the Johnson Space Center.

Save Your Next Trip

There are several strategies you can use to keep yourself feeling great during your next trip.

Avoid strong odors and foods that unsettle your stomach. Alcohol is out, too. Drink enough, and you'll produce symptoms similiar to motion sickness without even leaving the house.

You can also forestall motion sickness by taking a drug before you travel. The antihistamine Dramamine is a common nonprescription drug that works for most people. Prescription drugs also are available for this purpose.

Be aware that all of these drugs can cause drowsiness and remember to check any drug label for specifics.

Also available by prescription are skin patches that you attach behind your ear for a steady 72-hour supply of scopolamine. Scopolamine's side effects inlude drowsiness, disorientation, dry mouth, and blurred vision.

If you prefer a natural remedy, powdered ginger was found to be more effective than Dramamine in a study reported in *Lancet*.

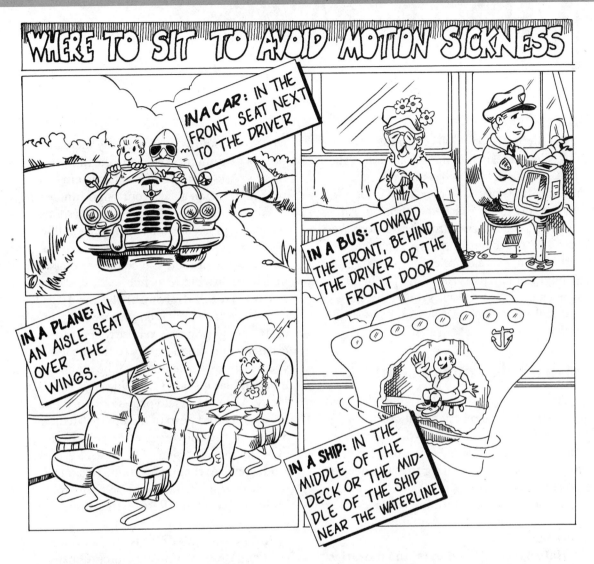

Daniel B. Mowrey, Ph.D., coauthor of the study, personally takes two capsules of 450 milligrams each, 10 minutes before setting out on a trip and more as needed. If you try ginger, be sure to take it in capsule form so you don't burn your esophagus.

Ginger is an old remedy for stomach disturbances. It doesn't cause drowsiness, since it works in the gastrointestinal tract rather than in the brain.

If you've done all the right things and you still end up with motion sickness, here's how to alleviate it.

"Fixate on an object in the distance that's more stable," says Dr. Bungo. "If you're in a boat, focus on the horizon, rather than on all the swirling and tilting motion."

Although it's more effective if taken beforehand, you can still take medication during a bout of motion sickness, says Dr. Bungo.

Deborah Grandinetti

295

MUSCLE CRAMPS

At night, the pain jolts you awake. The silent scream is coming from your calf, or at least, from what *was* your calf muscle. In its place is a rock-hard knot. Or maybe you've just finished exercising. All of a sudden, pain burns through your foot. You reach for the source of the pain and find a tight ball of dense muscle.

Night or day, foot, calf, thigh, or hand—when a muscle or muscle group tenses suddenly and involuntarily, you have a *cramp*.

Stalking the Cramp Culprit

Any number of things can spur the complex physical reaction that creates a painful muscle cramp—dehydration, use of diuretics, mineral deficiencies, overuse of a muscle, even just switching to lower-heeled shoes.

The best way to determine what's causing your cramps is to ask yourself these four questions.

Have I recently begun taking diuretics? "People who take diuretics, a medication for high blood pressure, can be potassium deficient—and that deficiency can cause cramps," says James Knochel, M.D., chairman of the Department of Internal Medicine at Presbyterian Hospital in Dallas and professor of internal medicine at Southwestern Medical School of the University of Texas. But not all diuretics have the same effect; some cause potassium retention. That's

why you shouldn't automatically increase your potassium intake if you take diuretics, he says. Ask your doctor or pharmacist how your medication affects your potassium level.

Potassium is one of the minerals responsible for helping your muscles recover following exercise. If you get a muscle cramp following a workout, you could be potassium deficient, says Dr. Knochel.

Do I stretch thoroughly before I exercise? "I can't overemphasize the value of stretching prior to exercise to increase elasticity and blood supply to the tissues. If you warm the tissue up, you'll be much less likely to tear it than if it's cold," says Edward Percy, M.D., associate professor of orthopedic surgery and head of the Sports Medicine Section at the University of Arizona College of Medicine.

He believes that many cramps stem from muscle overuse, which can lead to microtears in the muscle tissue. Resting the affected muscle will help speed healing.

Am I dehydrated? This is an all-too-common cause of muscle cramps. Outside temperatures are high, you've been active, and now you're sweating profusely. The fluid loss disturbs your body's balance of certain minerals (called electrolytes) and decreases blood flow, says Dr. Knochel.

"A lot of people have the idea that they shouldn't consume any salt at all. Your sweat contains, on average, one-third the amount of salt contained in the blood," he says. So if you are going to be active when the temperature climbs past 75°F, make sure to use some salt in your food, he advises.

Be extra careful when the humidity is high. If it's 80°F and humid outside, overdoing it could cause heat exhaustion and nasty cramps in your arms, legs, back, or stomach.

Have I exhausted the muscle? "If you're running out of fuel to supply the muscles, all the chemical processes that regulate contraction fail," says Dr. Knochel.

The best way to prevent cramps caused by exhaustion is to respect your limits.

When Pain Comes at Night

In addition to the known causes of cramps, there is one type of cramp that remains a mystery—night cramps. "Nobody knows what causes them," says Dr. Knochel. "We assume it's the decreased blood flow at night."

The fastest route to pain relief is to forcefully stretch the muscle in a direction away from the cramp. Aspirin can help interrupt the pain signals, says Dr. Knochel.

Typically, muscle cramps last no longer than about 10 minutes, says Dr. Knochel. If yours seem unusually severe and last for an hour, call your doctor.

You'll also want to consult your doctor if you get cramps regularly or if they're common in your family. Certain rare muscle diseases that have cramping as a symptom are inherited.

Deborah Grandinetti

How Charley Got His Name

Did you ever wonder where the term *charley horse* originated? So did we. And the annals of baseball had our answer.

It turns out that there really was a horse named Charley. He worked at Ebbets Field, the home stadium of the Brooklyn Dodgers before the team moved to Los Angeles. Charley was the horse that dragged a chain-link fence around to smooth the infield between innings.

As the years went on, poor old Charley grew lame. And someone had the bright idea of labeling any athletic injury that led to lameness a charley horse. The phrase caught on.

The problem is, the phrase never really got specific. Charley horse has been applied to any number of muscle injuries, from tendinitis to muscle strains and tears. So if you want people to know what you're talking about, retire poor old charley horse from your vocabulary and use the more specific term *cramp.*

MUSCLE CRAMPS

Unclamping Cramps

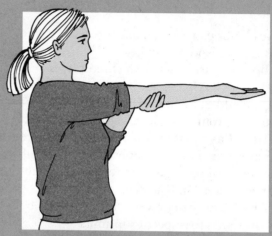

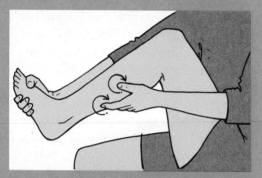

To relieve a calf muscle cramp, bend your leg at the knee and pull your toes and the ball of your foot toward the kneecap. Hold your foot in place as you massage the cramped calf muscle. This will promote increased blood flow to the muscle.

If you have a cramp in your biceps, the upper arm muscle that allows you to rotate and bend your forearm, flex your tricep muscle to relieve it. To do this, put your hand on the elbow of the affected arm to keep the elbow from moving. Then straighten the cramped arm.

Foot cramps are pretty common. Often, the muscles responsible are the interossei muscles, the long muscles that hold the toes down. Stretch these muscles by pulling up on the toes. You always want to stretch the cramped muscle in the opposite direction.

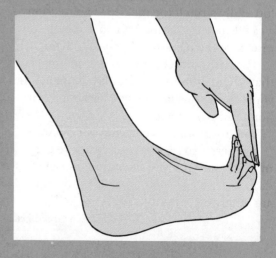

NAIL PROBLEMS

Want to know where you can get a great thumbnail sketch of your health history? That's right. On your own thumbnail.

Discoloration, ridges, and funny shapes have an uncanny way of reflecting specific disorders. How this happens is unknown. But somehow, information about your physical condition gets translated to the nail matrix, the root from which the nail grows.

The telltale nail has problems of its own, too, most of them preventable. Here's how to cope with some common nail problems.

Fingernail infections are common, says Paul Kechijian, M.D., chief of the nail section of the New York Univerity Medical Center.

Cutting or pushing back the cuticle, which functions like a bacteria shield, can put you at risk. Using nail wraps or polish can also lead to infection if moisture, bacteria, and yeast get trapped between the nail and nail bed, says Dr. Kechijian.

You can prevent this type of infection by leaving your cuticle intact and avoiding nail wraps. And if you have your nails done at a salon, "make sure they sterilize their instruments and use a clean basin and new liquids each time," he says. The only way to treat this infection is with antibiotics.

Toenail infections can result from athlete's foot. To prevent these infections, keep your feet as dry as possible because fungi grow best where it's damp, says Dr. Kechijian. Changing your shoes every day might also prove to be of some help.

Any number of things can make nails brittle—aging, dry heat in winter, frequent immersion in water, or repeated use of strong nail polish removers. If yours are brittle, dab moisturizer on the nail bed frequently.

Sometimes brittleness isn't the cause of a broken nail. Normal nails that are long can crack or tear more easily with everyday use or trauma, says Dr. Kechijian. If you are plagued by brittle, breaking nails, try trimming them a little shorter and apply a moisturizer each time you wash your hands.

Deborah Grandinetti

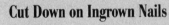

Cut Down on Ingrown Nails

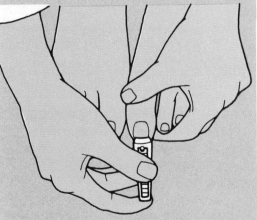

To avoid ingrown toenails, cut your nails straight across with a clean clipper. It's best to clip right after a bath or shower, when nails are softer.

NAIL PROBLEMS

Fingernail Diagnosis

Ridges, discolorations, unusual shapes— fingernails provide a fascinating set of clues about your medical condition.

Remember, though, only a physician can convert these clues into a confirmed diagnosis.

 If your nails are unusually wide or squarish, you may be suffering from thyroid disease.

 Nail plates that are unusually narrow and long suggest a pituitary hormone deficiency.

 "Clubbed" nails, which curve around your fingertip, may point to emphysema, tuberculosis, cancer, or cardiovascular disease.

 Blue spots or nail beds suggest impaired circulation, diabetes, heart disease, Raynaud's syndrome, or spasms of the arteries in the fingers.

 "Spoon" nails may be flat or may look scooped out. Doctors say they may indicate iron deficiency anemia.

 "Yellow nails" syndrome might point to diseases of the respiratory system. However, normal nails come in a wide variety of hues.

 "Beau's lines," depressed furrows across the nail plate, result from emotional disturbances, severe illness, or infection.

 Vertical red streaks in the nail bed, "splinter hemorrhages," signify bleeding of the capillaries. They may be a sign of psoriasis.

 "Mee's lines," vertical white streaks, may indicate arsenic poisoning, kidney failure, heart attack, or sickle-cell anemia.

 Pitting in rows that makes nails resemble hammered brass, frequently occurs as a result of psoriasis or alopecia areata.

 "Terry's Nails," the condition in which the nail bed has a dark pink to brown band near the tip, may indicate cirrhosis.

 Chronically chipped, sawtooth nails may suggest damage resulting from exposure to household or occupational chemicals.

 "Half and half" nails, in which the half near the tip appears brown, may point to kidney failure.

 Brown or black discoloration that spreads from the nail bed to surrounding finger tissue, may signify malignant melanoma.

NECK AND SHOULDER PAIN

Neck and shoulder pain go together like the sniffles and a sore throat—have one, and there's a good chance you have the other.

There are probably several hundred different specific causes of neck and shoulder pain, but some causes are more common than others. Among the culprits: poor sleeping posture, injuries, tension, nerve problems, sudden overexertion, muscle overuse, bursitis, and arthritis. And yes, the computer terminal appears in the lineup, too.

"Often, people with neck and shoulder stiffness are people who make their living sitting at computer terminals," says Robert Harrison, M.D., director of the Occupational Medicine Clinic at the University of California in San Francisco. "If the computer terminal is sitting too low (forcing the user to hunch forward and look down) or too high (forcing the user to lean back and look up), there are going to be problems," he says. Setting up your work station properly will go a long way toward relieving your discomfort. (See the chapter on eyestrain on page 187 for tips.)

But don't stop there. How you relax, even the way you sleep, affects muscle tension.

"Although stress is a common cause of neck and shoulder pain, we see more people with injuries or poor sleeping habits," says Margaret Avery, a licensed massage therapist and owner and director of the Desert School of Healing Arts in Tuscon, Arizona. "People sleep on one side of their body for years. And they develop a shoulder problem because of that."

So you try a better sleeping position and make sure your computer terminal is at eye level. What if you *still* have neck and/or shoulder problems?

Ice It, Rest It, Move It

Many people find that a heating pad relieves persistent pain. If the pain is the result of injury, however, applying an ice pack may bring relief.

An over-the-counter anti-inflammatory drug is a good adjunct to ice, Dr. Harrison says. But, he adds, rest is also important. You may simply have to take it easy for a while.

Exercises can also help. One easy exercise for shoulder soreness is the shoulder shrug. If you wish, you may want to add some light weights—say 2 to 5 pounds—to this exercise. If so, hold the weights in your hands while raising your shoulders. Hold the position for a moment. Then lower your shoulders and relax. Do this ten times.

Finally, neck and shoulder pain may warrant medical attention. If you've been in an accident, see a doctor. Don't merely endure, or worse yet, try to ignore, persistent neck or shoulder pain.

Don Wade

NECK AND SHOULDER PAIN

Unkink Those Knotted Muscles

You don't want to take the passive approach and virtually drop out of life for fear that any activity will leave you with a literal pain in the neck or with an aching shoulder. So what are you going to do?

Move!

- Take breaks from desk work and spend a few minutes stretching your arms across the front of your body, then to the side, and straight up over your head.
- Roll your shoulders in a big rowing motion. Bring them up toward your ears and then squeeze them together in front of you. Then drop your shoulders. Last, pull your shoulders back and try to touch your shoulder blades together.
- Carefully tilt your head forward as far as possible. Then move your head backward as far as possible.
- Slowly turn your head from side to side.
- Tilt your right ear toward your right shoulder while keeping your shoulder still. Straighten, then lean toward the other shoulder.

Maybe your job—be it working at a computer terminal or hoisting cases of beer—makes some neck and shoulder pain just about inevitable. You can protect yourself by regularly practicing the following exercises. *(1)* Begin by standing straight with your feet comfortably spread apart and your arms stretched upward. Feel the stretch from your heels up through your legs, back, shoulders, neck, and arms. *(2)* Next, let your upper body fall forward from the hips. Hang as loose and limp as a rag doll. Keep your knees slightly bent. Allow your head, arms, and shoulders to droop for about 30 seconds. *(3)* Shake your head and let your arms and shoulders dangle freely. Then slowly raise your body. Enjoy the warm wave of relaxation that moves through your shoulders and neck. You may do the exercise as slowly as you want. And if you choose to stay bent over longer, that's fine, too. Concentrate on feeling the differences as you move your body from one position to another. Repeat the entire sequence several times.

2.

3.

1.

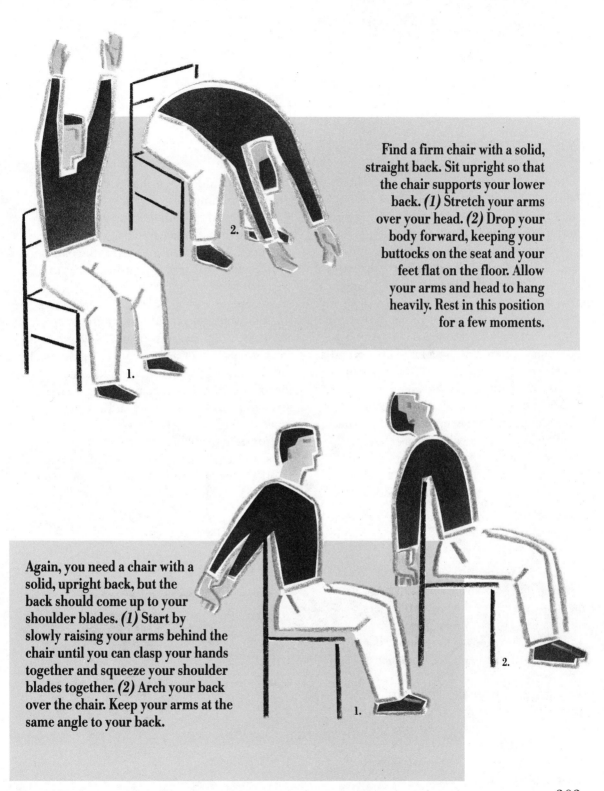

Find a firm chair with a solid, straight back. Sit upright so that the chair supports your lower back. *(1)* Stretch your arms over your head. *(2)* Drop your body forward, keeping your buttocks on the seat and your feet flat on the floor. Allow your arms and head to hang heavily. Rest in this position for a few moments.

Again, you need a chair with a solid, upright back, but the back should come up to your shoulder blades. *(1)* Start by slowly raising your arms behind the chair until you can clasp your hands together and squeeze your shoulder blades together. *(2)* Arch your back over the chair. Keep your arms at the same angle to your back.

Soothe Sore Shoulders

You are tempted to think it's too good to be true. Something that feels so good—a massage—is actually good for relieving neck and shoulder pain. But it is true.

"There are multitudes of muscles connecting the neck and shoulders that support the shoulder girdle like clothes on a hanger," says Margaret Avery, a licensed massage therapist and owner and director of the Desert School of Healing Arts in Tuscon, Arizona. "There are also a lot of nerves and a lot of arterial blood flow. So the neck can respond quickly to massage."

Massage is equally effective for many shoulder problems, Avery says, noting that many people with neck pain also have shoulder pain and vice versa.

For massaging shoulders, the "receiver" should lie down. If that is not practical, the receiver should sit in a chair with the "giver" standing behind.

"Be careful to keep the fingertips away from the throat area when you're massaging the neck," Avery cautions. "Use the palms to walk down the back. If your hands get tired, you can also use your elbows or forearms."

Whenever using any massage technique, be it for the neck, shoulders, or elsewhere, heed the body's warning signs. "If you [the person receiving the massage] feel pain, back off," Avery says. "If you have frequent headaches or experience numbness in the extremities, avoid massage and see your doctor."

But such problems are not likely, Avery says, adding, "Massage is an excellent way to soothe away tension and really enhance the function of your muscles."

The area of the neck pictured here is often a chief point of soreness. To relieve pain, use the tips of the first two fingers of each hand to apply firm pressure at the point where the neck and lower back ridge of the skull meet. Apply pulsing pressure for up to 3 minutes. Or, if you prefer, apply a more steady, but firm pressure for 10 seconds, then release for a few seconds and apply pressure again. You can do this for up to 3 minutes as well. Finish with light strokes to relax the back of the neck.

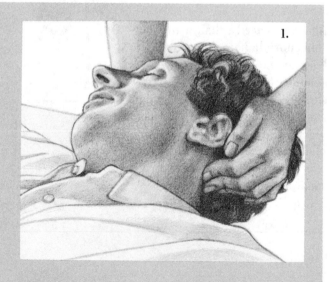
1.

Position one hand over each shoulder with the thumbs on the back side and the fingertips on the front side. Using firm pressure and a gripping motion, move back and forth from the end of the shoulder to the base of the neck. As you massage, try to vary the position of your thumbs to cover as much of the person's upper back as possible. Though in this illustration the person receiving treatment is lying down, this massage is also very effective when the receiver is sitting upright in a chair.

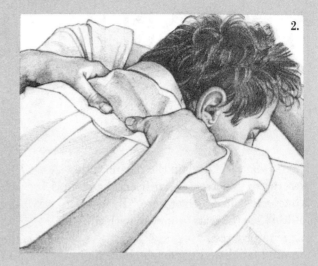

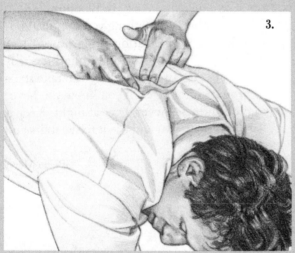

Sometimes the area between the shoulder blades feels like it's bearing the burden of all the world's problems. Tension somehow gravitates there. To relieve pain and tension in this area, use two or three fingers of each hand and make circular motions or stroking movements between the spine and the shoulder blades, from the bottom point of the shoulder blade to the base of the neck. Again, you will want to use firm pressure and perhaps vary the position of your fingers to cover a wide area.

Here's another common trouble spot, where tension and pain have a tendency—like in-laws—to stay and stay and stay. But fortunately, massage can hasten their departure. Begin by standing at the receiver's left side and placing both hands over the left shoulder blade with your fingertips just under the inner edge. Apply pressure along the entire inner edge of the shoulder blade. After a couple of minutes, switch sides and place both hands over the right shoulder blade. Repeat as needed.

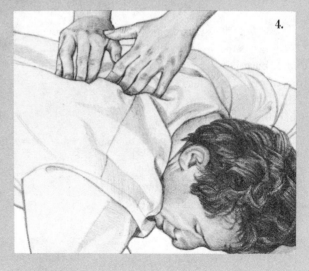

NIGHT BLINDNESS

It was scary standing in the theater aisle, trying to find a seat. Your friend had found hers and called, "Over here." But you couldn't see the seats, not even with the movie in progress.

Sound familiar? People who have night blindness find themselves "in the dark" more often than most people. No one can see in total darkness; however, a person with night blindness is unable to see with the help of low levels of illumination that are adequate for a person with normal vision, says Alfred Sommer, M.D., director of the Dana Center for Preventive Ophthalmology at Johns Hopkins Hospital in Baltimore.

Basically, what's causing the problem is that your eyes' rods—the light-sensitive, specialized nerve cells that enable you to see in dim light—are not operating properly.

"Go and have your eyes examined if they're troublesome," says Merrill J. Allen, O.D., Ph.D., professor emeritus of optometry at Indiana University in Bloomington. There might be something you can do about it with proper medication or glasses."

People who have true night blindness may not be able to cure it, but they can take steps to protect themselves. If you know you have night blindness, never drive at night. Keep a flashlight with you and use it to see stairs and curbs.

Bejou Merry

Blinded by the Night

How well does your night vision measure up? Use this chart, based on research findings of highway safety consultant David Preusser, Ph.D., and colleagues, to help determine whether you should be driving at night. Can you see a traffic signal or road sign in plenty of time to react? How far away can you see a bicycle with reflective lights? Be aware that distances can change when environments change.

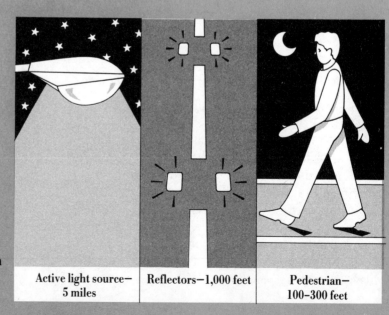

| Active light source—5 miles | Reflectors—1,000 feet | Pedestrian—100–300 feet |

NOSEBLEED

Both the nose and Florida are warm and humid with centrally located activity centers. In Florida it's Walt Disney World, and in the nose it's the Kiesselbach's area.

Located in the front of the septum, the partition separating the two nasal cavities, Kiesselbach's area houses a confluence of large blood vessels and many small superficial blood vessels. "It gets hit easily (especially by children's fingers) and is easily injured. It can also get dried out," explains William S. Gibson, Jr., M.D., otolaryngologist at Geisinger Hospital, Danville, Pennsylvania.

When the lining of the nose dries, a crust forms over this blood-rich, vessel-dense area. Dislodging the crust breaks vessels, causing nosebleeds.

Using a humidifier or applying petroleum jelly or similar ointment to the nasal septum can help prevent drying.

"Dry, cold air, nosepicking, constant nasal discharge, respiratory infection—all of these lead to irritation and erosion of the septal mucosa," states Linda Brodsky, M.D., otolaryngologist at Buffalo's Children's Hospital.

An adult who experiences frequent nasal stuffiness and nosebleeds might have what's known as a deviated septum. This condition requires medical attention. In fact, any nosebleed that does not respond to applied pressure should be brought to the attention of your physician.

Bejou Merry

How to Stop a Nosebleed

To stop a nosebleed, sit upright. Pinch your nostrils together tightly and squeeze for 5 minutes, breathing through your mouth. Keep your head tilted down so the blood won't flow down your throat. Applying ice is unnecessary. Avoid any activity that might disturb the crust that forms—including blowing your nose or overexertion. Keep your mouth open if you sneeze. If the bleeding doesn't stop after 5 minutes, consult a physician.

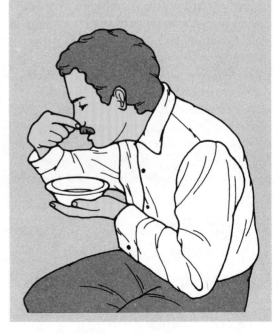

NUTRITIONAL GALLERY OF HEALING FOODS

P-s-s-st! Over here! Shut that medicine cabinet and come into the kitchen. Feast your eyes on this: fresh poached salmon, herb-seasoned brown rice pilaf with lentils, oven-roasted onions, an avocado garnish.

And check out this lunch spread: steaming minestrone soup, a white-meat turkey and tomato sandwich on oatmeal bread, a salad of scallion, cauliflower, and romaine dressed with tangy low-fat yogurt, and melon for dessert.

Hungry? Good. Just let your imagination savor the delicious appeal of foods that have the power to heal. Here in the kitchen, you can really have fun with your take-charge attitude toward health. That's because the right foods, eaten in the proper combinations, can help your body repair physical damage and prevent the onset of disease.

As the above fare shows, "good for you" doesn't have to mean "grin and bear it." The salmon dinner with all the fixings is rich in nutrients like omega-3 fatty acids, which have been shown to help lower blood cholesterol levels. The scrumptious soup, salad, and sandwich combo is low in fat, low in salt, and rich in potassium—ideal for anyone concerned about high blood pressure.

Mounting Evidence That Nutrition Counts

Consider some of the more recent findings about the healing power of food.

Eating soybeans may help guard against breast cancer. That's the inference University of Alabama researchers have drawn after noticing that people in countries with very low rates of breast cancer are big soybean consumers. Soybeans apparently contain a substance similiar to a drug used to treat breast cancer in humans. Researchers have not studied the impact of soybeans on human cancers, but one researcher noted, "I would assume it wouldn't hurt for a woman to add them to her diet."

Nor is that the only hot nutrition news from the anti-cancer front. Raw coleslaw may be a better bet than baked stuffed cabbage if you want to ward off stomach and colon cancer. (Ditto for other cabbage-family vegetables such as brussels sprouts, cauliflower, and broccoli.) According to Canadian scientists, the raw vegetables contain a higher concentration of a compound that's been found to prevent the formation of tumors.

Cancer is not the only disease under study, either. Vitamin E, a substance that's plentiful in nuts and wheat germ, may delay the onset of atherosclerosis, according to researchers at the University of Kentucky.

And on it goes. Scientific inquiry in recent years has focused on the link between the immune system and various nutrients—amino acids, vitamins A, B_6, C, and E, and the minerals zinc, iron, copper, and selenium.

Vitamin E, for instance, appears to enhance the ability of white blood cells to engulf and destroy bacteria and to control inflammation.

Each nutrient, it seems, has a unique set of talents. Combined intelligently, specific nutrients can help foster recovery, as doctors at Shriners' Burns Institute in Cincinnati, Ohio, discovered. When they replaced the standard formula given to burn patients with one containing fish oil, zinc, and vitamins A and C, the patients developed far fewer infections and required a shorter hospital stay.

Learning to make intelligent use of food, whether in a hospital room or your own kitchen, makes good sense. After all, even healthy bodies are in a state of constant renewal and repair. New cells replace old cells. Torn tissues knit together. Yesterday's cut becomes today's scab. The blood endures endless rounds of purification.

What fuels these healing processes? The food you eat. How can you help your body speed the job? By taking in the right amounts of essential nutrients. Ultimately, the choices you make in the supermarket and cafeteria line today can profoundly affect your health and well-being months and even years from now. Small changes, such as adding two or three servings of fish each week, can add up to big long-term benefits.

A Variable You Can Control

Of course, diet isn't the only factor that contributes to your state of health—

environment and genetic inheritance play a part, too. But while you can't change the fact that the men on your side of the family tend to get colon cancer, for example, you may be able to overcome your own susceptibility by taking a shine to broccoli, cauliflower, and foods rich in vitamin C and beta-carotene, two nutrients linked to lower rates of cancer.

The first step in creating a healing diet is to strive for balance. Replace fatty foods, such as doughnuts and french fries, with foods that are low in fat and high in complex carbohydrates, such as whole grains, fruits, and vegetables. Make sure that some of the fruits and vegetables are yellow and red, so you can be sure to get your beta-carotene and vitamin C.

And include two to three servings of fish per week, which will provide you with the omega-3 fatty acids that can help bring your cholesterol level down.

To fine-tune your diet, consult the chapters in this book that deal with your specific health concerns.

Here are some other tips: To boost your immunity, choose from the foods in our superfoods list that provide vitamins A, B_6, C, and E, the omega-3 fatty acids, iron, selenium, folate, and zinc.

To keep your cholesterol down, build your meals around low-fat foods that are good sources of soluble fiber, such as oat bran, fruit, and vegetables.

Deborah Grandinetti

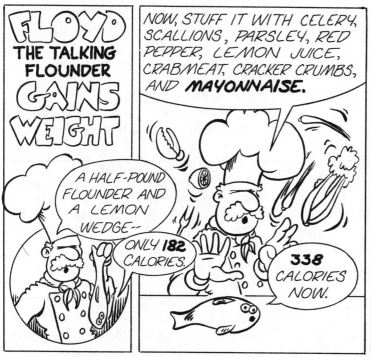

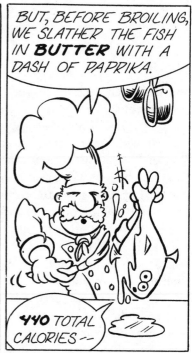

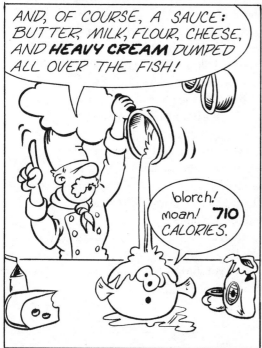

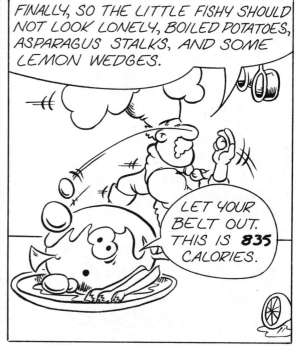

Fifty of the Best Healing Foods

You eat for pleasure. But you also eat for energy and healing. How can you be sure that you've made the best possible choices from the wide array available to you in the aisles of your local supermarket? What do you select when the restaurant menu teases you with dozens of delectable alternatives?

Let our list of 50 superfoods simplify your decision making for you. Scientists have studied each of the foods on this list and found them to contain amazing disease-preventing, health-giving nutritional factors—factors such as dietary fiber, omega-3 fatty acids, and beta-carotene. Many of these 50 superfoods are also low in calories and fat.

We call them superfoods because each does triple duty or better in the disease-prevention category. Choose a banana over a couple of cookies as your afternoon snack, for instance, and you supply yourself with essential nutrients that researchers have linked to lowered incidence of hypertension, increased protection against cancer, and enhancement of the immune system. You won't have to worry that the banana will push up your blood cholesterol level, either; only 4 percent of a banana's calories come from fat.

If you slice that banana into some low-fat yogurt, you add calcium, a mineral that may help you guard against osteoporosis.

Introducing the Superfoods Champs

Low-fat yogurt and broccoli happen to be the champions of the superfoods list. Why?

Their nutritional content makes them valuable allies against cancer, high blood pressure, high cholesterol, obesity, heart disease, stroke, and osteoporosis.

Of course, broccoli and yogurt do not a complete diet make. Each food has its strong points.

Cover all your nutritional bases by eating a variety of these foods each week.

If you take care to prepare these foods right, you can catapult them from super to superlative.

Here are some tips.

- Eat your foods as fresh as possible. Even a few days in the refrigerator will cause loss of vitamins and minerals.
- If produce doesn't look absolutely fresh, buy frozen fruits and vegetables.
- Slice vegetables, fruits, and meats as close to cooking time as possible. Minimize the cutting surface. For example, cut carrots into coins instead of making large diagonal slices. Cut surfaces promote loss of vitamins.
- Mackerel is best cooked the day you buy it. Other fresh fish will keep for up to two days if you wrap it in plastic and store it in the coldest part of the refrigerator.
- Good cooking methods include steaming, baking, broiling, grilling, and stir-frying in small amounts of oil. Or use a microwave or nonstick pan without fats.
- Baste turkey with fruit juice or stock instead of fatty pan liquids.

NUTRITIONAL GALLERY OF HEALING FOODS

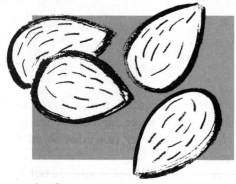

Almonds (unsalted)

You'd be hard-pressed to find a healthier, more portable protein snack. Almonds offer magnesium, which your heart needs to function properly, calcium for your bones, and plenty of vitamin E, a nutrient touted for its disease-fighting prowess.

Apples

Apples have been a power food since the Garden of Eden. They're low in calories, rich in fiber, and a source of boron, a mineral your mind may require for mental alertness and your body uses to maintain sufficient levels of calcium.

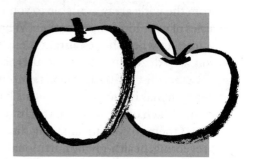

Apricots

Tart yet sweet, apricots are a storehouse of beta-carotene, a nutrient that helps protect against many types of cancer. Three raw apricots or ten dried halves will give you your daily quota of this nutrient.

Asparagus

This elegant spear-shaped vegetable offers three potent nutrients that help defend against cancer—carotene, vitamin C, and selenium. Asparagus also contains modest amounts of fiber, the kind that lowers cholesterol.

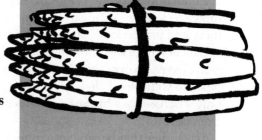

Avocados

Here's one creamy food that can help lower your cholesterol—by as much as 9 to 43 percent, according to one study. Avocados are also rich in potassium and magnesium, two minerals your muscles rely on.

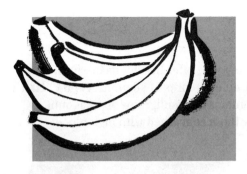

Bananas

The banana is the world's best natural, low-fat source of vitamin B_6, a nutrient that helps make antibodies to fight disease. Eat just one banana, and you'll have taken in one-third of the U.S. Recommended Daily Allowance of B_6.

Barley

This rib-sticking grain is low in fat and sodium and rich in B vitamins and minerals, including calcium. It also offers some protein and fiber. Whole-hulled or "flaked" barley is more nutritious than pearl barley.

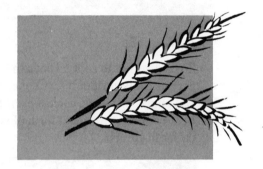

Broccoli

Broccoli can help you build strong bones, fortify your blood, and prevent cancer. A single cup serving will give you even more than the Recommended Dietary Allowance for vitamin C and offers plenty of calcium, iron, and beta-carotene to boot.

Brown Rice

Brown rice offers more fiber, iron, magnesium, zinc, and vitamins E and B than white rice. It's also a good source of selenium, a mineral that may help protect against lung cancer.

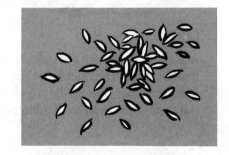

Cabbage

This fiber-rich vegetable is practically bursting with nutrients like vitamin C, which can reduce your chances of developing certain cancers and help prevent the spread of cancer once it has developed in the body.

313

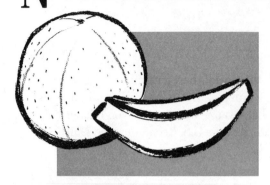

Cantaloupe

What does cantaloupe offer besides its luscious, summery taste? Ample amounts of vitamins A and C. Half a cantaloupe contains 825 milligrams of potassium, a real bonus for those concerned with high blood pressure.

Carrots

To cook or not to cook? That's the question. Raw carrots contain vitamin C. Cooked carrots have less. But ounce for ounce, cooked carrots have more beta-carotene—the plant form of vitamin A—and it's easier to absorb.

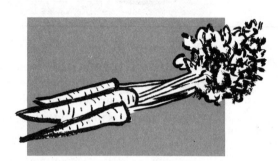

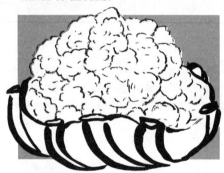

Cauliflower

To derive the most benefit from this fiber-rich vegetable, steam it. Don't overcook. One cup will give you 100 percent of the Recommended Dietary Allowance for vitamin C and provide you with potassium, too.

Celery

At 6 crunchy calories per stalk, celery is a tried-and-true diet food. The fiber helps you feel full. Meanwhile, you're treating your cardiovascular system to potassium and your bones to 14 milligrams of calcium.

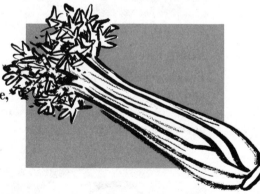

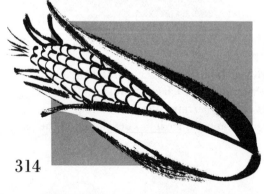

Corn

If you're on a low-sodium diet, take another look at corn. It has only 28 milligrams of sodium per cup. Yet a single ear will provide you with protein, fiber, vitamin B$_6$, folate, zinc, and potassium.

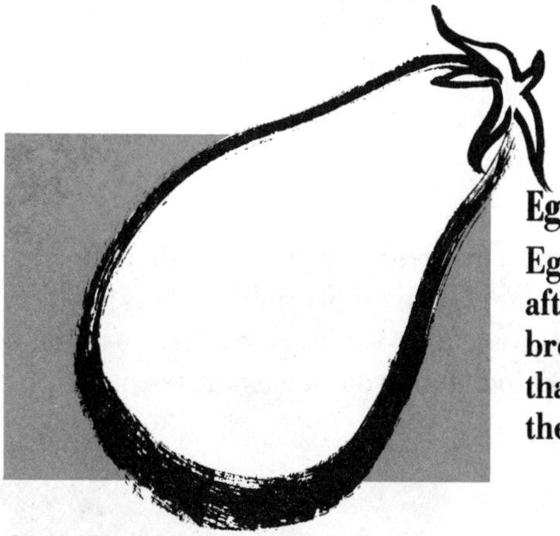

Eggplant

Eggplant may be a good base for parmesan cheese after all. An Austrian study suggests that eggplant breaks down in the intestine into various components that bind with excess cholesterol and escort it out of the body.

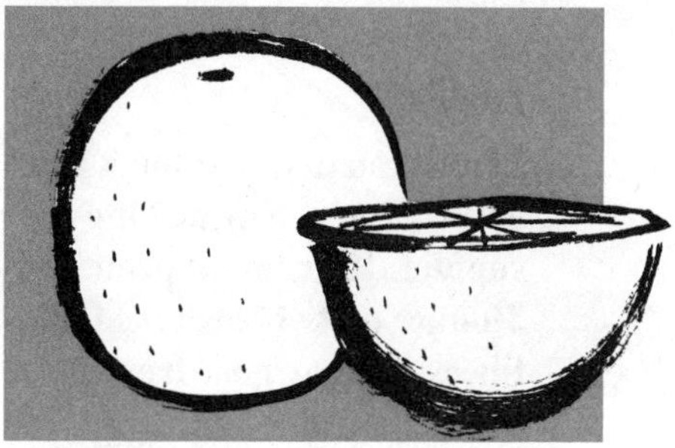

Grapefruit

A fruit this golden has to be bursting with vitamin C. It is. A medium-size grapefruit contains 50 percent more vitamin C than the Recommended Dietary Allowance. Try flavoring it with cinnamon instead of sugar.

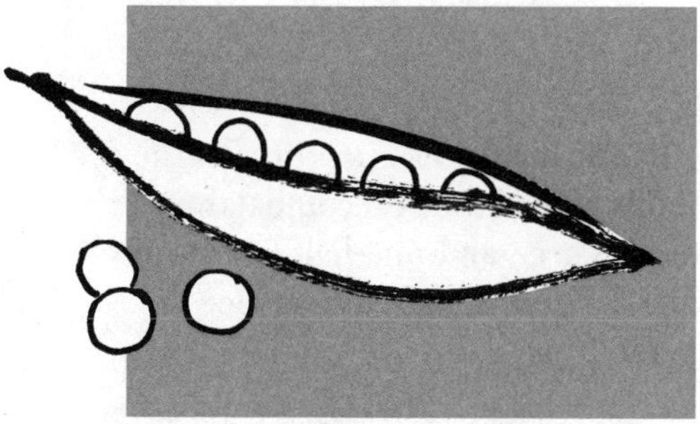

Green Peas

Nature packs a lot of goodness into the tiny pea. Three-quarters cup of peas provides 645 units of vitamin A, 6 grams of protein, plus thiamine, riboflavin, niacin, calcium, iron, phosphorus, and potassium.

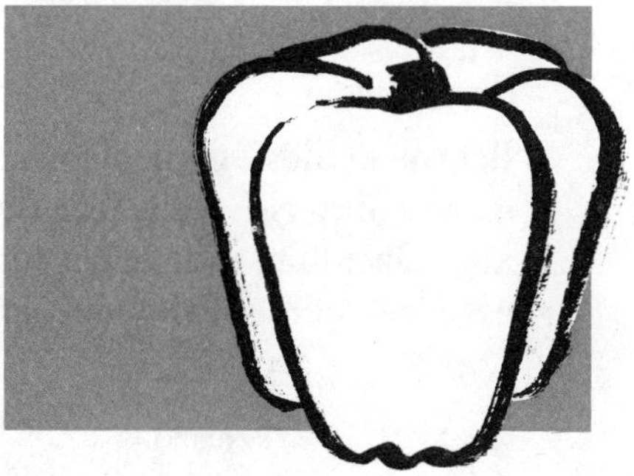

Green Peppers

Bell peppers have more nutrients per calorie than many other green vegetables. In fact, a single pepper has more vitamin C than a cup of orange juice! Instead of frying them, try roasting peppers to get rich flavor.

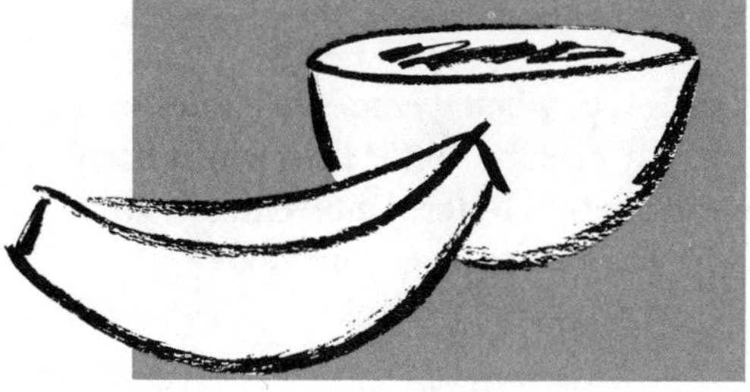

Honeydew Melon

Fragrant and inviting, this juicy melon packs a vitamin C wallop. You can also count on it for potassium, a mineral you need in sufficient amounts to keep your muscles from cramping. Let your sweet tooth indulge.

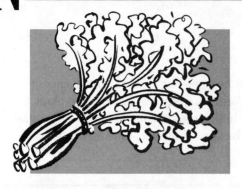

Kale

Hail to kale, a nutrient-packed green that offers you vitamins A and C and plenty of fiber. This low-fat, low-calorie vegetable is recognized as one of the best you can eat to defend yourself against cancer.

Lentils

Lentils can help you meet your protein needs as you cut back on red meat. One cup of cooked lentils supplies 16 grams of protein, 1 gram more than a 3-ounce patty of lean beef. Plus, lentils are high in fiber and almost fat-free.

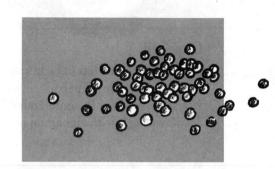

Mackerel

You can't beat Atlantic mackerel as a source of the potent omega-3 oils, one of the best combatants against cholesterol. Three-and-one-half ounces of mackerel supplies 2.5 grams, more than twice the amount you'd get in tuna.

Nectarines

Bet you wouldn't think of the nectarine when asked to name a fiber-rich fruit. Yet a single nectarine has even more fiber than a whole banana. Nectarines are also an excellent source of vitamin A and potassium.

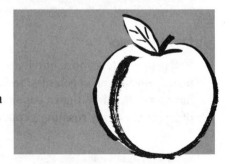

Oat Bran

This form of fiber is tops when it comes to cholesterol-busting ability. It may even be better than wheat bran. Oat bran surrounds the cholesterol molecules in your intestine and eliminates them from your body.

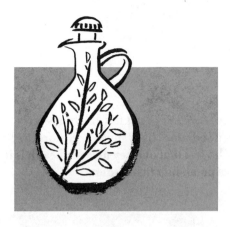

Olive Oil

Take a daily dose of olive oil—2 to 3 tablespoons on a salad—as a protection against heart disease. The oil contains the kind of fat that has been found to lower the harmful variety of cholesterol but leave the good kind intact.

Onions

Your breath may protest, but your stomach will thank you. Researchers in China found that a diet heavy in onions—and related vegetables such as garlic, scallions, and Chinese chives—may lower your risk of stomach cancer.

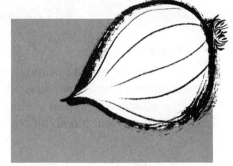

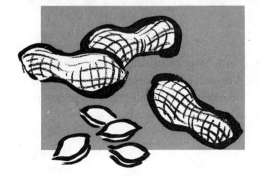

Oranges

Sure, the orange is synonymous with vitamin C. But did you know it's also a source of calcium? A medium-size orange gives you as much calcium as an ounce of Brie, though it has 30 fewer calories and none of the sodium.

Peaches

Keen on peaches? Well that's peachy keen because this source of vitamins A and C will satisfy your sweet tooth without overloading you with fat. Pick fresh peaches over canned to get the maximum fiber benefit from this fruit.

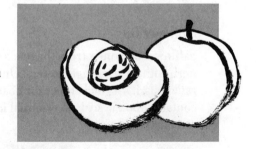

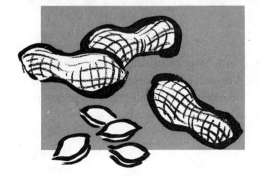

Peanuts (unsalted)

Unsalted peanuts are actually good for your arteries. One-quarter cup of peanuts contains as much mono-unsaturated fat as a tablespoon of olive oil. Monounsaturated fats have been shown to lower blood cholesterol.

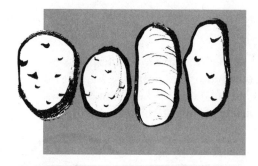

Potatoes

A baked potato without the salt has 130 times more potassium than sodium. That's super, according to researchers who feel that one key to heart health is to consume more potassium than sodium.

Prunes

If you've never eaten a prune, you're in for a moving experience. Prunes are nature's best-tasting laxative. They contain a great deal of fiber, making them great for lowering your blood cholesterol level as well.

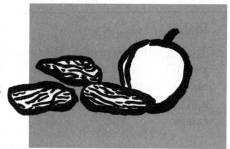

Raisins

Want a portable, storable, sweet source of iron and potassium? Reach for a package of raisins. One-half cup will supply you with 545 milligrams of potassium, a nutrient that can help keep you feeling energetic.

Safflower Oil

Safflower oil comes from the seeds of the safflower, an herb with large orange flowers. One of the polyunsaturated oils, it's a good choice for heart health. It contains linoleic acid, an essential fatty acid our bodies can't make.

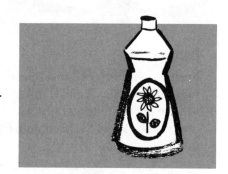

Salmon

Don't spurn salmon if you're fishing for a nutrient-packed entree. A 3-ounce steak supplies you with lots of vitamin B_{12} and calcium, 319 milligrams of potassium, and 1.7 grams of omega-3 fatty acids.

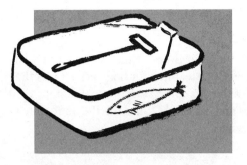

Sardines

Sardines are so loaded with calcium that a single 3-ounce serving will give you almost 20 percent more calcium than an 8-ounce glass of milk. Go easy on sardines, however, if you're on a low-sodium diet.

Skim Milk

Choose skim milk over whole milk, and you say goodbye to about half the calories and most of the fat. Yet you'll still get all the calcium, riboflavin, B$_{12}$, magnesium, thiamine, and vitamin A that make milk supernutritious.

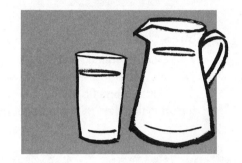

Spinach

You *know* spinach is good for you, but do you know why? This low-calorie, leafy green vegetable is a good source of vitamins A and E and potassium. Potassium works with sodium to regulate the water balance in your body.

Strawberries

Say "fiber" and you immediately think of heavy foods such as bran, right? Well, strawberries contain fiber, too; the soluble kind that slows digestion of foods so you feel full longer. Count on them for vitamin C, too.

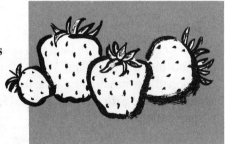

Sunflower Seeds

Don't let the size of the sunflower seed fool you. Nature has crammed these little seeds with calcium, copper, iron, magnesium, phosphorus, potassium, zinc, and vitamin E, which may protect you from lung cancer.

319

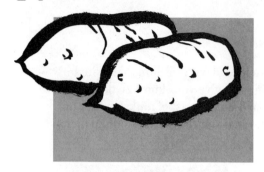

Sweet Potatoes

You might like them for their creamy texture and their just-sweet-enough-taste, but your body recognizes the sweet potato as the vitamin A storehouse that it is. A single cup will give you eight times the Recommended Dietary Allowance.

Swiss Chard

This quaintly named leafy green vegetable is high in vitamin C and beta-carotene (the plant form of vitamin A) and also offers fiber. You can prolong its shelf life for up to five days by wrapping it in perforated plastic.

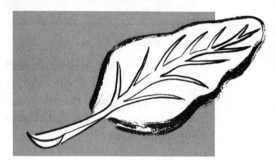

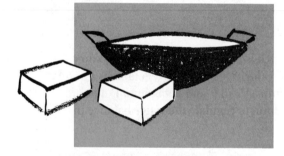

Tofu

If dairy products are on your list of foods to avoid, consider tofu. Four ounces will give you 232 milligrams of calcium per serving. Use it as a cheese substitute in a dish such as manicotti, to help cut your cholesterol.

Tomatoes

The simple tomato can help you meet your requirements for vitamins C and A in so many pleasing ways: chopped raw in salsa or gazpacho; sun-dried, sweet, and splashed with olive oil; cooked and seasoned as a spaghetti sauce.

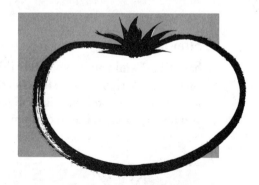

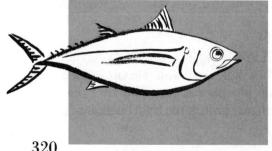

Tuna

The fish oil in tuna can help reduce inflammation from arthritis, according to a recent study. You'll benefit the most from fresh tuna steak or tuna packed in water. Avoid oil-packed tuna to keep your fat intake down.

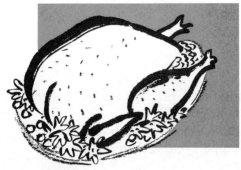

Turkey (white meat)

Good guys wear white, and turkey, a good source of niacin and zinc, is no exception. The white meat has fewer calories and less fat than the dark meat, although dark turkey meat is still more healthful than red meat.

Watermelon

Heaven can be had for just 152 calories a slice. But don't dismiss watermelon as a mere taste-pleaser. The vitamin C content of this juicy melon may help protect you against cancer of the esophagus and stomach.

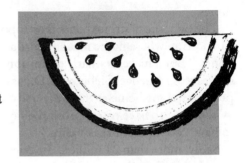

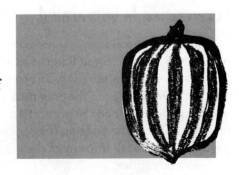

Whole-Grain Cereal

If you eat whole grains just for their fiber, think again. A morning cereal of whole grains will nourish you with vitamins B and E, protein, and minerals such as iron, magnesium, zinc, copper, manganese, and selenium.

Winter Squash

Choose butternut and hubbard squash over acorn to give you more than a day's recommended allowance of vitamin C, fiber, and beta-carotene. These three nutrients are in the spotlight as cancer protectors.

Yogurt

Can't tolerate milk? Yogurt is a fine source of calcium and B_{12}. If you eat it every day, you might find, as some recent studies did, that it will curb or completely eliminate those uncomfortable symptoms you get from other dairy foods.

OSTEOPOROSIS

Your skeleton supports you. But it's up to you to support your skeleton—to do all you can to build and maintain strong bones.

The opposite of strong bones is osteoporosis, a condition whose name means "porous bones." But a more dramatic definition comes from Michael Siebers, M.D., assistant professor of medicine at the University of Wisconsin. To have osteoporosis, he says, is to have "bones that break easily."

Sadly, more than 24 million Americans fit that description. And most of them are women. That's because the hormone estrogen acts like a dam to hold bone mass in the body. When menopause hits and estrogen all but disappears, so does bone—at the rate of about one percent a year.

Forewarned Is Forearmed

Knowing that you are at increased risk for osteoporosis may help you find the motivation to take the steps necessary to protect yourself. Women are not the only ones who need to pay special heed to preventive measures. Check the table on the opposite page to see if you fall into any of the other high-risk categories.

Whether you are at high risk or low risk, aging will change your bone formation. In children, teenagers, and even young adults, the body builds bone faster than it loses it. In the young adult, for example, 15 to 30 percent of the skeleton is renewed each year. Total bone mass remains relatively stable

during adulthood, but after age 35, bone loss exceeds bone growth.

How can you prevent this bone loss—how can you support your skeleton? Bone up by reading on.

Building Bone

For young people, the anti-osteoporosis strategy is to build as strong a skeleton as possible. Consider it an insurance policy. The stronger your bones are when you're young, the less affected they'll be by your changing body as you age.

For older people, the strategy is to slow the rate of inevitable bone loss through preventive action.

For both young and old, calcium is the key player in this bone-protection program—study after study has confirmed that a lack of calcium is a crucial factor in developing osteoporosis.

Unfortunately, "a lot of people have gotten away from drinking milk [an excellent source of calcium]," Dr. Siebers says. Many women and adolescent girls are getting less than half the recommended 1,200 milligrams of calcium each day, according to the National Osteoporosis Foundation. Many doctors even suggest that women get up to 1,500 milligrams each day.

"It's not just because I'm from Wisconsin, the dairy state," Dr. Siebers says. "People should be drinking more skim or 1 percent milk."

Nor is milk the only food that delivers a

322

valuable payload of calcium. An 8-ounce glass of skim milk contains 302 milligrams of calcium, but 4 ounces of part-skim ricotta cheese provides 337 milligrams.

Other calcium-rich foods: 2 cups of raw broccoli, cooked and drained, 356 milligrams; 3 ounces of canned-in-oil sardines, drained, including bones, 329 milligrams; 1 cup of green soybeans, cooked and drained, 262 milligrams, and 1 ounce of part-skim mozzarella, 183 milligrams. Plain, low-fat yogurt is an excellent source of calcium as well—8 ounces supplies 415 milligrams. Getting enough calcium is only part of the picture, however.

The ability to absorb calcium, like the ability to build bone, declines with age. This makes getting adequate vitamin D even more critical among older people. Vitamin D aids calcium by both increasing absorption in the intestines and raising reabsorption through the kidneys.

You should strive for a minimum of 200 international units (IU) of vitamin D each day. An 8-ounce glass of low-fat fortified milk provides you with 102 international units of vitamin D as well as a healthy dose of calcium. Tuna, salmon, and sardines are also good sources of vitamin D. So, too, is the sun, though depending on where you live,

Are You at Risk?

High Risk	Low Risk
Smoker	Black
Northern European heritage	Mediterranean heritage
Family history of osteoporosis	Dark skin
Fair skin	Dark hair
Red or blond hair	Exercise regularly
Heavy alcohol use	Adequate calcium intake
Low-calcium intake	Big-boned frame
Small-boned frame (petite)	Large muscles
Small muscles	Overweight or obese
Underweight or thin	Nondrinker
Lack of exercise	Nonsmoker

you can't count on it all the time. "Vitamin D levels in people living in northern climates tend to wax and wane with summer and winter," says Dr. Siebers. Even people living in sunshine states may not get enough of the sunshine vitamin, especially if they let the heat drive them indoors to the comfort of air-conditioned (and sunless) rooms.

People who suspect that they have trouble getting enough calcium may want to consult their doctor about taking a calcium supplement. Several are available, but Dr. Siebers recommends trying calcium carbonate first because it is usually the least expensive and offers the most calcium per tablet.

Calcium Plus Exercise Equals Stronger Bones

If you choose to lead a sedentary lifestyle, you can probably count on the bone-depletion process that occurs naturally as you age to flip into fast forward.

"We expect people diagnosed with osteoporosis who are now active walkers to continue that activity—it helps bone formation," says Joseph E. Zerwekh, Ph.D., associate professor of medicine at the University of Texas Southwestern Medical Center.

There is growing evidence to support exercise as a bone-builder. A recent study from the U.S. Department of Agriculture Human Nutrition Research Lab at Tufts University compared postmenopausal women who walked 45 minutes a day, four days a week, with a similar group of nonwalking women. Over a year, the walking women showed about a 3 percent increase in bone

density, while the inactive women showed an average reduction in bone of about 10 percent.

Really, bones aren't so different from the muscles in your arms or legs—with exercise they grow stronger. And walking is the ideal exercise for people most at risk for osteoporosis. "Work into it gradually," Dr. Siebers advises, "and aim for four times a week."

Having osteoporosis does not necessarily mean leading a more passive life. In fact, it may mean doing more—with your doctor's guidance, of course—than you had done previously.

What Else Can I Do for My Bones?

For some people, treatments such as estrogen replacement therapy may be appropriate. If this is appropriate for you, your doctor can fill you in on the details.

Screening tests for osteoporosis have become popular, but they are expensive and the National Osteoporosis Foundation does not endorse mass screenings. Still, for women at high risk, screening is worth considering, says Dr. Zerwekh.

In lieu of embracing sophisticated tests and therapies, you might want to do a little bet-hedging on your own. Don't smoke—some studies indicate you just puff away your youth and bring on early menopause. Limit your use of alcohol and caffeine and go easy on the salt. Heavy use of alcohol, caffeine, and salt have been linked with osteoporosis; they may increase the amount of calcium lost in the urine.

Don Wade

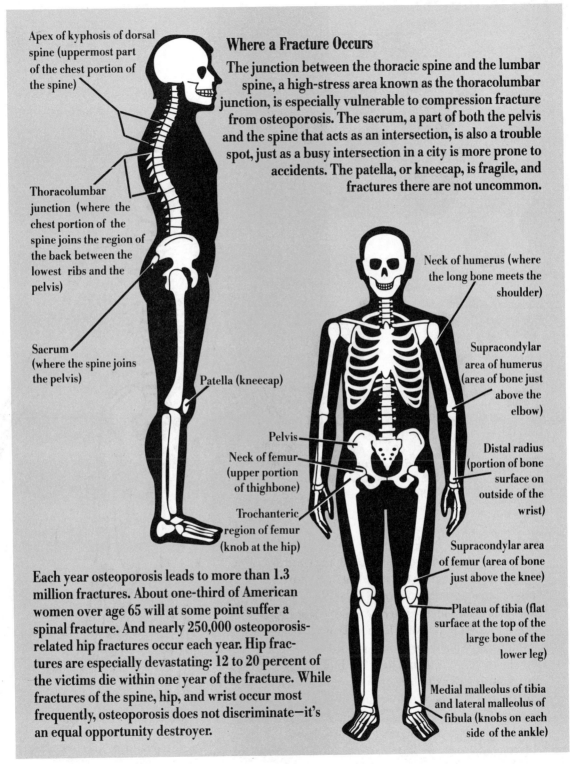

Apex of kyphosis of dorsal spine (uppermost part of the chest portion of the spine)

Thoracolumbar junction (where the chest portion of the spine joins the region of the back between the lowest ribs and the pelvis)

Sacrum (where the spine joins the pelvis)

Patella (kneecap)

Where a Fracture Occurs

The junction between the thoracic spine and the lumbar spine, a high-stress area known as the thoracolumbar junction, is especially vulnerable to compression fracture from osteoporosis. The sacrum, a part of both the pelvis and the spine that acts as an intersection, is also a trouble spot, just as a busy intersection in a city is more prone to accidents. The patella, or kneecap, is fragile, and fractures there are not uncommon.

Neck of humerus (where the long bone meets the shoulder)

Supracondylar area of humerus (area of bone just above the elbow)

Distal radius (portion of bone surface on outside of the wrist)

Pelvis

Neck of femur (upper portion of thighbone)

Trochanteric region of femur (knob at the hip)

Supracondylar area of femur (area of bone just above the knee)

Plateau of tibia (flat surface at the top of the large bone of the lower leg)

Medial malleolus of tibia and lateral malleolus of fibula (knobs on each side of the ankle)

Each year osteoporosis leads to more than 1.3 million fractures. About one-third of American women over age 65 will at some point suffer a spinal fracture. And nearly 250,000 osteoporosis-related hip fractures occur each year. Hip fractures are especially devastating: 12 to 20 percent of the victims die within one year of the fracture. While fractures of the spine, hip, and wrist occur most frequently, osteoporosis does not discriminate—it's an equal opportunity destroyer.

OSTEOPOROSIS

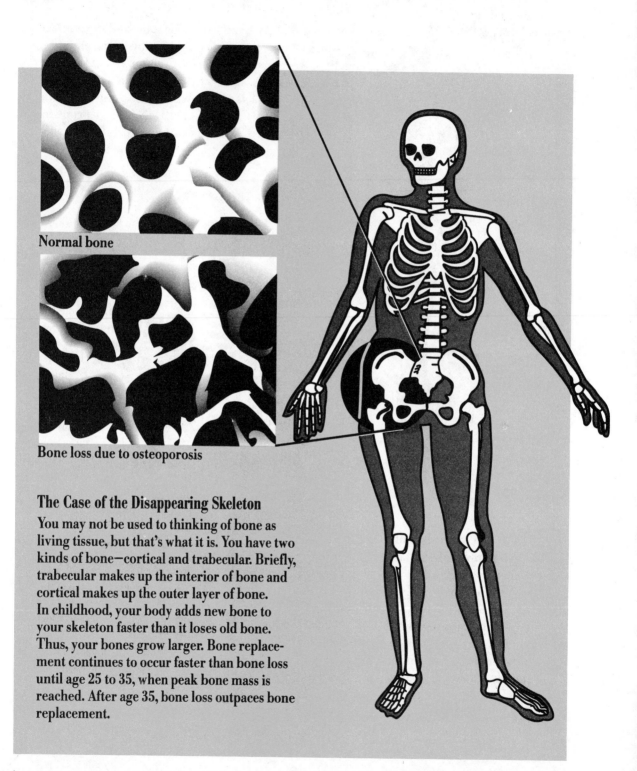

Normal bone

Bone loss due to osteoporosis

The Case of the Disappearing Skeleton

You may not be used to thinking of bone as
living tissue, but that's what it is. You have two
kinds of bone—cortical and trabecular. Briefly,
trabecular makes up the interior of bone and
cortical makes up the outer layer of bone.
In childhood, your body adds new bone to
your skeleton faster than it loses old bone.
Thus, your bones grow larger. Bone replacement continues to occur faster than bone loss
until age 25 to 35, when peak bone mass is
reached. After age 35, bone loss outpaces bone
replacement.

OVERWEIGHT

For years, cheesecake cried out to Sonja Connor each time she opened the refrigerator door. She knew she shouldn't eat it, but she couldn't resist.

Connor, a registered dietitian, is associate professor in the Department of Medicine at the University of Oregon Health Sciences Center, coauthor of *The New American Diet*, and a specialist in heart disease and obesity research. Even she—despite her specialty—knows what it feels like to get hung up on a specific food.

"Cheesecake was a big deal to me," she says. "I just couldn't stop wanting to eat it. And then, one day, I decided not to buy it again."

The same mind-set—making a firm commitment to change an eating habit—gets results if you want to lose weight. "If people get to a certain point where they are *ready* to make changes, they will have less of a problem losing weight," she says. "But don't call this method of weight loss a diet. Call it an eating style."

She and her husband, William E. Connor, M.D., a professor in the Division of Endocrinology, Metabolism, and Nutrition at the University of Oregon, studied 233 families over five years, charting successes and failures at lowering their fat intake. Through this study the couple discovered what they consider the two important secrets to losing weight and maintaining a healthy body weight: (1) gradual changes that lead to (2) new habits.

The Dieting Dilemma

The problem with diets, says Connor, is that they are often self-defeating. When dieters don't learn new eating habits, they return to old behavior patterns when the diet is done. Some dieters lose the game before they even begin to play because they try to change too many behavior patterns at once—and they tire quickly of all the restrictions. The dieter runs into enough barriers without constructing additional obstacles by trying to overdo.

"In our society, there's little support for eating low-fat foods. You have to work hard to go to the grocery store and buy low-fat food. You have to look hard for the recipes that encourage low-fat eating," she says. "And everything in society pushes us to be less active: valet parking, elevators, escalators."

Quick weight-loss schemes are doomed, too, according to Kelly Brownell, Ph.D., obesity researcher at the University of Pennsylvania in Philadelphia.

Severe dieting actually makes dieting more difficult because it reduces the body's natural calorie needs, says Dr. Brownell. Your body thinks you're starving, so it stays busy storing up fat to get you through what it perceives as the next famine. Your metabolism slows down and tries to conserve every calorie you eat.

What happens is that the first time you diet, you lose weight easily. But then, if you are what's known as a yo-yo dieter, you gain the weight back. You diet again, but your second effort at calorie cutting takes longer to achieve the same weight loss. What's worse, studies show, you gain the weight back again more rapidly than ever.

Victuals for Victory

To be successful, you have to slowly integrate good eating habits into your life. "You need to develop a whole new lifestyle," says Connor.

And whether you are a winner in that new eating behavior may hinge simply on how many new recipes and new foods you are willing to try. The winning foods are low in fat and high in fiber and definitely include fresh fruits and vegetables. Don't give up in your search for foods that satisfy you while slimming you down.

"You don't like all the high-fat recipes you try, so you shouldn't expect to like all the low-fat recipes you try," says Connor. "Most people don't really care if what they eat is high in fat or low in fat, they just look for taste. So, if you incorporate the low-fat recipes you do like into your life, pretty soon the high-fat recipes and low-fat recipes will be equal in number. And eventually the low-fat recipes will outnumber the high-fat recipes. Just find low-fat, high-fiber foods you like to eat and make them a permanent part of your weekly menu."

Exercise is another important ingredient in the successful weight control equation, says Jane Moore, Ph.D., a registered dietitian who is a nutrition consultant with the Oregon Health Division. In a nine-month study conducted by Dr. Moore, women learned new nutrition habits and gradually incorporated them into their lives. They also gathered three times a week to walk for 40 minutes.

At the end of the nine-month study, the average weight loss was 11 pounds. Participants found that 95 percent of the weight lost was fat tissue. Dr. Moore attributes the loss of fat rather than muscle tissue to the regular exercise along with a low-fat diet that reduced calories only moderately.

"What's most important to learn from this is that people need to change their eating *and* exercise behaviors and not necessarily peg their success to what their scales say," says Dr. Moore.

Hurdling the Overweight Obstacles

You have a battle ahead of you, but with the right strategy, you are bound to win. Here are a few more weapons for your fat-fighter's arsenal.

While you are gaining control over your weight, learn to plan meals ahead so you can shop thoughtfully—from a list. Don't ever go to the store hungry. And if you must buy fattening foods for other family members, buy them treats you don't like.

At home, store high-calorie items in hard-to-reach places. Eat only at the kitchen or dining room table. Concentrate on what you are eating and how much food your body wants; don't eat while watching television, reading, or talking on the phone.

Eat meals slowly. It takes about 20 minutes for your body to signal that it's full, so eating quickly may fill you beyond what is necessary to satisfy your appetite. Experts

How to Figure Body Fat

How much fat are you carrying around? Find your percentage of body fat with this chart. To calculate your body fat, use a ruler to line up your measurements. Men, line up your waist measurement (taken at belly button level) with body weight. Women, line up your hip measurement (taken at the widest point) with height. Your ruler will pass through the "percentage of fat" line at your personal reading. Men above 17 percent and women above 24 percent are considered plump.

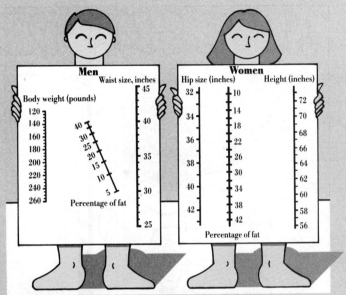

Note. From *Sensible Fitness*, Second Edition (pp. 31–31) by J. H. Wilmore, 1986, Champaign, Ill.: Leisure Press. Copyright 1986 by Jack H. Wilmore. Reprinted by permission.

suggest laying down your fork between bites and chewing your food thoroughly as two ways to fill the time.

And don't fool yourself into thinking that eating on social occasions will help cut calories. People eat 44 percent more food when they eat in a group than when they eat alone, according to a study at Georgia State University. Researchers found that when people eat alone, they eat smaller meals and their meals are lower in fat and higher in carbohydrates.

Stalling at the 10-Yard Line

As you near your weight goal, your weight loss may stall 5 or 10 pounds shy of the finish line. That's all right, say the experts. Congratulate yourself on your success. Then take a vacation from dieting and work on your maintenance plan.

For every pound you have lost, you'll burn 10 calories fewer per day, just because you are lighter. That means that to maintain your lower weight, you may be able to eat more than you did while dieting, but never as much as you did at your peak weight. After a 30-pound loss, for instance, your calorie intake will have to be 300 calories fewer per day than the calories you ate at your starting weight.

After you've maintained your new weight for three to six months, tackle the remaining pounds by eating a moderately reduced high-carbohydrate diet and by brisk walking for an hour or so each day. Your goal will be within your grasp.

Claudia Allen

WHY STAN'S DIET DIDN'T WORK...

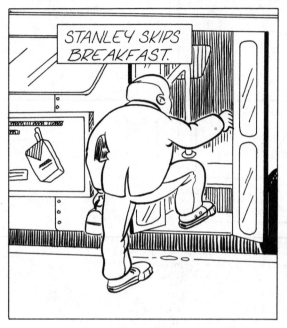

STANLEY SKIPS BREAKFAST.

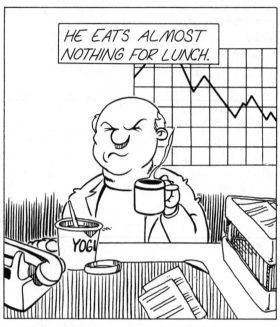

HE EATS ALMOST NOTHING FOR LUNCH.

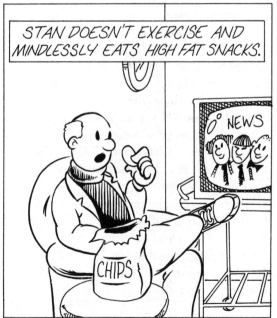

STAN DOESN'T EXERCISE AND MINDLESSLY EATS HIGH FAT SNACKS.

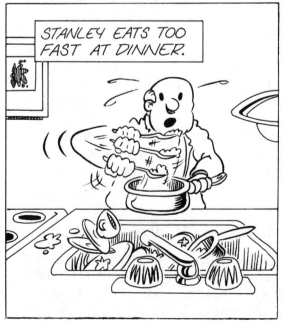

STANLEY EATS TOO FAST AT DINNER.

AND STELLA'S DIET DID!

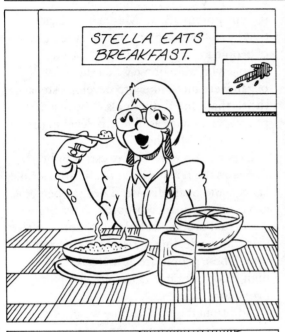

STELLA EATS BREAKFAST.

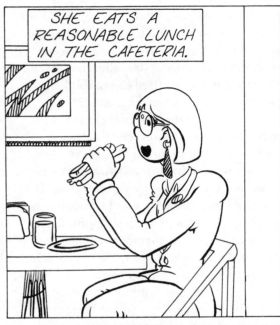

SHE EATS A REASONABLE LUNCH IN THE CAFETERIA.

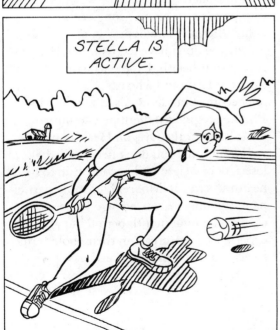

STELLA IS ACTIVE.

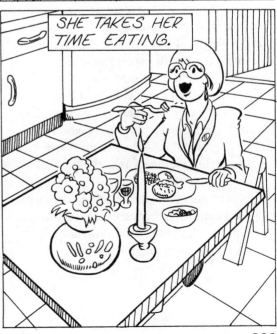

SHE TAKES HER TIME EATING.

OVERWEIGHT

Additional Burdens on the Overweight Body

Pick up a 10-pound bag of sugar and carry it around for a while. Climb stairs with it against your hip. Hold it tightly when you stoop to pick up laundry. Balance it across your shoulders during your afternoon stroll.

Does it make you tired just to think about carrying that extra weight around?

Well, think of that bag of sugar as the saddlebags you carry on your thighs, the spare tire around your middle, the padded cushion on your hips. You may not notice those extra pounds, but your body does. If you don't shed the extra weight, you may pay a steep price in increased health problems.

Studies show a disturbing relationship between body weight and medical problems. For every extra pound you carry, your risk of problems multiplies disproportionately.

For instance, people who are 15 percent overweight have a 40 percent better chance of having a digestive disease than someone at normal weight. The chance of digestive disease increases 150 percent in someone who is 25 percent or more overweight.

Because diabetes is so closely linked to obesity, some medical researchers have combined the two words into one: "diabesity." Experts say that if Americans simply weighed what they should, nearly two-thirds of all cases of diabetes would disappear.

Doctors also link obesity and osteoarthritis —a joint condition that can make walking or standing painful in the knees and ankles. They go so far as to suggest that excess weight may cause the condition. In the famous Framingham, Massachusetts, study that has followed the health of large numbers of people for years, researchers found that people who were obese when the study began were more likely to develop osteoarthritis than slim individuals. The heaviest people were twice as likely to develop the disease as the slimmest.

Experts also warn that excess weight increases the possibility of death from stroke, cancer, and heart disease. They say being fat can cause pregnancy problems, sterility, menstrual problems, kidney stones, varicose veins, and a decline in testosterone production. Obese people are at increased risk of high blood pressure. They are also more prone to accidents.

Additionally, experts note weight control may prevent gallstones, congestive heart failure, hernias, and depression.

Yet, you don't have to go on a crash diet to regain your health. People who learn to eat the right foods and who exercise regularly *can* become fit individuals, says Jane Moore, Ph.D., a registered dietitian and nutrition consultant for the Oregon Health Division.

"I found that you don't necessarily have to lose a lot of weight and become thin to be healthy," says Dr. Moore. Her study participants not only lost an average 11 pounds each over a nine-month period but also experienced a decrease in their cholesterol levels and blood pressure readings.

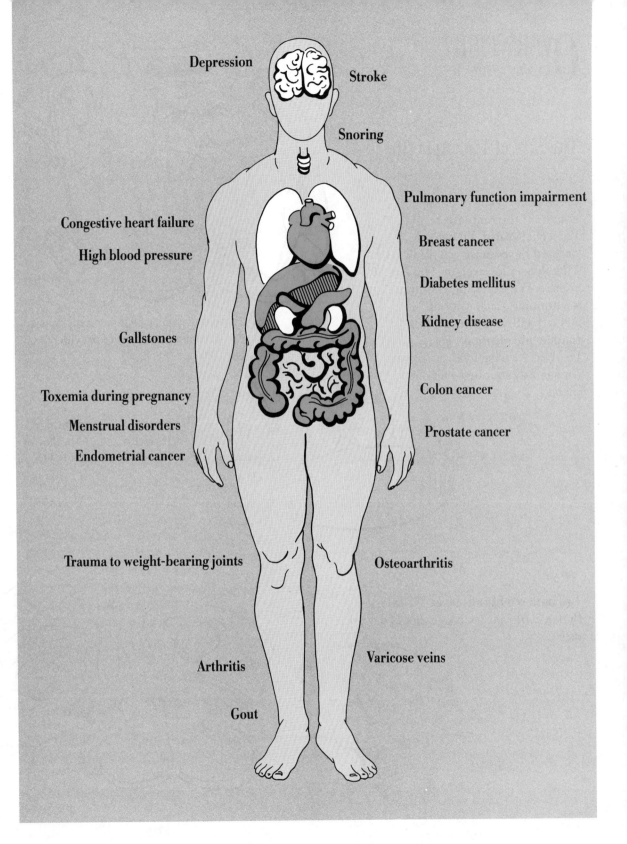

OVERWEIGHT

The Size of Your Appetite

Weight loss would be ever so much easier if only foods would announce their intentions: "Hi, I'm a chef's salad. I'll bet you ordered me because you think I'll help you lose weight. Ha! Fat chance. With dressing I contain a whopping 1,500 calories." Armed with a calorie counter (and an imagination), you *can* begin to see what food can do for (or against) your best-laid diet plans.

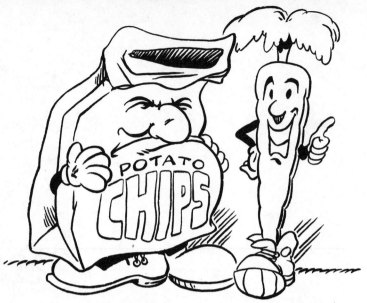

Munching a mere 20 potato chips costs you 228 calories. A carrot provides only 30.

Ice cream . . . mmmmmm. At 254 calories a cup . . . ughhh. Plain yogurt is 113.

Two buttered biscuits boast 278 calories. Better, at 61 calories, is one slice of dry rye toast.

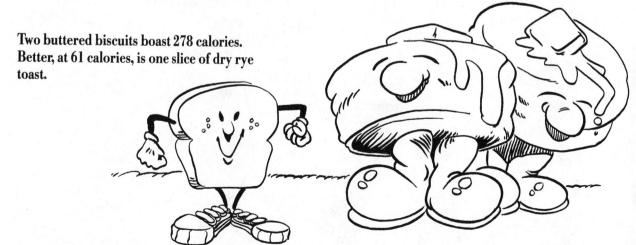

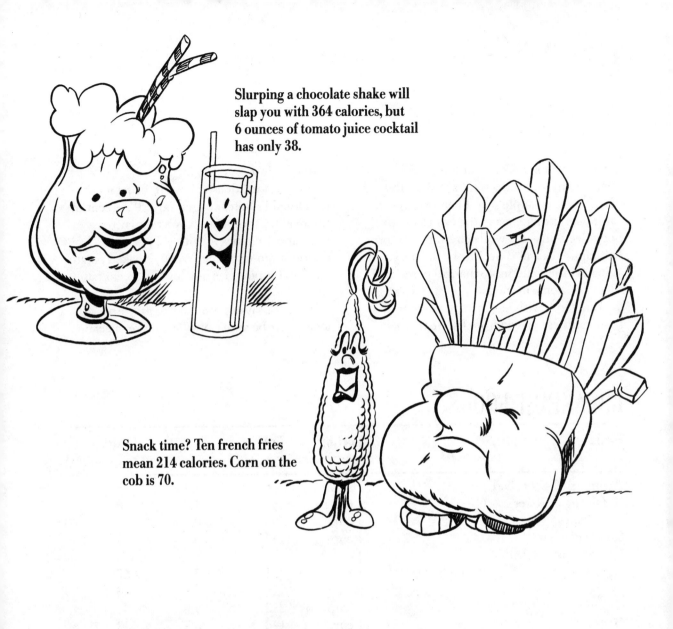

Slurping a chocolate shake will slap you with 364 calories, but 6 ounces of tomato juice cocktail has only 38.

Snack time? Ten french fries mean 214 calories. Corn on the cob is 70.

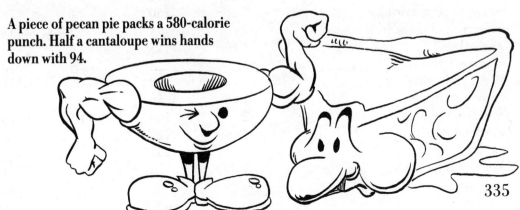

A piece of pecan pie packs a 580-calorie punch. Half a cantaloupe wins hands down with 94.

335

Count Those Calories

Got a yen for a bacon double cheeseburger with fries and a vanilla shake? Topped off with a fried apple pie? Then prepare to eat in one sitting most of the calories your body needs in a day while consuming more fat than is healthy. That meal will cost you 1,363 calories, and more than 50 percent of them will come in the form of fat. Experts say that foods with less than 30 percent of their calories derived from fat are the best hedge against overweight.

But fast food doesn't have to be fat food. McDonald's hotcakes get only 20 percent of their calories from fat. Roy's regular roast beef sandwich logs in with a 28 percent calories-from-fat rating. Wendy's baked potato with no toppings earns a low 7 percent fat rating.

No one's saying you have to give up fast food—just be aware of what you're ordering.

BREAKFAST FOODS

Food	Portion	Total Calories	Fat (g)	Calories from Fat (%)
Bacon, fried or broiled	1 slice	36	3.1	77
Bagel, egg or water	1 (2 oz.)	163	1.4	8
Corn flakes	1 cup	98	0.1	1
Cream of wheat	1 cup	143	0.6	3
Egg, raw or poached	1	79	5.6	63
Egg, scrambled with milk and butter	1	95	7.1	67
Egg substitute	¼ cup	25	0.0	0
Granola	½ cup	252	9.8	35
Grits	1 cup	146	0.5	3
Instant breakfast drink	1 cup	280	8.0	26
Oat cereal, O-shaped	1 cup	91	1.1	11
Oatmeal	1 cup	145	2.4	15
Pancakes (from mix)	1	58	2.1	32
Rice cereal, crispy	1 cup	109	11.9	11
Rice cereal, puffed	1 cup	56	0.1	2
Sausage links, low-fat	2	160	11.5	66
Shredded wheat	1 cup	116	0.6	5
Waffles (from mix)	1	205	8.0	35
Wheat germ, toasted	1 tbsp.	26	0.8	25

FAST FOODS

Food	Portion	Total Calories	Fat (g)	Calories from Fat (%)
Arby's				
Bacon 'n Cheddar Deluxe	Average	526	35.7	61
Fish fillet sandwich	Average	580	30.9	48
Roast beef sandwich	5 oz.	350	15.0	39
Burger King				
Bacon Double Cheeseburger	Average	510	31.0	55
Chicken sandwich	Average	688	40.0	52
Onion rings	Regular	274	16.0	53
Vanilla shake	Regular	321	10.0	28
Whaler	Average	488	27.0	50
Whopper	Average	630	36.0	51
McDonald's				
Big Mac	7.6 oz.	562	32.4	52
Chef's salad	10 oz.	231	13.6	53
Chicken oriental salad	8.6 oz.	141	3.4	22
Garden salad	7.5 oz.	112	6.8	55
Fillet of fish sandwich	Regular	442	26.1	53
French fries	Regular	220	11.5	47
Hamburger	Regular	257	9.5	33
Quarter pounder with cheese	Average	517	29.2	51
Soft-serve cone	3 oz.	144	4.5	28
Roy Rogers				
Chicken breast	Average	324	18.0	50
Taco Bell				
Bean burrito	6.7 oz.	357	10.2	26
Beef burrito	6.7 oz.	403	17.3	39
Taco	Regular	183	10.8	53
Taco, light	6.7 oz.	410	28.8	63
Taco salad	21 oz.	941	61.3	59
Wendy's				
Baked potato	8.8 oz.	250	2.0	7
Baked potato with broccoli and cheese	12.9 oz.	500	25.0	45
Big Classic Double	Average	680	39.0	52
Chef's salad	11.7 oz.	180	9.0	45
Chicken sandwich	Average	430	19.0	40
Taco salad	27.9 oz.	660	37.0	51

DELI FOODS

Food	Portion	Total Calories	Fat (g)	Calories from Fat (%)
Bagel with cream cheese	2 oz.	361	21.2	53
Bologna, pork	1 oz.	70	5.6	72
Chef's salad	Average	722	56.1	70
Chicken salad	Average	509	39.0	69
Coleslaw	½ cup	127	11.1	79
Corned beef	1 oz.	71	5.4	68
Egg salad	Average	425	41.0	86
Greek salad with feta cheese	Average	377	21.5	51
Grilled cheese sandwich	Regular	440	31.0	63
Ham, baked	1 oz.	52	3.0	52
Ham and cheese loaf	1 oz.	73	5.7	71
Ham and cheese sandwich on rye with mustard and mayonnaise	Regular	615	37.7	55
Hero sandwich on roll	4.75 oz.	1,154	62.2	49
Liverwurst	1 oz.	93	8.1	78
Macaroni salad	Average	286	25.1	79
Olive loaf	1 oz.	67	4.7	63
Pastrami, beef	1 oz.	99	8.3	75
Pastrami, beef, sandwich on rye	Regular	541	36.0	60
Pastrami, turkey	1 oz.	40	2.1	46
Pimiento and pickle loaf	1 oz.	74	6.0	73
Potato salad with mayonnaise	¾ cup	288	18.9	59
Reuben, grilled, on rye	Regular	835	59.5	64
Roast beef sandwich on rye with horseradish	Regular	444	18.8	38
Roast beef sandwich on rye with lettuce, tomato, and mayonnaise	Regular	576	35.1	55
Salami, cooked, beef	1 oz.	72	5.7	72
Salami, hard	1 oz.	116	9.6	74
Tuna/cheese melt	Regular	640	48.2	68
Tuna salad	⅓ cup	306	26.1	77
Turkey	1 oz.	37	1.4	36
Turkey club sandwich	Regular	626	33.5	48
Turkey club sandwich on whole wheat	Regular	357	14.3	36
Turkey sandwich on whole wheat	Regular	297	11.6	35

PET CARE

They win us over with their enthusiastic tail-wagging, frolicking, slobbery kissing, nuzzling, cuddling, and pur-r-r-ring. But while a dog or a cat can bring laughter, love, and cheer into our lives, it also brings responsibilities.

"Caring for a dog or cat is much like caring for a young child. It is clearly a relationship in which someone totally depends on you," says Richard H. Pitcairn, D.V.M., Ph.D., veterinarian (and father) in Eugene, Oregon, and author of *Dr. Pitcairn's Complete Guide to Natural Health for Dogs and Cats.*

Just like being a good parent, being a good guardian for a dog or cat requires both wisdom and knowledge. On the following pages you'll find lots of tips to help you take care of your pet. Mix with plenty of love, and you'll be well on your way to having the healthiest and happiest animal on the block.

Nibbles beyond Kibbles

Walking the pet food aisle of your local supermarket, you could easily be overwhelmed by the enormous selection of dried and canned meals for pets. How do you choose what's best? That's easy, says Dr. Pitcairn—turn around, walk out the door, and go home. "I promote a home-prepared diet. My experience is when people do this, they have much healthier pets," he says.

The problem with commercial pet foods is that they are often loaded with preservatives, artificial colorings (to make them look good to humans), and meat by-products that are generally somewhat below standards for human consumption and questionable even for animals, says Dr. Pitcairn. So, what's better? "Fresh meat, dairy products, fish, eggs, grains, legumes, and vegetables," he says.

In other words, our pets thrive on a varied, wholesome diet just as we do. The main difference between us and our pets is that dogs and cats need more protein and calcium, says Dr. Pitcairn. For sufficient protein, provide foods like meat, dairy products, eggs (dogs and cats needn't worry about cholesterol), and nuts.

For more calcium, consider supplements—it's hard for dogs and cats to get what they need in their diets.

Dogs need about 115 milligrams a day per pound of body weight, says Dr. Pitcairn. That's a lot of calcium—a 20-pound dog would need more than 2 quarts of whole milk. Cats need a total of 200 milligrams per day, or the equivalent of 1½ cups of low-fat cottage cheese.

If your life is too hectic to prepare doggie dinners, Dr. Pitcairn recommends that you use one of the alternative brands of pet food generally sold in health food stores. Although a bit more expensive, they tend to be of higher quality.

Whether you buy pet food in a health food store or in a supermarket, it should always be marked "nutritionally complete and balanced." And try to steer away from the generic or store-brand foods. Some of these have been found to be nutritionally inadequate.

Slim Down Tubby Tabby and Flabby Fido

How *much* you feed your pet can be as important as *what* you feed your pet. Overfeeding may very well be the most common pet-care mistake people make. Keep an eye on your dog or cat's weight, and control how much he eats accordingly. Fat cats and dogs are more likely to suffer from joint disorders, heart disease, and other ailments.

The way to tell if your pet is overweight is by looking and feeling, says Amy Marder, V.M.D., clinical assistant professor at the Tufts University School of Veterinary Medicine. A trim dog or cat looks lean and firm. He should not have a sagging tummy. A dog should have a clearly defined waistline behind the rib cage. Feel the ribs along the underside of the torso to detect flab, says Dr. Marder. If you can easily feel each rib, that's good. If you can't feel any ribs at all, that's bad.

If your pet does have a weight problem, make an appointment to see the veterinarian, says Dr. Marder. He or she can rule out any serious health problems that may be causing your pet's puffiness. Then your vet can help you develop a kitty or doggie diet plan.

It's best to divide your pet's total allocation of chow into two or three small meals rather than one big one. Your little guy won't feel so hungry and will be less inclined to beg at the dinner table. Try not to give your pets snacks throughout the day. If you feel you must, Dr. Marder suggests offering something low in calories, like a carrot for your dog or a teaspoon of fat-free cottage cheese for your cat.

"Dogs require quite a bit of exercise. It's in their nature. That's how they evolved," says Dr. Pitcairn. Determining what constitutes the right amount of exercise for your dog will depend on the breed. Most dogs need at least half an hour a day to stretch their muscles and get their hearts pumping.

Besides, exercising your dog becomes a good incentive to exercise yourself. You may want to plop down in front of the TV, but it's impossible to resist the plea in those big brown eyes. Fulfilling your responsibility means taking him on walks or runs in the park, having him chase balls or retrieve sticks, or giving him the opportunity to romp with fellow pups.

These activities also satisfy a great psychological need. "Dogs have simple mentalities. It's hard for us to comprehend how exciting it is for them to walk around checking out smells. It's like our going to the movies or visiting friends. They love it," says Dr. Pitcairn.

Cats are another story. They don't have the stamina to romp around for long periods of time the way dogs do, says Dr. Pitcairn. Cats tend to get the exercise they need in shorter spurts, he says. You can help your little tiger stay fit and happy by playing games with him for 10–15 minutes a day. Cats get a kick out of chasing lightweight balls and playing with toys on strings. Having two kitties so they can wrestle with each other is also a good way of providing exercise.

Remember that whenever your animal ventures into the great outdoors, a host of dangers can present themselves, including fights with other animals, poisons on grass or in trash, and run-ins with motor vehicles. Protect your vulnerable friends by keeping a careful eye on them. Fences and leashes protect dogs—and people, too.

What a Pretty Pooch!

Bathing and brushing your pet makes him look and smell his best. But proper grooming is also important to an animal's health, says Dr. Pitcairn. Daily brushing is ideal for dogs and cats, he says. Monthly baths for dogs are also a good idea, as are baths for cats several times a year.

Bathing and brushing not only remove dead skin, loose hairs, burrs, and blades of grass, they also help to remove the pollutants that animals pick up as a result of living in a human's world.

And whisking away pollution isn't the only benefit to grooming. "It's also a good time to check your animal for tumors, wounds, and other things that, if not detected early, can mean trouble," says Dr. Pitcairn. You should also be checking for parasites such as fleas and ticks that attach themselves to your pet's skin.

Roll Over, Casanova

Neutering your pet will prevent him or her from reproducing and adding to the pet overpopulation problem. It also offers numerous health benefits, even if your dog or cat is confined and never allowed to come into contact with other animals, says Dr. Marder.

Spaying, which is the removal of the entire uterus and both ovaries in a female animal,

will protect her from potentially fatal uterine infections and tumors. It also drastically reduces the incidence of breast cancer.

Castration, the removal of the male's testicles, reduces the incidence of roaming, mounting, urine marking, and aggression with other males. Your male pet, once neutered, will be less likely to fight with other animals or to get hit by cars while roaming around looking for a date. Neutered males are also much less likely to develop prostate disease and some types of tumors, says Dr. Marder.

Get Your Pet to the Vet

Your pet probably doesn't like going to the vet any more than you like going to the dentist. Take him anyway. Regular vet care, a yearly exam at the least, is an important way to keep your pet healthy.

During the annual exam, your veterinarian can detect diseases in their early stages—before they get too serious. He or she will also see to it that your pet is up-to-date on all of his vaccinations.

However, pets with allergies or immune problems should probably not be receiving these vaccinations. Let your veterinarian know if your pet has a history of allergies.

Russell Wild

341

Give Your Pet a Quick Checkup

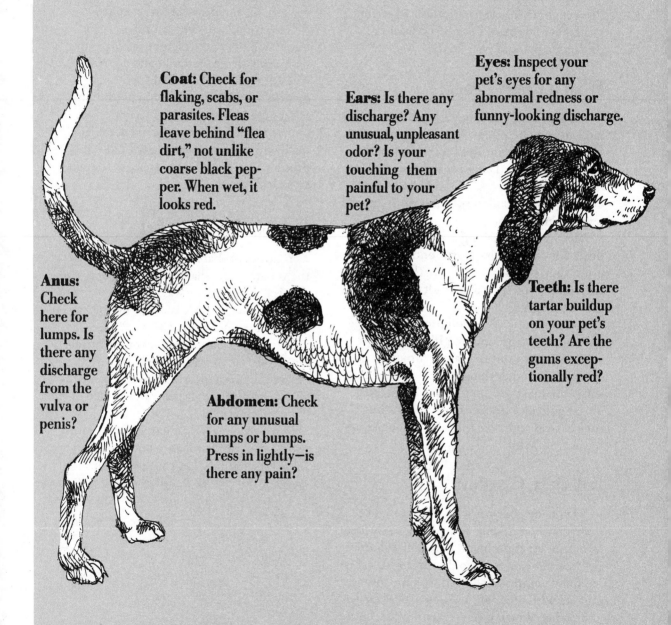

Coat: Check for flaking, scabs, or parasites. Fleas leave behind "flea dirt," not unlike coarse black pepper. When wet, it looks red.

Ears: Is there any discharge? Any unusual, unpleasant odor? Is your touching them painful to your pet?

Eyes: Inspect your pet's eyes for any abnormal redness or funny-looking discharge.

Anus: Check here for lumps. Is there any discharge from the vulva or penis?

Abdomen: Check for any unusual lumps or bumps. Press in lightly—is there any pain?

Teeth: Is there tartar buildup on your pet's teeth? Are the gums exceptionally red?

How to Tell If Your Pet Is Sick

Even without a medical degree, you can often tell when people are in poor health: they slouch, they drag, they cough, they're always tired. But what about dogs and cats? Early detection of health problems can lengthen your pet's life—if you know what to look for.

There are a host of symptoms that signal poor health in both dogs and cats.

Despite those cat food commercials that star finicky cats, such behavior is quite abnormal. "A normal, healthy cat is not a finicky cat," says veterinarian Richard H. Pitcairn, D.V.M., Ph.D., of Eugene, Oregon, author of *Dr. Pitcairn's Complete Guide to Natural Health for Dogs and Cats.* One of the most common signs of feline health problems is the cat that at first looks happy and excited when you put his dish down, but then turns up his nose and whiskers at first sniff of his food. Such a cat may be on his way to developing liver or thyroid problems or other internal disorders and should have a medical checkup.

While healthy cats like to eat, they don't generally drink, says Dr. Pitcairn. "Cats get just about all the water they need from the food they eat—healthy cats rarely drink, maybe once a week," he says. If your cat is drinking every day, it's an alert that something may be wrong. Ask your vet.

Dogs show ill health in different ways than cats. Typical warning signs of a sickly pup are constant scratching, dandruff, and a "scaly look," says Dr. Pitcairn. Similarly, a bad smell, a "musty" or "corn-chip kind of smell," are signs of an unhealthy dog.

Excessive licking, especially of the front paws, is also a cue. Licking or gnawing on his paws is a dog's way of telling the world, "I don't feel so hot."

Hip problems are a common health problem, particularly in breeds such as German shepherds. How do you recognize hip problems? "Observe them running," says Dr. Pitcairn. "They'll keep their rear feet together kind of like a bunny might hop. If it isn't a hip problem, it might be a spine problem. In either case, see your vet."

Another thing to check is the ears. If the ears smell bad, if they tend to produce a lot of a dark brown or black waxy matter, if they are red or itchy or cause your dog to shake his head, it's a sign of trouble. Get to the vet.

Vet Alert Symptoms

Some symptoms, whether found in your dog or your cat, indicate health problems. One of the most common is a change in weight, especially if your pet is eating normally. Weight loss may signal a gastrointestinal or metabolic disorder such as hyperthyroidism, a condition common in older cats. A loss of 1 pound in a cat or small dog or 2 to 3 pounds in a larger dog is reason to consult your vet. Sudden weight gain can also spell trouble. Also take heed if your pet seems especially lethargic.

Other signs of pet disease that warrant visits to the doctor include visible discomfort or pain, repeated vomiting or diarrhea lasting for more than a day, constipation, blood in the stool, coughing, excessive sneezing, and excessive urination.

PET CARE

Grooming Your Pet

Many cats, and some dogs, do a fairly good job of keeping themselves clean. Nevertheless, they still need human help to keep looking—and feeling—their best. In fact, grooming is an important part of an animal's preventive health program. It helps keep the skin, ears, and teeth in top condition. And grooming sessions are a perfect time for performing the quick checkup illustrated here and on the opposite page. Proper grooming also includes lots of touching, which will strengthen the bond between you and your pet. If possible, long-haired animals should be groomed daily, and short-haired weekly.

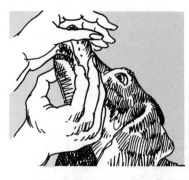

To clean and inspect your dog's teeth, you'll first have to open his mouth. But your pooch can be mighty obstinate. Try holding the lower jaw firmly with one hand while blocking the nostrils with the other.

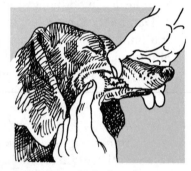

Using a toothbrush—firm or soft—can possibly hurt your pet's sensitive gums. So instead of a brush, use a damp cotton ball, a damp washcloth, or a gauze pad to remove any surface debris.

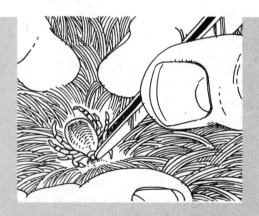

Tackling a Tick
Ticks, yuck. With fingernails or tweezers, grab 'em as close to the animal's skin as possible. You want to make sure the pest's head is not left behind, so rather than jerking, pull slowly with a slight twist. Wash your hands when finished.

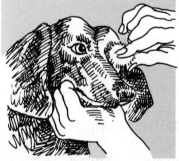

For cleaning the eyes, you'll need a moist cotton ball. Loose hairs, eyelashes, dirt, and mucus can be cleaned away with gentle wiping. Use a fresh cotton ball for each eye.

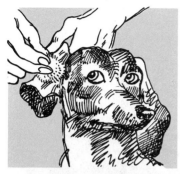

Ears should be wiped regularly, especially big, droopy ears, such as those of spaniels and dachshunds. Use a fresh cotton ball moistened with a little alcohol or vegetable oil to remove any dirt and excess wax.

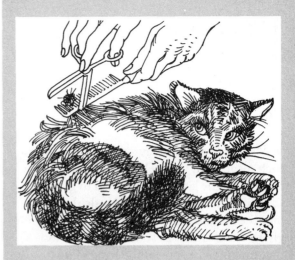

How to De-Mat

Grip the mat with your fingers and begin to separate the hairs. Tease the rest of the mat out with a wide-toothed comb. Once you get the mat far enough out from the skin to keep from injuring your pet, snip it off with scissors.

Your Good Grooming Tool Kit

Keeping your pet well groomed shouldn't require a warehouse full of utensils. The ones you will probably find most helpful are *(1)* cotton balls, *(2)* a seamstress's stitch remover to remove knots, *(3)* a metal comb with wide teeth, *(4)* a fine-toothed flea comb, *(5)* a slotted spoon to clean cat litter, *(6)* toenail clippers, *(7)* a chamois cloth, *(8)* a fine-toothed comb, *(9)* a rubber brush with nubbles, *(10)* and a stiff-bristled brush.

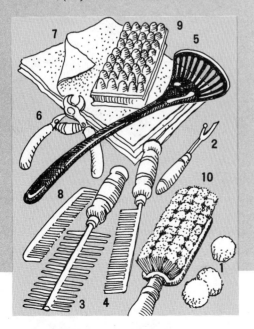

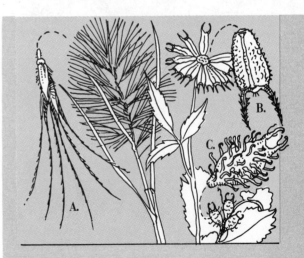

Plants That Hitch a Ride

Removing burrs from your pet's fur requires patience—and maybe scissors. Watch for the plants that can cause problems, including: a. foxtail, b. beggar-tick, and c. cocklebur.

345

PET CARE

How to Give Medications

The vet says, "Give him two of these after each meal," and you feel a sudden terror. You remember the last time you tried to give your little darling a pill—and little darling mouthed it and spit it out, 23 times. But giving medications to your pet isn't really that tough, once you get the hang of it. Below are some tips from veterinarian Richard H. Pitcairn, D.V.M., Ph.D., on making the pills and liquid medicines go down smoothly. If administering a liquid is easier than a pill, you can always grind the pill and mix it with water.

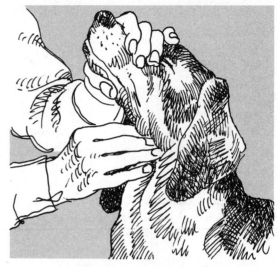

2. You next want to keep the head tilted back slightly so that the medicine will flow down the throat. Gently stroking the throat will encourage your pet to swallow. Gently hold the mouth closed as you massage. Your dog or cat may not appreciate this, so be firm.

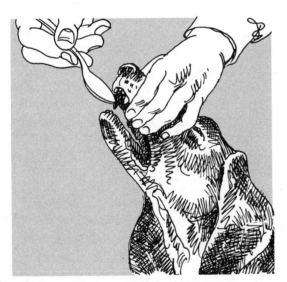

1. The first step in giving a liquid medication is to hold your pet's head up, pry the mouth open with your thumb and forefingers, and pour the medicine between the front teeth, using either a spoon or a dropper. If your pet resists, pull out the lower lip to form a pocket.

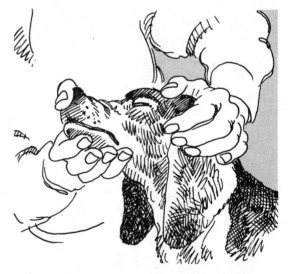

3. If your dog or cat is determined not to swallow his medicine, you can induce swallowing by gently putting your thumb over the nostrils for a brief moment. This will almost always do the trick with even the most stubborn animal.

346

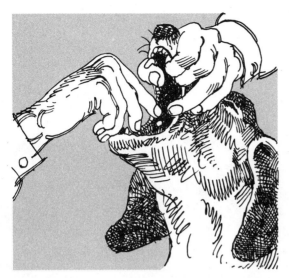

4. Giving your pet a pill should not be a major task, either. Hold the animal's head up. Pry the mouth open and place the pill on the back of the tongue and quickly push it as far back as you can. Hold the muzzle shut and massage the throat to get your pet to swallow.

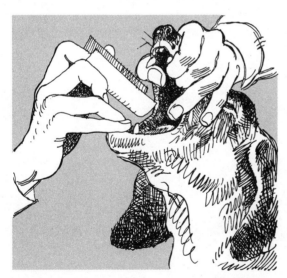

5. To administer a powder or a crushed pill, start by making a crisp fold in a small clean sheet of paper. Pour the medicine onto the paper and then let it slide from the paper directly onto the tongue. This will eliminate the possibility of your pet spitting the medicine out.

The Art of Wax Removal

Dogs and cats get wax in their ears, just as humans do. And as with human ears, you should *not* use a cotton swab to get the wax out, except perhaps around the outer parts. Veterinarian Richard H. Pitcairn, D.V.M., Ph.D., suggests using warm (not hot!) olive oil. The oil loosens and dissolves the lodged wax and helps bring it out. You may want to enlist a friend's help in holding your pet still — if he's free to shake, you're likely to get warm olive oil all over your clothes!

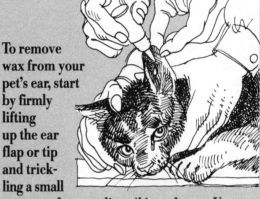

To remove wax from your pet's ear, start by firmly lifting up the ear flap or tip and trickling a small amount of warm olive oil into the ear. Use either a dropper or a squeeze bottle.

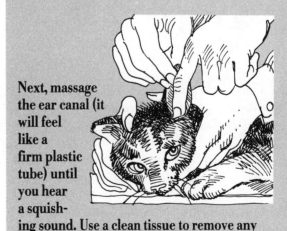

Next, massage the ear canal (it will feel like a firm plastic tube) until you hear a squishing sound. Use a clean tissue to remove any excess oil and debris that works its way out.

CPR: It's Not Just for Humans

You've probably heard of CPR (cardio-pulmonary resuscitation) saving human lives. With a few modifications, this same technique can be used to help animals in distress. In fact, if your pet's heart stops, your knowledge of CPR could make all the difference in whether he lives or dies.

While performing CPR on an animal requires some coordination, the technique can be learned. Don't wait until you're confronted with an emergency. A little study and practice ahead of time will prepare you for the worst.

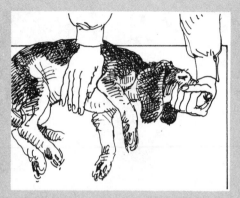

2. Cup the animal's mouth and nose with one hand and blow into the nostrils three times. Then use the other hand to press down on the chest six times, allowing 1 to 2 seconds between pumps. Alternate breaths and pumps until you get to the clinic.

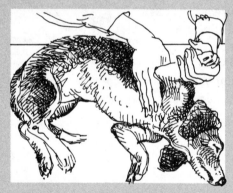

1. Your first step is to immediately lay the animal on its side on a firm surface. Check for a heartbeat by pressing the lower side of the chest, just behind the elbow. If you can't detect a heartbeat or breathing, begin CPR. Extend the head and the neck. Pull the tongue out to make sure you have an open airway.

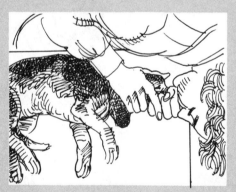

3. If there is another person available, one of you can blow into the animal's nostrils once every 4 seconds while the other applies both hands to the task of pumping the chest once every second. On a smaller animal use the fingertips to pump the chest.

How to Bandage a Leg

Your dog ran for the ball, but wound up colliding with the picket fence. Yelp! He's bleeding. You can take him to the veterinary hospital, or—if the cut is a small one—you can take care of him at home.

Most wounded animals will bite when approached. You might want to muzzle even a beloved pet before you begin. Apply pressure with clean gauze to slow the bleeding before you begin bandaging. While your animal is being bandaged, check for swelling, drainage, or signs of continued pain.

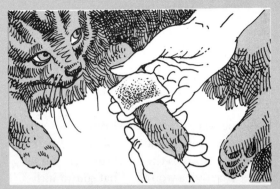

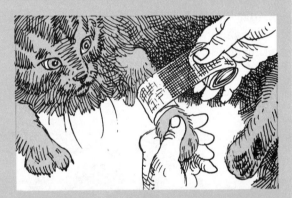

(2) Apply a first-aid cream, preferably an antibiotic ointment. Place sterile gauze over the wound and hold it securely in place. This should stop any bleeding.

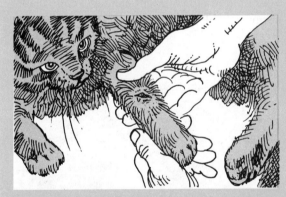

(1) Find the wound. If it is not clean, wash it out thoroughly with gentle soap and water or hydrogen peroxide. Snip hair from the edges of the wound. Dry the wound if possible.

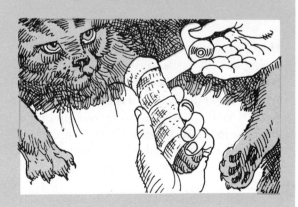

(3) Third, roll several layers of gauze snugly, but not tightly, around the wound area. Leave the tips of the toes uncovered.

(4) Finally, apply tape directly over the gauze, not the fur. Make sure the tape is not too tight. While your pet is bandaged, check for any signs of puffiness, which can indicate the wrapping is too tight or an infection is forming.

How to Bandage the Chest

A wound to the chest or stomach area can be serious. It is critical to wrap the chest and rush the animal to the vet if you hear sucking noises through a wound. That sound indicates the chest cavity has been penetrated. If it's going to take a while to get to the veterinarian, the first thing you'll want to do is stop the bleeding by pressing with clean gauze. When the bleeding slows, you can apply a bandage, as shown here. Such a bandage is also helpful if your dog has fresh stitches and you want to keep him from biting and scratching.

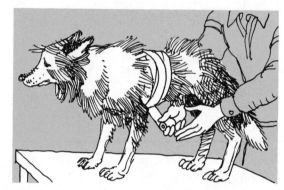

Step 2: Begin taping with nonadhesive tape across the gauze pad so it will be held securely against your pet's body. As you wrap the tape around the chest, take care not to bandage your pet too tightly. Tight bandages can create serious problems later on.

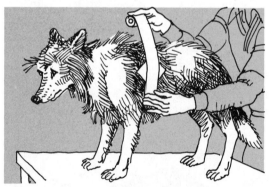

Step 1: Apply pressure to the wound for a full 5 minutes with sterile gauze. If the bleeding continues, press a fresh piece of gauze in place over the other piece. Do not remove the first piece. Even the most beloved pet can nip in the panic following an accident. If possible, you might want to muzzle your animal. Once you stem the flow of blood, you can proceed to step 2.

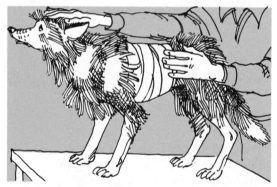

Step 3: Continue wrapping your pet until you feel that the gauze won't budge. The tape should extend several inches on either side of the gauze pad to ensure that it stays in place and remains clean. Make sure the wrapping isn't so tight as to interfere with your pet's normal breathing. Tie the tape securely in a place where your pet can't reach it with his teeth.

350

How to Apply a Splint

Scre-e-e-ch. Your dog has been hit by a car. If a limb is dangling or looks distorted, it's possibly broken. You need to get your pet to the hospital, says Genye Hawkins, D.V.M., a veterinarian in Orlando, Florida, and coauthor of *The Pet First-Aid Book*. But before you put your beleaguered pooch in the car, you can place a splint on his injured limb to keep it from getting further traumatized. If your pet won't cooperate, put him in the car without the splint.

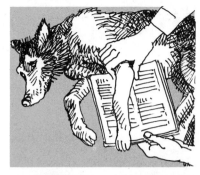

Step 1: Place your pet on his side opposite the side of the hurt leg. Straighten the leg by bracing it at the elbow—do not pull on the paw. Find a fairly thick magazine and place it gently under your pet's injured leg.

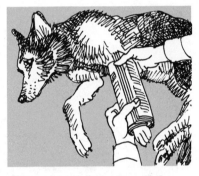

Step 2: Then fasten the rolled-up magazine with a piece of tape. Loosely roll the magazine around the animal's leg. You might want to apply a muzzle during this procedure. The animal is sure to be upset.

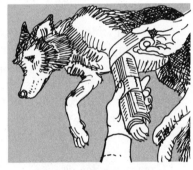

Step 3: Your next step is to wrap the magazine in tape so that the splint remains securely attached to the leg. It's best to start above the elbow and work your way down. If someone is available, have him call the vet.

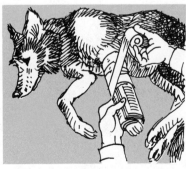

Step 4: Continue wrapping until you cover the entire length of the leg. Do not cover the toes. This entire procedure should take only a few minutes—it's important to get your animal to the vet as soon as possible.

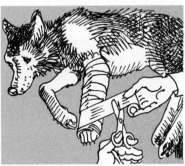

Step 5: When you reach the bottom of the magazine, make sure the toes are still visible. Cut the end of the tape with scissors. With the splint in place, gently lift your dog and lay him as comfortably as you can on the seat of the car.

POISON IVY

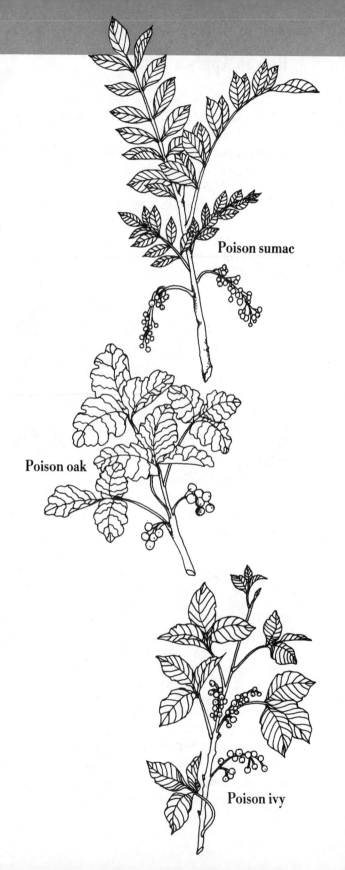

Poison sumac

Poison oak

Poison ivy

Yow. You've done it. Gotten into poison ivy. You didn't mean to but, armchair naturalist that you are, you didn't realize that seemingly harmless stick with white berries is what poison ivy looks like in the winter. Now you know. But what can you do to keep from breaking out into an itchy, ugly rash?

Got any fingernail polish remover or Scotch tape handy?

"If a woman has fingernail polish remover in her purse, she could use that to take off the oleoresin [the irritating oil in the plant] immediately," says Jere Guin, M.D., professor and chairman of the Department of Dermatology at the University of Arkansas. "If you have Scotch tape, you can remove a lot of the surface dead skin that contains the oleoresin on the surface, but it's not a very practical way to treat it.

"Anything you do in the first 5 minutes in the way of soap and water or even just plain water is going to beat what you do 30 minutes later," he adds.

If you are unaware that you've been contaminated, the telltale itchy rash will soon appear to let you know. Over-the-counter lotions containing calamine or zinc oxide can help relieve itching. Some products, however, should not be applied on oozing blisters; none should be used for more than a week. Read labels carefully. Severe cases require medical attention. Treatment probably will include cortisone.

Recognition remains the best prevention.

Bejou Merry

PREGNANCY

Your breasts are heavy and tender. Your body is tired. Your favorite food flip-flops your stomach. Your head does a whirly-twirly tango while your feet stand still. You don't need a medical test to tell you. You're going to have a baby!

Inside your uterus, a microscopic egg and sperm have joined. In nine very short months, you'll nuzzle a sweet-smelling baby in your arms—the reward for the vitally important work that you have ahead of you.

Your responsibility over the next nine months is to ensure that this person-in-the-making has the best possible start in life—and that you come through the process in tip-top shape, too.

"Ideally, a pregnancy is a planned event," says Lawrence Devoe, M.D., obstetrician/gynecologist at the Medical College of Georgia in Augusta. "A woman will have had a checkup prior to her pregnancy to be sure there are no medical problems that might interfere."

However, most women don't see their doctor until they suspect they already are pregnant. If you haven't seen your doctor prior to conception, make that first appointment early within the first two months of pregnancy, says William N. P. Herbert, M.D., professor in the Maternal and Fetal Medicine Division of the Department of Obstetrics and Gynecology at the University of North Carolina School of Medicine.

The first three months are especially important to fetal development and the most critical period is "weeks four to ten," Dr. Devoe says. So the sooner you make your first appointment, the better it will be for your baby. Plan to see your doctor at least once a month in the beginning of your pregnancy and more frequently toward your due date.

Future Perfect

To make sure your baby arrives in tip-top shape, you'll have to live a near-perfect lifestyle. Your doctor will advise you to give up smoking and drinking. You'll also have to get your doctor's permission to take any over-the-counter medications, even aspirin.

Cigarette smoking has been shown to increase the chance of having an underweight or small baby—a condition that has been linked with learning problems in school later in life. Also, smokers may give birth to asthmatic children.

Alcohol is, of course, out of the question. Even a social drink may put unborn babies at risk for minor malformations of sex organs and the urinary tract as well as increase the risk of growth retardation, say researchers at the National Institute of Child Health and Human Development.

Another lifestyle factor that can influence the size and health of your baby may not be as apparent as cigarettes or alcohol, Dr. Devoe says. That factor is stress.

"Stress is hard to identify," Dr. Devoe says. "Trying to burn the candle at both ends, working two jobs, trying to raise a family and work full time. Those are all stress factors. Sometimes stress can put a woman at risk for preterm birth."

Some stress factors—such as working full time—may be unavoidable. But perhaps you can recruit your family to help with housework or negotiate with your employer for rest breaks to lessen stress.

All pregnant women should take a rest break *before* becoming fatigued and plan to lie down during the lunch hour, resting on the left side to allow the free flow of blood through the large blood vessel in the right side.

Neonatal Nutrition: The Mommy Menu

Good nutrition is another building block for the physical and mental development of your baby. It also builds your strength for labor, delivery, and breastfeeding. Daily menus should contain fresh fruit and vegetables and whole grains. Rather than fried dishes, enjoy baked, poached, or broiled foods.

Now that you're "eating for two," don't think you should eat twice as much, counsels the American College of Obstetricians and Gynecologists. The average woman should gain between 24 and 30 pounds, says Dr. Devoe.

But no matter what your prepregnancy weight, don't put yourself—or your unborn baby—on a diet. Severe caloric restriction can be dangerous, increasing the risk of low birth weight and certain birth defects.

"In someone who is overweight, we are more concerned about her nutritional intake than we are about her actual weight gain,"

according to Dr. Herbert.

Your obstetrician will probably prescribe a vitamin supplement. Be sure to take it. A study reported in the *Journal of the American Medical Association* notes that pregnant women who take a multivitamin with folate before and during early pregnancy are less likely to have babies with a defective spine and brain.

Certain nutrients—omega-3 fatty acids, calcium, magnesium, and zinc—are especially important. Nutritionists advise that foods high in omega-3 fatty acids, such as fish and green leafy vegetables, are important to the development of the child's brain and nervous system. Two preliminary studies show pregnant women who take a 1,500-milligram calcium supplement daily lower their blood pressure by 5 to 6 percent. Sufficient amounts of zinc may make for a smoother delivery. A study at Case Western Reserve University shows women with insufficient levels of zinc in their blood experience more cases of mild toxemia, vaginitis, and late deliveries. They also experience more complications during pregnancy than women with adequate zinc levels. A Swiss researcher found that women who take magnesium supplements are less likely to hemorrhage, have cervical problems, or retain fluid than pregnant women who don't get extra magnesium. The babies of women who take magnesium are more likely to be normal in size and be more responsive at birth.

Weathering the Worst of Pregnancy

In the beginning of your pregnancy, morning sickness may well be your major discomfort. So here's a bit of good news to remember while you're hanging over the porcelain. Studies show that women who vomit during pregnancy are less likely to miscarry or deliver prematurely than women who do not.

Morning sickness is usually limited to the first two or three months of pregnancy. If yours goes on and on, make sure to mention it to your doctor. "Women who have an excessive amount of morning sickness may be at higher risk for small babies," says Dr. Devoe. "But typical morning sickness is reasonably benign."

You'll weather morning sickness a little better if you employ a few simple tricks. Eat several small meals throughout the day rather than two or three large ones. And eat your largest meal of the day at noon rather than in the evening. Drink plenty of fluids to neutralize stomach acids. The old advice to eat a dry saltine cracker in bed before you arise is good. Try to keep a carbohydrate in your stomach at all times. Also, a snack at bedtime may alleviate early morning sickness.

Heartburn is another problem that can plague you in the early stages of pregnancy as well as in the last trimester. Use the same tricks that work to prevent morning sickness. Also, sleeping propped up in bed may be helpful. Relieve some of the burn by lying in bed with your arms over your head. Try an antacid only on a doctor's recommendation.

Water retention, especially in the last few months of your pregnancy, can be another worry. Your ankles and feet may swell from excess fluid in your tissues. This is often just a common pregnancy problem, but it can be a symptom of a disease, so it is important to mention any water retention to your doctor. It's especially important to see your doctor if you experience swelling in your hands or face. You can prevent some of the bloated look by resting with your feet up as often as possible and by wearing support hosiery.

Varicose veins are a common problem during pregnancy because the increased weight of the womb presses against the pelvic veins, blocking the return of blood from the legs to the heart. If you have this problem, regular rhythmic walking and leg exercises may help push the blood along. Wearing support hose, elevating your feet, and getting plenty of rest also may help prevent varicose veins.

Maintaining good posture can be a problem as the extra weight pulls at the front of your body. Poor posture can increase strain on your back, causing lower back pain. To avoid strain, try to stand with your back straight, fanny tucked under, and abdominal muscles contracted. Distribute your weight evenly between both feet when you stand to prevent leaning too far forward. When you sit, be sure there is no gap between your lower back and the chair back.

Poor posture also can worsen stretch marks, which result from the breakdown of elastic fibers in the skin as it stretches over your growing abdomen and breasts.

Having a baby is one of the most wonderful things that can happen to a woman. Your marriage, too, may benefit from this addition to the family. One survey shows that 40 percent of new mothers and 55 percent of new fathers say parenthood made them "more in love" with their mates.

Claudia Allen

PREGNANCY

Getting out of Bed

Bugs buzz on their backs in tiny circles, working up the momentum to flip over. Turtles claw at the air to rock their shells until they finally tumble. Pregnant women probably think about bugs and turtles a lot, particularly when they try to get out of bed. So, how do they hoist themselves out? Here is the safe and easy method. You'll probably want to use it again after the baby is born, while you get your muscles back into shape.

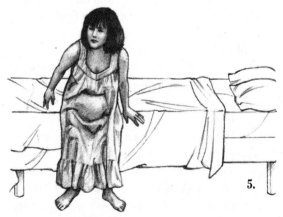

Now push yourself up to a sitting position on the bed. Rest for a moment to keep from becoming faint as your circulation adjusts.

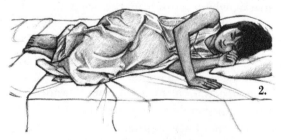

Lying on your back, first pull your knees up so that your feet are flat against the mattress to give you leverage.

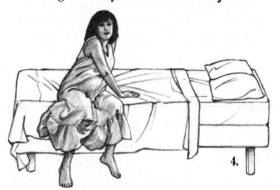

Swing your legs off the bed and put your feet flat on the floor. Lean forward slightly. Continue to support yourself with your hands.

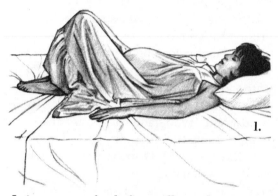

Next, roll onto one side, knees together. One arm should be bent with your hand out to catch you.

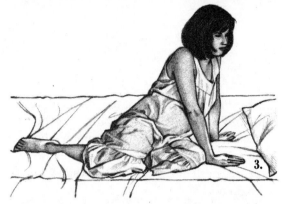

Now stand up. Use your hands if you need to push yourself off a soft mattress.

356

How to Sleep with a Tummy

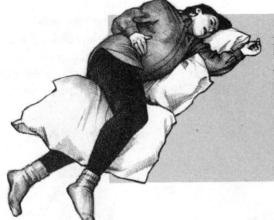

As your weight increases, lying on your back may make you feel faint or uncomfortable. Doctors advise lying on your left side, propped up with pillows. This position will ease pressure on the large blood vessel in your right side while offering comfort. Use a cushion between your legs for additional support.

A pillow tucked under your thighs and knees will help flatten the hollow of the back. It will also relax your joints without cutting off circulation. If you feel faint, switch to another position.

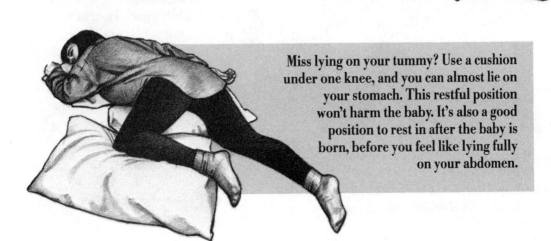

Miss lying on your tummy? Use a cushion under one knee, and you can almost lie on your stomach. This restful position won't harm the baby. It's also a good position to rest in after the baby is born, before you feel like lying fully on your abdomen.

Pregnancy

Training for Delivery

It feels like the tenth round and you're wishing for a knockout . . . your own!

Labor, like boxing, requires enormous stamina—and the fitter you are, the better you'll do. You don't have to take up road-work or the heavy bag to get results. Here are a few exercises that will give you the strength you need to have a safe and successful delivery.

Lie flat on your back with your knees bent, your pelvis tilted up, and your spine flattened. Holding your pelvis tilted so your lower back remains flat on the floor, slide on your heels until your legs are stretched out straight. Holding this position will help strengthen your abdominal muscles.

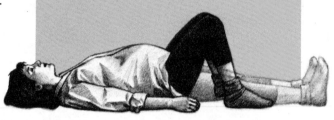

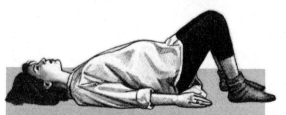

Lying on your back with your knees bent and your back flat against the floor, bring your chin to your chest and smoothly fold forward, curling halfway to your knees. Carefully lie back down.

Take the opportunity to elevate your feet with your calves supported whenever you can. While sitting, do foot stretching and rotating exercises to aid circulation in your legs. Kick off your shoes and sit with your legs slightly apart. Then turn your feet first in a clockwise movement, then back in a counterclockwise movement.

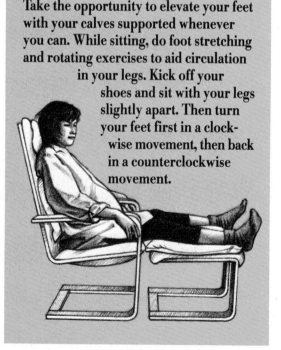

Lying on your back, knees bent, roll your pelvis up by flattening your lower back onto the floor. Contract your abdominal muscles on an outward breath and tighten the buttock muscles, then relax.

Practice your pelvic tilt by getting into the "cat" position. *(1)* Kneel on the floor with your hands directly under your shoulders, knees under hips. Keep your back straight and don't let your spine sag. *(2)* Then pull in your abdominal muscles and buttocks and press up with your back. Hold for a few seconds before relaxing back into the straight-backed position.

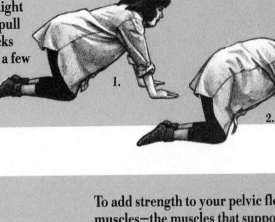

To add strength to your pelvic floor muscles—the muscles that support the weight of the developing baby—try this exercise. *(1)* Lie on your back with your knees bent and feet flat on the floor. Tighten your buttock muscles and hold the position. *(2)* Then slowly extend one leg at a time, returning it to the starting position before extending the other leg.

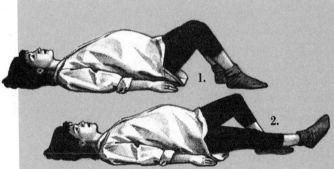

Here's another easy-to-do exercise that will improve muscle tone and circulation. It's especially handy for women who must spend a lot of time in a sitting position. *(1)* Sit with the small of your back pressed against the back of a chair and your heels resting on the floor. Bend your feet up so your toes point toward the ceiling. *(2)* Then point your toes down, flexing the muscles in your feet.

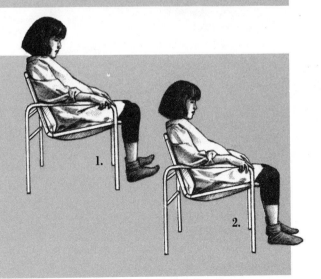

Postpartum Rest (You've Earned It)

Here's one useful bit of advice commonly passed from mother to daughter: When the baby naps, you nap. After delivery, use pillows to help take the strain off your lower back.

By placing pillows under your hips and lying on your tummy, your stitches won't bother you and you'll relieve back strain. The abdominal wall is relaxed. You can also use this position for practicing the pelvic floor contractions and pelvic tilts that you learned on pages 358 to 359.

Rest in these positions at least twice a day for an hour or so. If you wish, you can nap. It's important to use a pillow because mattresses aren't usually firm enough to support your back properly.

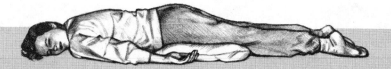

Lying on your stomach without a pillow under your hips puts undue strain on your back and abdominal muscles. Instead, use a pillow under the hips to create the correct pelvic tilt. This position will raise your pelvis, flatten your back, and relax your abdominal muscles. And it feels so-o-o good.

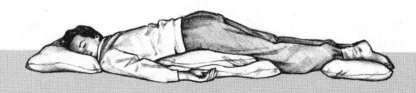

Extra pillows under your head and feet, with an additional pillow under your hips, keep your pelvis positioned correctly while relieving pressure on your breasts. Note the pillows are under the hips, not under the central abdomen. If the pillows are too high, you'll feel discomfort in your stomach and back.

RAYNAUD'S DISEASE

aynaud's disease—isn't that something you get from driving tiny French cars? No. The cars are Renault. The disease is Raynaud's, named after the French physician who described the condition in 1862. It rhymes with "Drano" and pertains to fingers and sometimes toes that lose normal blood flow because of cold or emotional stress.

The first episode may occur as early as the teens, although the onset can happen at any age. Far more women than men get Raynaud's, although doctors don't know why. During an attack, small arteries of the fingers (also sometimes the toes and occasionally the nose and ears) suddenly contract. This produces a numb or tingly feeling in the distressed area. Sometimes fingers change color. First they turn white as the blood leaves the affected arteries, then become red as the blood returns.

An attack can last a few minutes or an hour or two. Depending upon what caused the attack, it ends when either the hands are warmed or stress is alleviated. Raynaud's may be associated with other conditions, such as arthritis, so it's important to let your doctor know about it.

"Cold avoidance and care of the hands are probably the best treatments," says Eric I. Friedman, M.D., general surgeon with Surgical Oncology Associates of Portland, Oregon. "Because nicotine constricts blood vessels, we ask people to avoid cigarette smoking."

Bejou Merry

A "Warm-Up" Exercise

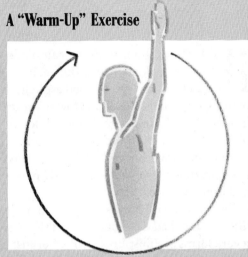

To warm chilled hands, use this "windmill" exercise conceived by Donald McIntyre, M.D., a Vermont dermatologist. Swing one arm at a time behind your body and then upward at about 80 revolutions a minute.

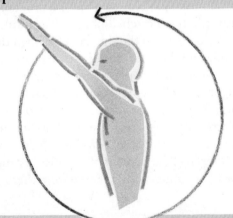

You may find it more comfortable to swing your arms in the other direction. Again, do one arm at a time, keeping your elbow, wrist, and fingers straight. Aim for 80 circles a minute. Don't attempt this exercise if you have shoulder pain.

361

SHINSPLINTS

His rhythmic, high-stepping gait made the miles look effortless. But each time Budd Coates's feet touched asphalt, pain sliced through his shin. It wasn't until he collected his time—good enough for 14th place overall in the prestigious Boston Marathon—that the world-class Pennsylvania marathoner knew how much damage he had done to his leg.

Diagnosed with a stress fracture in his left tibia, Coates had developed one of the most severe forms of shinsplints. Still, after just four weeks of rest and the addition of an orthosis, a small plastic device inserted in shoes that corrects the angle of the foot, Coates was able to resume training. He hasn't had a problem since.

Most nonathletes aren't at risk of suffering shinsplints—a catchall phrase that simply describes pain in the shin area between the ankle and the knee. But if you've recently begun an exercise program that includes vigorous walking, jogging, aerobics, or bicycling, you may have experienced them. According to one study, shinsplints account for 12 to 18 percent of running injuries. A whopping 28.6 percent of aerobics instructors in another study suffered from them.

Your Leg Versus the Pavement

Tendinitis and stress fractures develop in some runners as a result of a simple law of physics: Irresistible force (your leg) meets immovable object (the earth).

With each stride, the muscles and bones of the lower leg, called the tibia and the fibula, are forced to absorb the impact of the body's weight slamming against the ground, says Gary Gordon, D.P.M., director of the running and jogging program at the University of Pennsylvania's Sports Medicine Center. For weak muscles and bones, it's a matchup comparable to Pee Wee Herman taking on Hulk Hogan, the heavyweight wrestling champ. "When your muscles aren't strong enough to absorb that pounding—which is actually three to four times your body's weight—you get tendinitis. When the bone is weakened by the pounding, you develop stress fractures," Dr. Gordon says.

Although it sounds like a broken bone, a stress fracture is actually a weakening of a spot on the bone. But continue to run on a stress fracture and, just like a piece of metal that's been bent too many times, it may break, says David R. Webb, M.D., associate director for the Center for Sports Medicine in San Francisco.

Olympic track star Mary Decker-Slaney at one time suffered from compartment syndrome, considered by some doctors as the most serious shin ailment. Essentially, Decker-Slaney had pain because the flow of blood through the muscle in her shin was restricted.

Doctors theorize that Decker-Slaney's enlarged leg muscles prevented proper blood flow out of the muscles. To ease the pain and allow the blood to circulate properly, surgeons sometimes snip open the fascia, or

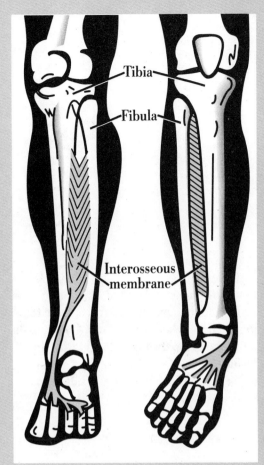

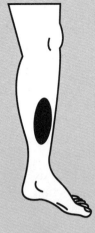

The Many Causes of Shin Pain

Shinsplints mean a lot of things to a lot of different athletes. Generally, the term describes several specific ailments that cause pain in the area of the leg between the ankle and the knee. Culprits are overuse, poor conditioning, or even the effects of running on hard surfaces.

The most serious cause of shin pain, compartment syndrome, is thought to develop when the flow of blood to the front of the shin is reduced by leg muscles that are enlarged from exercise. Tendinitis often occurs when a runner's foot repeatedly lands hard while running downhill. This movement pulls the tendon at its attachment to both the tibia and the interosseous membrane, resulting in painful inflammation. Stress fractures, the nearly invisible yet painful spot-weakening of the tibia or fibula, are frequently caused by running or jumping on hard surfaces.

casing, of the muscle, says Ted Percy, M.D., chairman of the University of Arizona's Sports Medicine Progam.

Old Shoes, Hard Floors

Choosing the right athletic shoe can help save your shins from injury, but even that's not enough—constant hammering against the ground pounds the support out of a shoe. If you run 25 miles or more a week, replace your shoes every two to three months, regardless of how much tread is left on the sole. If your training program is less than 25 miles a week, replace your shoes every four to six months.

Aerobics buffs also need to be mindful of the condition of their footwear. Those who take aerobics two times a week should replace their shoes every three months. Six-day-a-week trainers should get new shoes every two months, Dr. Gordon says.

Running and jumping surfaces should also be chosen carefully. Asphalt and concrete are much harder on the shins than crushed gravel, wood floors, or dirt. Both massage and certain types of exercise can also help soothe and strengthen the shins.

Brian Kauffman

363

SHINSPLINTS

Power Away Pain

Shin pain is often caused by weakness of muscles in the shin area. A new exercise program can often cause discomfort. But, by incorporating several lower leg-strengthening and stretching movements into your new program, you can avoid shinsplints in the future. Consult your doctor before beginning any exercise program. If shinsplint pain persists, see your doctor immediately.

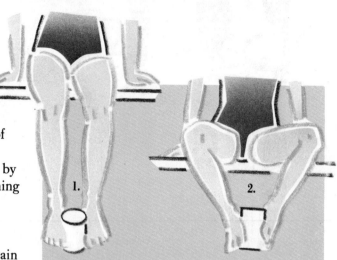

Place the bucket in front of a table that's just high enough to prevent your feet from touching the floor when you sit on it. *(1)* Sit on the table and grasp the paint bucket with the insides of your feet. *(2)* Bending your knees, bring the can toward your chest. Repeat several times.

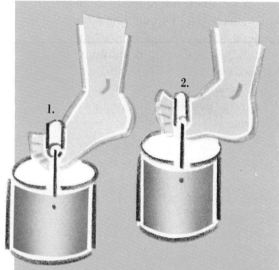

Here's the first-ever health-related use for a paint bucket. Sit on a table with your legs dangling over the edge. *(1)* Hang a paint bucket over your foot. *(2)* Flex the foot upward without moving your leg for 2 to 3 seconds. Repeat several times and then switch legs.

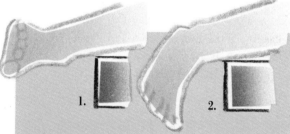

Some shin-strengthening exercises don't require any equipment. *(1)* Lie on your side in bed or on a table. Allow your top foot to hang off the edge. *(2)* Move your foot toward the floor. (Your foot will move only slightly.) Repeat several times. Turn over and repeat on the other side.

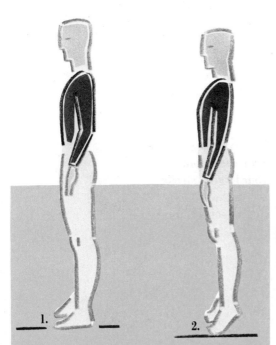

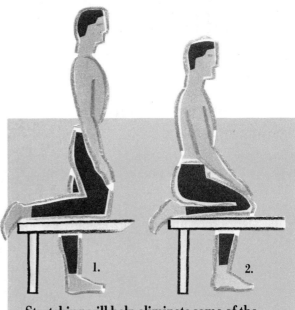

Strong calf muscles are essential for any vigorous activity. This exercise will help build them. *(1)* With your shoes off, stand erect. *(2)* Slowly raise onto your toes and hold for a few moments. Repeat several times. If that's too easy, stand with the balls of your feet on a step.

Stretching will help eliminate some of the soreness caused by shinsplints. In addition, stretching each day before beginning any exercise program is important. *(1)* Stand with one leg resting from knee to foot on a bench. *(2)* Carefully sit on your foot for a few moments. Repeat with the other leg.

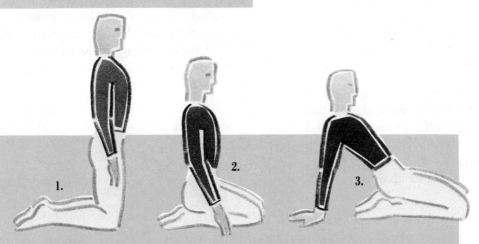

This stretch should prepare you for your exercise program. *(1)* Kneel on the floor. *(2)* Carefully sit on both feet. *(3)* Slowly lean back on your hands until you can feel the stretch in your shins and thighs. Maintain the stretch for a few moments.

365

SHINSPLINTS

Four Ways to Rub Out Shinsplint Pain

This may be the only redeeming quality of shinsplints: They make you legitimately eligible for massage once a day. Deep massage of the shin area helps eliminate fatigue of the lower leg muscle, where the tendons attach to the shin bone. Calf tension that sometimes causes shin tightness also will disappear. Make sure the person doing the massage is gentle—the area may be tender.

Grasp the bottom of his foot with one hand and locate the tendons on the outside top of the foot with the other. With the tips of your fingers, stroke across the tendons. Repeat several times.

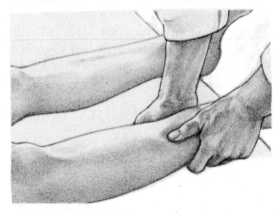

The person receiving the massage should lie on his back. Stand at his feet and grasp the inside of his right calf with your right hand. Then, using the thumb of your left hand, press into the shin and stroke back toward your fingertips. Move your hands down the leg.

The person receiving the massage should lie on his stomach. Locate the tendons that attach the calf to the back of the knee. Using your fingertips, gently massage across the tendons for about 10 seconds. Repeat several times and then switch legs.

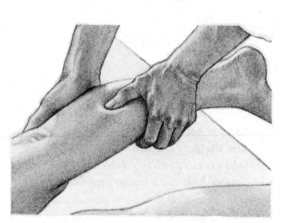

Have the person receiving the massage lie on his stomach. Grasp the right leg at the knee with your right hand. With the thumb of your left hand, begin stroking across the leg from the outside to the inside, just above the Achilles tendon. Press deeply.

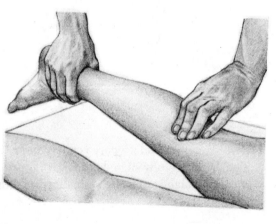

SIDE STITCHES

On November 5, 1989, Ken Martin finished second in the New York City Marathon. It was his fastest marathon ever and the fastest American performance in almost six years. He did it side-stitch-free.

"In a couple of marathons I got side stitches late in the race, around mile 16. In another marathon I got one as early as mile 6."

Even athletes in top physical shape have to learn how to deal with this nuisance. Side stitches are the lost socks of exercise: They happen to everybody, but nobody knows why.

"Why a side stitch occurs is a mystery," says well-known cardiologist and runner George Sheehan, M.D.

Experts theorize that side stitches result from lack of oxygen to the diaphragm caused by insufficient blood flow. The oxygen deprivation, they speculate, produces a painful spasm. Other possible causes include weak abdominal muscles, wheat and milk food intolerances, eating too much before exercising, drinking carbonated beverages, intestinal gas, or liver congestion.

No matter what brings on these inconvenient pains during exertion, one thing is certain, you don't have to let them keep you from exercising. Practice the technique illustrated below for quick relief.

Bejou Merry

How to De-Stitch Your Side

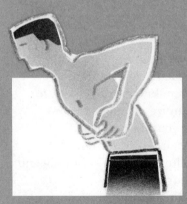

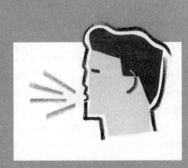

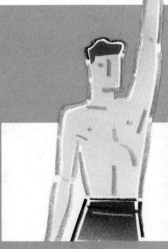

When the pain of a side stitch strikes, stop, bend forward slightly, and press your fingers into the painful area.

Inhale deeply, then exhale through pursed lips as you continue to push on the cramped area.

Lift your rib cage by raising the arm on the affected side. You might also try bending backward.

SINUSITIS

You wake up at dawn with pounding pain in your head—everywhere: Your eyes, your nose, your forehead, even your teeth hurt. Your nose is so stuffed up you'd need a power drill to unplug it, and thick, vile-tasting fluid drips down your throat.

A cold turned killer? Close. What you probably have is *sinusitis*—inflammation and usually infection of one or more of the eight small cavities within your head called the para-nasal sinuses.

"Sinusitis is simply an inflammation of the membranes lining the sinuses that can interfere with normal drainage," says J. R. B. Hutchinson, M.D., president of the American Academy of Otolaryngic Allergy.

Sound simple? That's because it is. The big question: Why does such a simple condition cause so many problems?

The mucus produced in our sinuses normally flushes out germs and debris that might otherwise cause infection. When the sinuses become inflamed, drainage stops. When drainage is interrupted for any reason, problems can develop.

Each of the sinuses drains into one small outlet about the size of the open tip of a ballpoint pen, explains Richard Mabry, M.D., clinical professor of otolaryngology at the University of Texas Southwestern Medical Center in Dallas. "The nose is very easily plugged up, and when that happens, the trapped fluid becomes the perfect medium for bacterial growth, usually leading to infection."

Produced in your nose and sinuses, mucus contains substances that attack and kill marauding bacteria that happen to land in your respiratory tract.

How do you tell a bad cold from sinusitis? The key distinction is the course of the infection. "A cold normally starts to get better after about 72 hours," explains Dr. Mabry. "It may drag on for a week, but most of us notice improvement starting around the third day. Sinusitis is the exact opposite: It gets worse after two or three days and continues to worsen."

The message here: If your cold gets worse after three days, or you notice a key symptom of sinusitis—increased pain, fever, or a change in nasal discharge—see your doctor.

Preventing Sinusitis

There's really no way to armor yourself perfectly against sinusitis. But there's a lot you can do to make that armor less vulnerable. For one, stay away from smoke. If you smoke, stop. If you live with a smoker, request that all smoking be done outside. Also, try to minimize dust, pollen, and pollution. Keep your house clean to minimize dust in the air. Avoid the outdoors during peak pollution hours—morning and evening rush hours.

Keeping the air conditioner on during allergy season may also help prevent sinusitis. But remember to check the filter regularly to make sure it doesn't harbor any mold.

It's also a good idea to humidify the air.

368

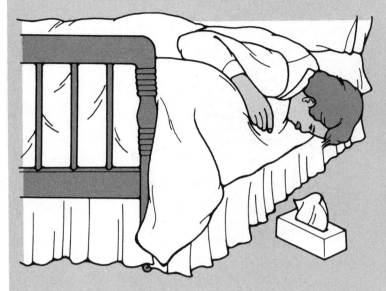

The Gravity Cure

Clogged sinuses? Get gravity working on your side. Hanging your head over the edge of the bed for 3 to 5 minutes can promote drainage of the maxillary and sphenoid sinuses. Normally, when you're standing in an upright position, these sinuses have to drain uphill before they drain downhill—a difficult thing to do.

"Keeping the air between 45 and 65 percent humidity is really important, especially in the winter," says Dr. Smith. Reason: A dry nose is vulnerable to infection.

Finally, drink lots of fluids. One of the most effective ways to prevent infection is to keep the mucus flowing. It won't flow if you're dehydrated, so make a point of drinking several glasses of water per day and getting plenty of other fluids, such as soup.

Plugging the Drip

If it's already too late for preventive measures, what can you do to clear your clogged head? You can use drugs, but use them wisely. Treatment for allergy-related chronic sinusitis usually consists of deconges-

tants to permit easier breathing and keep the sinuses draining properly. Your doctor may prescribe antibiotics to treat infection, usually caused by bacteria that are frequently present in the nose.

Over-the-counter decongestants are fine, but don't abuse them. "Don't exceed the limit on the bottle," warns Dr. Hutchinson. "You can actually end up with more inflammation instead of less if you do."

Don't use antihistamines, Dr. Mabry cautions: "Antihistamines reduce swelling and let you breathe a little easier, but they also dry up the nose and thicken the mucus—exactly the opposite of what you want to do. Drainage is what you want, not dryness."

Kim Anderson

369

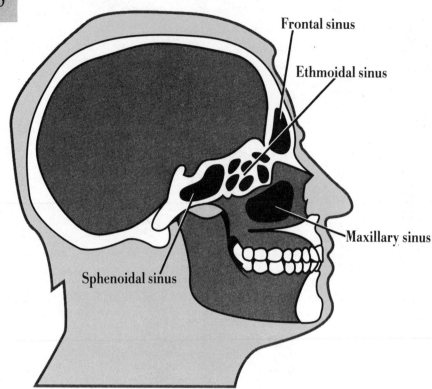

Frontal sinus

Ethmoidal sinus

Maxillary sinus

Sphenoidal sinus

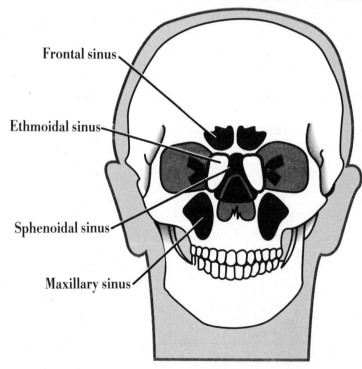

Frontal sinus

Ethmoidal sinus

Sphenoidal sinus

Maxillary sinus

Why We're All a Little Empty-Headed

When we talk about the *sinuses,* we're actually talking about four different pairs of sinuses, the bony air spaces in the skull around the nose and eyes. There are frontal sinuses, behind your forehead; maxillary sinuses, behind your cheekbones; ethmoidal sinuses, between your eyes; and sphenoidal sinuses, more or less right in the middle of your head. Why do we have these bony cavities? Scientists aren't entirely certain. But one thing is clear: To those with sinusitis, they are causes of great aggravation.

Acupressure Points

Acupressure—acupuncture without needles—is an ancient oriental healing method that gets an impressive amount of support from some thoroughly modern Western doctors. One of the ailments that responds well to acupressure is sinus trouble.

To press an acupressure point, use the tip of your index finger, your middle finger, or both, side by side. Generally, you'll know you've located the right point because it will be a bit more tender than the surrounding area. Apply pressure for a few seconds and repeat several times.

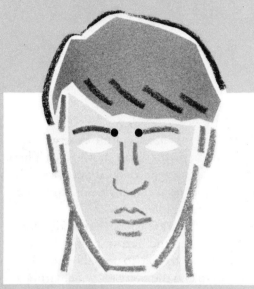

Found at the inside edge of each eyebrow, these points, when pressed for several minutes a few times a day, should give you relief within a couple of weeks.

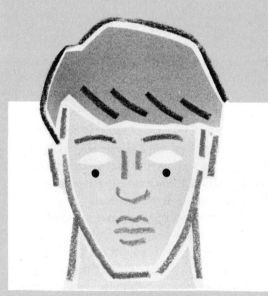

Acupressure points are generally found on both sides of the body. These two are located under the pupil of each eye, right under the lower rim of the eye socket.

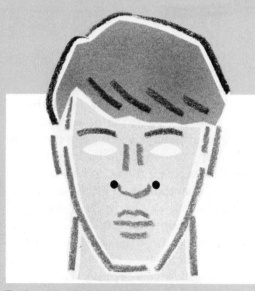

To the side of the nose are two points acupressure experts suggest you press to maintain clean sinuses. Do it after you've been exposed to pollens, smoke, or other irritants.

SNORING

Once and for all, let's put to rest two common myths about snoring: (1) There isn't a thing you can do about it and (2) snoring is just noise, laughable or annoying, of no medical significance.

In truth, there are effective remedies for nightly snorting and harrumphing. In some cases, you may be able to use self-care strategies to end the noise for good within a week. Plus, there are doctors (called somnologists) who can successfully treat snoring and other sleep problems. And snoring is not just benign clatter. One type not only raises the roof but signals a serious medical problem.

Why All the Racket?

About 45 percent of all adults snore occasionally; 25 percent snore habitually. Most snorers are men. What causes all the noise? An obstruction in the airway, usually the tongue. Most often when a snorer relaxes during sleep, his tongue falls backward against the rear of his throat. When he breathes, the air that enters his throat causes the tongue to vibrate against the throat tissues that it's resting against. The farther back the tongue drops, the more vibrating, or snoring, occurs.

For about 30 percent of heavy snorers, the tongue drops back so far that it winds up getting sucked into the airway "like a moist cork," in the words of Chicago snoring specialist Charles F. Samelson, M.D. The

floppy throat muscles collapse around the tongue, the snorer's airway is completely blocked (halting all sound), and he actually stops breathing for 10, 20, or 30 seconds or more. These frightening silences happen at regular intervals, often after long sequences of raucous snoring.

After breathing ceases, his survival instincts usually come to the rescue, and he awakens enough to move his tongue out of the airway so he can breathe again. As soon as he falls into another deep slumber, however, the process repeats itself.

This malady is called sleep apnea. Its cause is unknown, although some experts suspect that apnea victims have narrower airways than other snorers. In any case, doctors take the disorder very seriously for several reasons. For one, doctors suspect that 2,000 to 3,000 people die in their sleep every year because of sleep apnea. The deaths are usually caused by suffocation.

More often, victims of sleep apnea spend many of their days in a half-awake condition due to the lack of a good night's sleep. And all that nightly breath holding also takes a slow but steady toll on the heart.

Which antisnoring treatment is used depends on what's causing the snore, how much the snorer wants to stop a snoring problem, and how dangerous the snoring is. For a simple snoring problem, doctors often first recommend simple, noninvasive solutions like small changes in lifestyle. If these don't work, the snorer can opt for an antisnoring device or a surgical procedure.

Four Ways to Stop Snoring

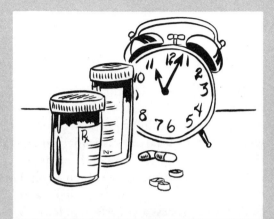

Avoid tranquilizers, sleeping pills, and anti-histamines before bedtime. These can cause the muscles in your throat to become too relaxed.

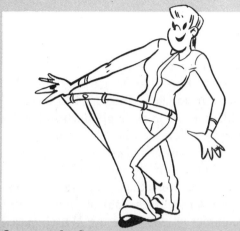

Lose weight. Snorers are notorious for being overweight, and there's a reason why. Added bulkiness in the throat can contribute to blocked airways, causing snoring.

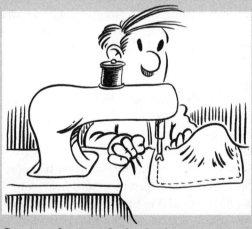

Sew a pocket into the back of your pajamas, then sew a tennis ball inside. It will force you to sleep on your stomach or side.

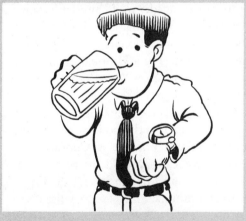

Stop drinking alcohol at least 3 hours before bedtime. Alcohol is a depressant that can have too relaxing an effect on your throat muscles.

Your nerves are stretched tight as bongo drums. Butterflies are dancing the hula in your stomach. And your bed sheets look like they spent the night on "tumble."

Diagnosis? Stress. Other common signs of stress include anxiety, depression, headaches, fatigue, tightness in the neck, itchy skin, poor appetite, overeating, indigestion, pounding heart, forgetfulness, lack of confidence, and hammer-headed bickering. What's more, medical researchers point to stress as a risk factor for serious diseases such as high blood pressure, heart disease, gastrointestinal disorders—even infectious diseases and cancer.

In fact, doctors generally agree that 50 to 70 percent of *all* illness is related to stress. The American Academy of Family Physicians, for example, reports that two-thirds of office visits to family practitioners are for stress-related illnesses. (For additional details, see "How Stress Distresses Your Body" on pages 380 to 381.)

Conversely, if you can manage stress, you can prevent much of the body-wide toil and trouble it inflicts. Think of it: Conquer stress, and you can say good-bye to nervous indigestion, pounding tension headaches, torturous insomnia, and a laundry list of other ills.

What Is Stress?

If you look up *stress* in Webster's dictionary, you'll find a couple of definitions. Stress may be defined as "a physical, chemical, or emotional factor that causes bodily or mental tension and may be a factor in disease causation." Having gallbladder surgery, for example, is physically stressful: Doctors put your body into a state of suspended animation and remove a vital organ. Breathing polluted air or drinking too much alcohol is chemically stressful: Your lungs, liver, and brain try to process an overload of toxic chemicals (which is why you probably feel pretty lousy after a night of partying in a smoke-filled room).

Emotional crises, such as going through a messy divorce or losing your job, attack your body from the inside out, triggering anger, resentment, jealousy, and other negative feelings. Strong emotions are much like toxic chemicals: They unleash powerful hormones and trigger other bodily changes. In fact, emotional stresses are no less harmful than physical or chemical stresses.

But even minor assaults on your body or psyche can be stressful, especially if life's little challenges occur one after the other, before you have time to adjust: Trying to cope with a checkbook that won't balance, a car that won't start, and a child who won't eat his cereal, all in one morning, can leave you as out of sorts as a polar bear in a hot tub. Throw in a sleepless night or two, and you can see how stress might, as Webster also puts it, "alter equilibrium."

How Do You Spell Relief?

Given the fact that stress is an inherent part of life, coping with stress is an essential life skill. A new breed of doctor—the stress-management expert—has evolved to help people learn new, twenty-first-century ways to prevent and relieve stress.

"Relaxation techniques like meditation, biofeedback, or progressive muscle relaxation are often prescribed generically as antidotes for stress," says Harold Steinitz, Ph.D., coordinator of the Stress Management Program at Sheppard Pratt Health Systems, Towson, Maryland. "Like Herbert Benson's Relaxation Response, they produce a decrease in blood pressure, a drop in oxygen consumption and metabolic rate, and an increase in emotional stability. Practiced 20 minutes a day, a relaxation technique produces immediate benefits. But the long-range results are also dramatic. People who practice some form of relaxation suffer fewer stress-related symptoms like headaches, stomachaches, fatigue, and irritability."

What works for one person may not work for another, though. "People respond differently to different approaches, so for stress management to work, the methods have to suit the individual," says Dr. Steinitz.

"Gazing at a fish tank may work wonders for one person, but if you get bored easily, you may feel tense. By the same token, a massage may not relax someone who's uneasy about being touched. The best strategy is to choose stress-management techniques tailored to your particular needs, likes, and dislikes," explains Paul Silver, Ph.D., assistant professor of psychiatry and psychology at the University of Texas Southwestern Medical Center in Dallas.

Here's what experts have to say about various coping techniques.

Turn Off Tension with Biofeedback

Biofeedback is a method of consciously influencing the bodily changes you experience under stress but don't ordinarily consciously control: blood flow, muscle tension, heart rate, brain waves . . . even how much you perspire. (Ever notice how your palms get clammy when you're nervous—that's a sure sign stress is on the scene.) To learn biofeedback, you're hooked up to a monitoring machine that measures one or more of these vital signs and translates them into audio or visual clues (beeps or a flashing light, for example).

John A. Corson, Ph.D., professor of psychiatry at Dartmouth Medical School, explains it this way: "Basically, what a biofeedback unit does is monitor a biological process that would otherwise be difficult or impossible for the person to detect. Changes in body function are then transformed into an easily understood signal, such as a tone or meter reading, so that the person can see exactly what a certain part of his body is doing from moment to moment."

"Changes in palm perspiration, for example, are very small and are measured in units called micro mhos. One type of biofeedback unit, the GSR 2, monitors the skin's micro-mho levels and emits a tone, which rises in pitch as more moisture is produced or drops

375

in pitch as the skin becomes drier," he notes.

Once you become an expert at noticing and controlling the physical end product of the stress response—in this case, sweaty palms—you become better able to control your reactions to stress in everyday life. In short, the machine has taught you how to keep your cool. You can also use biofeedback to help you monitor how well you're doing when you practice stress-control techniques such as deep breathing or the Relaxation Response.

"Biofeedback is also helpful for many kinds of stress-related problems—skin problems, memory problems, even headaches," says Dr. Corson.

Memory problems?

"Yes. When you're stressed, your memory can fail," he explains. "A lot of older people worry that they're losing their memory as they age, but many times, it's not only age—it's too much stress."

To find a licensed biofeedback professional in your area, send a stamped, self-addressed envelope to the Association for Applied Psychophysiology and Biofeedback, 10200 West 44th Avenue, Suite 304, Wheat Ridge, CO 80033.

Fed Up? Take a Walk

You don't necessarily need a lot of complicated machinery or weeks of training to relax, though. Robert Thayer, Ph.D., professor of psychology at California State University, Long Beach, has studied how a brisk 10-minute walk affects tension levels. He says that people felt less tense and more energetic after walking. Another study sug-

gests that *how* you walk can determine how relaxed you'll feel afterward. Sara Snodgrass, Ph.D., professor of psychology at Skidmore College in Saratoga Springs, New York, found that students who took long strides, while swinging their arms and looking forward, reported less fatigue and depression (two symptoms associated with stress) than students who walked normally or shuffled along looking downward. One theory says that when you swing your arms, the mechanical action relaxes muscles in the shoulders, neck, and back, areas that often tense up when we're under stress.

"My particular body stress signal is a feeling of tightness in my right shoulder," says David J. Fletcher, M.D., a specialist in occupational stress and corporate stress management. "To counteract stress, I regularly take long walks in the woods near my home, or otherwise exercise regularly."

Almost any kind of exercise that keeps you fit may act as a buffer against stress. Researchers at the University of Kansas in Lawrence compared aerobic exercise (running and brisk walking) with relaxation training (mental imagery and progressive muscle relaxation) as a method for counteracting depression triggered by stressful life events. The study involved 55 people. The researchers concluded that exercise worked better than relaxation training as an antidote to stress.

That's great news for people who'd rather whack a racquetball than sit and meditate. But Dr. Steinitz offers one caution for achievement-oriented people: If you're already pushing your limit, don't approach exercise as another challenge to conquer. "Biking, swimming, and running are okay as long as you aren't striving to shave seconds off your time, and as long as you don't make these activities stressful in other ways. If you do that, you're only trading one stress for another."

Do What You Love to Do

You may already be practicing stress management without realizing it.

"One of the first things I ask people when we discuss stress management is what they already do to relax," says Dr. Fletcher. "Reading, going to the movies, knitting, woodworking, even watching TV are forms of stress management. The idea is to disengage yourself from a sense of time urgency."

In other words, it's okay to goof off. Hobbies can *heal*. But whether or not a hobby is relaxing depends on how you approach it. "If you sit down at the piano and say to yourself, 'I'm doing this for me. I enjoy it,' and it gets you away from your obligations, good," says Dr. Silver. "But playing the piano is *not* helpful if you do it to impress company or to practice for leading a sing-along in two weeks. Each activity is open to that kind of interpretation."

"One common cause of stress is overemphasis on goals like getting good grades, a good job, a big raise, or a promotion, while neglecting personal relations, exercise, sports diversions, and, above all, those activities that you love to do," says John Larson, M.D., director of the Institute for Stress Medicine in Norwalk, Connecticut, and lecturer at the Yale University School of Medicine. "Striving toward goals is fine to a point. But you need to broaden the basis for your self-esteem by also doing what you love to do and spending quality time with people who love you. You'll be better off. For one thing, you won't be distressed if goals don't work out. But more important, the things we like to do are what reflect our inner being; they nurture us and make us feel good. Doing what you love to do, be it listening to music, writing poetry, decorating a room, gardening, or stamp collecting—is what makes you 'you'. Goal-oriented activities, which focus strictly on getting somewhere or getting something, just don't nurture. People who fixate on goals have heart attacks."

"A lot of the people we counsel are achievement-oriented, success-minded people who are striving toward a goal, making a lot of money, but missing the point," says Dr. Steinitz. "We teach them to define success in a broader way."

The Soothing Power of Music

Listening to music can be especially relaxing. In fact, music therapy is a growing field of medicine. A study published in the *Journal of the American Association of Nurse Anesthetists* found that the soothing strains of Brahms played through cassette headphones reduced the heart rate and blood pressure of patients under anesthesia. In another study, nurses taught recovering heart attack patients how to relax using soothing music (popular, classical, or nontraditional) combined with guided relaxation techniques (such as muscle relaxation). Compared to a group not receiving the training, patients taught relaxation experienced lower blood pressure and heart rate and less psychological anxiety, among other benefits. (Part of the reason these people got into such a fix was due to the inappropriate ways they dealt with stress. So learning a way to handle stress after they left the hospital was as important to their recovery as controlling other cardiovascular risk factors, such as watching their intake of saturated fat and not smoking.)

Some researchers suggest that for music to relieve stress, its beat should approximate your resting heart rate—60 to 70 beats a minute. Stress therapists often recommend soothing, nontraditional "New Age" tunes (such as *Healing Journey* by Emmett Miller) or classical works (such as the second movement of Bach's *Brandenburg Concerto No. 4*) to reduce tension. But personal taste also plays a part.

"If you don't like a piece, it won't relax you," says Dr. Silver. "I suggest people spend some time with their record collection. Rate the songs that affect you in a serene, relaxed way. Then make your own tape of those songs and use this play list when you need to relax."

Try to Develop a Stress-Resistant Attitude

In addition to teaching relaxation skills, stress counselors try to show people how to change the way they think about the events and circumstances that cause stress. Hans Selye, M.D., in his classic book, *The Stress of Life,* observes that the same stress that makes one person sick becomes the spice of life for another. The difference lies in their attitudes.

Step one in this attitude make-over: Go easy on yourself. A lot of stress is self-induced.

"We tend to send ourselves subtle but stressful messages," says Dr. Steinitz. " We tell ourselves 'Don't be late . . . Be perfect . . . I've got to get this right.' We try to live up to what we *think* other people expect us to be. And it takes a lot of courage and strength to move away from trying to meet those expectations. But we can learn to do it."

Step two: Slow down.

One of the classic signs of stress is the feeling that you have too much to do and not enough time to do it.

But doesn't everyone feel harried and overburdened these days?

"No, not everyone, although it seems that way sometimes," says Dr. Larson. "Stress is so prevalent, you start to think that feeling rushed is a normal way to go about all your daily activities. But it's not—it's pathological. The paradox is that feeling is never resolved by going faster, but by going slower. If you go faster, you lose contact with people, they become mere functionaries in your life, and you feel anxious. But if you slow down and make an effort to get back in touch with people, you feel less anxious."

To better illustrate why "slower is better," Dr. Larson talks about long-distance trips. "If you go as fast as you can, you'll feel anxious when you arrive with a sense of not having enough time, even though you're on time. But if you drive 10 miles an hour slower, you have time to talk to passengers, enjoy the scenery, or listen to music or educational tapes. You'll feel more composed when you arrive. The time it takes to make a 3-hour trip at 50 miles an hour is only 20 to 30 minutes longer than the time it takes at

60 miles an hour. So by driving fast, you don't save a heck of a lot in real time, and you create a sense of time urgency within yourself. By driving slower, you gain quality time."

"You can stay pretty healthy if you function at about 80 percent of your maximum potential," says Dr. Steinitz. "But if you're *always* functioning at maximum overdrive, you're depleting your emotional resources and compromising your health. That's why superhuman efforts are so often followed by a collapse. And if maximum overdrive becomes your norm, it erodes everything else."

One way to slow down to a less stressful pace is to concentrate on one task at a time. "Many people are also what we call polyphasic —always trying to juggle several things at

once," says Dr. Steinitz. "That results in brain overload and exacts a high emotional or physical toll. Instead, do one thing, do it well, then shift to the next task."

"Humor is a third option to the fight or flight response," says Arthur M. Nezu, Ph.D., director of the doctoral program in psychology at Hahnemann University in Philadelphia. "A sense of humor is especially helpful in coping with the aftereffects of a stressful event—preventing mild depression from becoming severe, for example. The few studies that do exist on this topic say that therapists should encourage patients to distance themselves from a crisis, to foster the client's ability to step back and look at a problem from a distance. And humor can do that."

Sharon Faelten

The Permanent Wave <u>Inside</u> Your Head

Your brain wave patterns change when you shift from an aroused, attentive state to a relaxed, serene state. Beta waves—rapid, shallow, and irregular wave activity— predominate as you go about your daily business. Switch your focus to a calming sound, however, and slower, higher, more rhythmic alpha and theta waves will predominate. (One stress-management counselor calls relaxation "alpha seltzer" for the mind.) Delta waves happen only during the total relaxation of deep sleep.

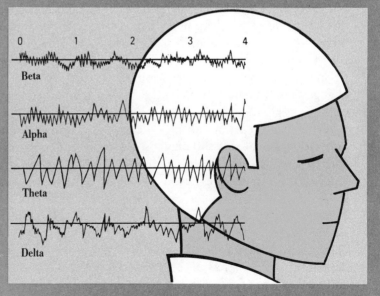

How Stress Distresses Your Body

Think about the last time you were startled, scared, or embarrassed. Maybe the phone rang at dawn. ("Bad news," you think.) Or a car pulled out in front of you. ("What an idiot!") Or you were called on to speak in public. ("People are staring at me.")

Did your heart begin to pound? Your mouth feel dry? Your palms perspire? These are all common, easily detectable reactions to a stressful incident. But stress is much more than a state of arousal: It's a three-stage bodywide reaction, a mosaic of measurable changes in virtually every organ of the body.

During the alarm phase, your adrenal glands (endocrine glands perched above your kidneys) discharge powerful hormones (such as cortisone) into your bloodstream. These hormones travel to distant organs such as your heart, brain, lungs, stomach, and kidneys, raising your blood pressure, speeding your breathing, tensing your muscles, and triggering other changes. (See the illustration on the opposite page.)

As the alarm reaction subsides, your body adapts to the stressful demand—or tries to, anyway—and the initial discomfort fades. The butterflies in your stomach settle down, your palms don't sweat as much, and you get through it. This stage—called resistance—is the opposite of the alarm stage and can last indefinitely, depending on how stressful the demand is and how well you cope with it.

But suppose you *never* get used to speaking in public? Suppose you grit your teeth as you battle teenage Ninja traffic warriors driving to work every day? Suppose bad news seems to grow every time the phone rings? Under continued stress, the body exhausts its supply of adaptive energy. During this stage of exhaustion the initial stress reactions—heightened blood pressure and so forth—reappear, but now they're nearly irreversible.

If you feel tired, jittery, or ill when you're under a lot of stress, it's no wonder: Unrelenting stress exerts wear and tear on almost every part of your body, from neurons in your brain to the muscles in your feet.

Stress can alter the way your body handles cholesterol in such a way that the heart can be damaged, for example. And it can weaken your immune system, leaving you vulnerable to infections (like the flu) or cancer.

Anxiety, depression, mouth ulcers, angina, heart arrhythmias, muscular pain, digestive problems, reproductive disorders, and skin ailments are other by-products of stress. In fact, Hans Selye, M.D., the stress research pioneer, said that much disease is caused not by germs or poison, but by failure to cope with stress.

Luckily, relaxation acts as an antidote for stress, counteracting it before it can sabotage your health.

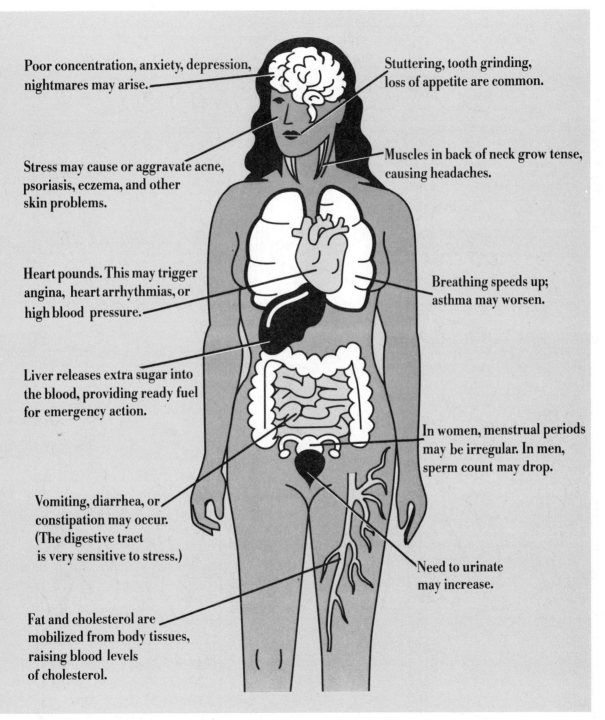

Poor concentration, anxiety, depression, nightmares may arise.

Stuttering, tooth grinding, loss of appetite are common.

Stress may cause or aggravate acne, psoriasis, eczema, and other skin problems.

Muscles in back of neck grow tense, causing headaches.

Heart pounds. This may trigger angina, heart arrhythmias, or high blood pressure.

Breathing speeds up; asthma may worsen.

Liver releases extra sugar into the blood, providing ready fuel for emergency action.

In women, menstrual periods may be irregular. In men, sperm count may drop.

Vomiting, diarrhea, or constipation may occur. (The digestive tract is very sensitive to stress.)

Need to urinate may increase.

Fat and cholesterol are mobilized from body tissues, raising blood levels of cholesterol.

3 WAYS TO HANDLE STRESS (BUT ONLY ONE IS GOOD)

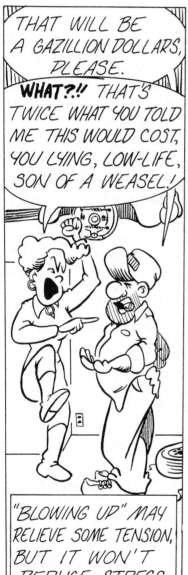

THAT WILL BE A GAZILLION DOLLARS, PLEASE.

WHAT?!! THAT'S TWICE WHAT YOU TOLD ME THIS WOULD COST, YOU LYING, LOW-LIFE, SON OF A WEASEL!!

"BLOWING UP" MAY RELIEVE SOME TENSION, BUT IT WON'T REDUCE STRESS.

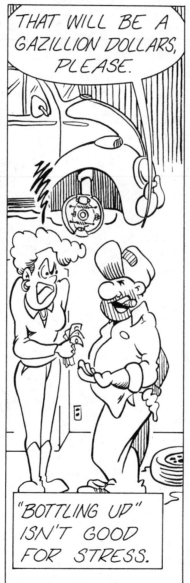

THAT WILL BE A GAZILLION DOLLARS, PLEASE.

"BOTTLING UP" ISN'T GOOD FOR STRESS.

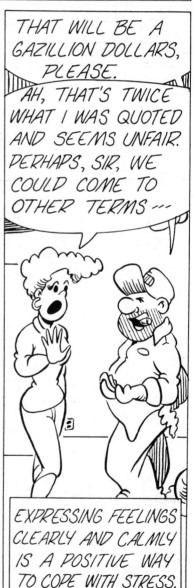

THAT WILL BE A GAZILLION DOLLARS, PLEASE.

AH, THAT'S TWICE WHAT I WAS QUOTED AND SEEMS UNFAIR. PERHAPS, SIR, WE COULD COME TO OTHER TERMS ---

EXPRESSING FEELINGS CLEARLY AND CALMLY IS A POSITIVE WAY TO COPE WITH STRESS.

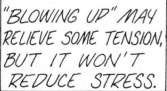

Relax and Unwind

You don't have to "get away from it all" to relieve stress. The following relaxation routine takes 20 minutes, tops. Practiced daily, it can relieve tension and help you stay calm under pressure. Choose a quiet, comfortable place to do the technique.

4. Imagine that your shoulders are very heavy. Press them down to the floor. Hold briefly, then relax.

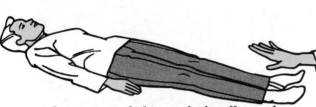

1. Loosen your clothing and take off your shoes. Lie on your back with your arms at your sides and your feet together. Close your eyes.

5. Extend your arms to each side, stretching your fingers outward. Tense the muscles in both arms, concentrating on the feeling of tension. Then let your arms go limp.

2. Crinkle up your face, tensing the muscles in your forehead and around your eyes, your nose, and your mouth. Then relax.

6. Bracing yourself with your feet and shoulders, raise your buttocks 2 inches off the floor. (You'll be able to feel your spine stretch.) Then relax and lower yourself to the floor.

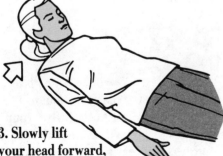

3. Slowly lift your head forward, pointing your chin toward your chest. (Be careful not to clench your jaw or tense your neck muscles.) Then gradually lower your head back down.

7. Keeping your feet together, point your toes and stretch your legs. Then relax. Rest quietly for 2 or 3 minutes. You should feel relaxed from head to toe.

STRESS

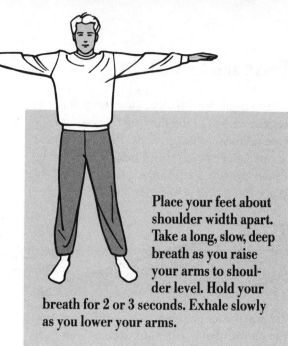

Exercise Loosens Tension

Taking a few minutes from a hectic schedule to stretch your neck, shoulders, back, arms, and legs can relieve mental and physical tension. Before you get started, close your door and play some soft music to help take your mind off your work or other concerns. After exercising, just sit quietly with your eyes closed for a few minutes. You'll feel refreshed and rejuvenated. (Besides the exercises shown here, you may want to take a brisk, 10-minute walk or jog in place for a couple of minutes.)

Place your feet about shoulder width apart. Take a long, slow, deep breath as you raise your arms to shoulder level. Hold your breath for 2 or 3 seconds. Exhale slowly as you lower your arms.

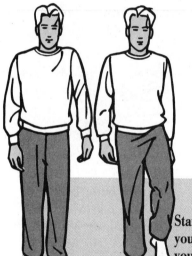

Stand erect with your arms limp at your sides like a rag doll. *(1)* First shake your right wrist, then your forearm and arm. Then shake your left wrist, forearm, and arm. Next, lift your right foot slightly and shake your foot, lower leg, and thigh. Place your foot on the floor. *(2)* Now repeat the procedure with the other leg.

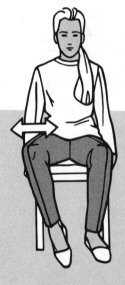

Sit in a chair with a firm seat and back. Be sure your feet reach the floor. Place your feet about 6 inches apart. Lift your heels. Swivel your right leg back and forth 10 or 12 times. (If your legs feel very tense, knead the muscles in your thighs to loosen them.) Then swivel your left leg back and forth 10 or 12 times.

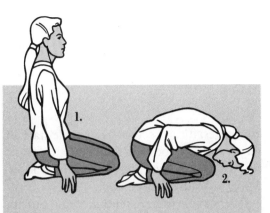

To work out tension in your back, try this. *(1)* Remove your shoes and kneel on the floor. It's best to do this on a soft carpet or mat. *(2)* Slowly bend your trunk forward as far as you can. Then straighten up slowly. Take three or four deep, relaxed breaths. (You can do this while you're listening to your favorite music.)

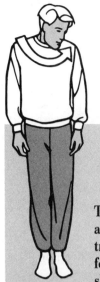

To unkink tension that accumulates in your neck, try this. Tilt your head forward, as shown. Then slowly rotate your head in a circle, first to your right until your right ear is over your right shoulder, then forward until your left ear is over your left shoulder. This is excellent for people who drive a lot or work at video display terminals or cash registers and don't have much opportunity to shift their position for hours at a time.

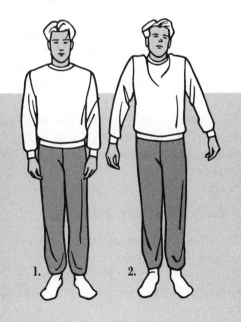

If you carry tension in your shoulders, add this maneuver. *(1)* Stand with your head erect and your arms hanging limply at your sides. *(2)* Shrug your shoulders, lifting them to your ears. Hold for a count of three, then relax. Repeat five times. You can also swing your arms from front to back, five or ten times, clapping your hands lightly each time. (These are good ways to relieve mid-day tension buildup if you work at a desk.)

385

TENDINITIS

You've been playing tennis for years, and except for a few lopsided losses you'd like to forget, the sport has been both enjoyable and pain-free. But now—win or lose—each match is no longer just good exercise but also an exercise in shoulder pain.

Oh, my aching serve!

Shoulder tendinitis, especially among tennis players, baseball players, and swimmers, is hardly rare. Nor is tendinitis rare among meat cutters (please excuse the pun), poultry processors, or electrical assemblers.

These sports and occupations all have something in common: years of repetitive motion. And tendinitis, the inflammation of a tendon, can be the unwanted by-product. In a word, the problem is *overuse*, says Robert Harrison, M.D., director of the Occupational Medicine Clinic at the University of California, San Francisco.

Tendinitis of the knee, for example, is no stranger to many distance runners, some of whom have had to abandon the sport. Running and jumping or direct trauma to the heel are common contributors to Achilles tendinitis (the Achilles tendon runs from a third of the way up your calf to your heel bone).

Tendons connect muscle to bone. And tendons—be they in the shoulder, knee, or elsewhere—can take only so much strain. Overhead motions, such as serving a tennis ball, throwing a baseball, or swimming, are especially stressful on the shoulder.

"While overuse is the cause of tendinitis in most cases, it can occur when people start an activity and do too much too quickly," says Roger Kalisiak, past president of the Illinois Athletic Trainers Association.

It is possible to have tendinitis and bursitis at the same time, but usually it's strictly a case of having one or the other. (See the chapter on bursitis on page 118.)

"Usually bursitis takes place more around a joint area," says Kalisiak. "Tendinitis is more related to a muscle. Tendinitis tends to ache while you're doing the activity. With bursitis, the pain stops [while you're doing the activity] and comes back later."

It's best to leave diagnosis to an expert. You want to make sure that tendinitis is, in fact, the problem and that a tendon hasn't ruptured or been badly torn. You also want to know the dos and don'ts of treatment. For example, many people automatically use heat to try and relieve pain. But heat will only aggravate pain in a shoulder with tendinitis.

Chronic tendinitis—in extreme cases—can eventually require corrective surgery. But usually more conservative measures will help a great deal.

Go Easy on Those Joints

For all types of tendinitis, rest from the tendinitis-causing activity must be part of the treatment plan, Dr. Harrison says. Of course, it's much easier to skip playing tennis for a few weeks than to skip going to your job. But even short, periodic rests ought to help some. If your tendinitis is job related, you might try performing your routine tasks using your muscles and joints differently.

Over-the-counter anti-inflammatory medications are good for controlling pain. Ice also remains a standard part of any treatment plan. Apply an ice pack for 20 minutes at a time, up to several times a day. But if you have circulatory problems, check with your doctor first.

Strengthening exercises also can be of great help. People with shoulder tendinitis sometimes are placed on a home rehabilitation program in which they use dumbbells weighing as little as 2 pounds to strengthen various muscles in the shoulder.

People with tendinitis in the knee often use a stationary bicycle to gain strength. And for people with Achilles tendinitis, Kalisiak recommends toe raises. Place the affected foot on the floor and the other one on a stair. Then lean forward over the leg on the stair and raise up onto the toes of the foot that's resting on the floor. Do the exercise slowly and work up to three sets of 15.

Massage can also be helpful in relieving the pain of tendinitis. First, locate exactly where your pain is. Then move your index finger *across* the tendon; don't rub lengthwise. For added support, place your middle finger on top of the index finger.

The first few treatments should last 1½ to 2 minutes, once per day, says Kalisiak. After a few days, stretch treatments to 2½ to 3 minutes and do them every other day. After the massage, stretch the area as far as you can in every direction. Then apply ice for 20 minutes.

Don Wade

Shoulder Exercises

1. Stand facing a wall about an arm's length away. Hold your body in a comfortable—not too tense—position. Then let your fingers do the walking—not through the telephone book, but slowly up the wall as high as you can reach. Once your fingers have walked up as far as they can go, slowly walk them back down.

2. Now stand at a right angle to the wall and repeat the previous exercise, again walking your fingers slowly. As your hand moves higher, step closer to the wall to allow your shoulder to experience the maximum reach.

3. Grasp the ends of a large bath towel behind your back. Then move the towel as though you were drying your back—reaching and pulling as far as possible in each direction. Repeat with arms in opposite positions.

TENDINITIS

The Right Stroke

Often you hear tennis players talking about their backhand being the weak part of their games. They can't get a comfortable stroke and find themselves hitting shots all over the place. *Bottom left,* In the faulty backhand stroke shown here, the player's front shoulder is up, his body is leaning backward, and the racquet is pointing down. These mistakes put great stress on the forearm muscles. *Bottom right,* But here the player is using good shoulder motion and correctly transferring his weight forward. The front shoulder is down and the elbow is firm, thus arm muscles are better protected. A two-handed backhand, a la Chris Evert, offers even more protection.

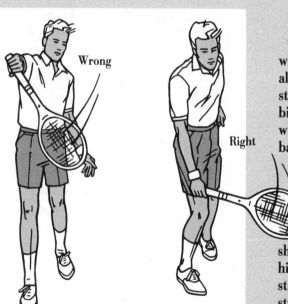

Top right, Employing the incorrect forehand technique will not only cost you sets and matches, it also will put your elbow under tremendous stress. The end result could be sharp, stabbing pain—tennis elbow. So let's look at what's wrong. Notice that the racquet hits the ball late—in front of the player's right hip. This, in combination with the player's weight being on his back foot, puts pressure on the elbow during the swing. *Top left,* In the correct forehand technique shown here, the player is smoothly shifting his weight forward. The wrist is firm and in a strong position. The player is prepared to strike the ball off the front foot and the forearm is in a comfortable position—the elbow is protected with this stroke. And it won't hurt your tennis game either.

TMJ PROBLEMS

Lynn heard a cracking sound whenever she moved her mouth—and it wasn't because she was eating peanut brittle. That disturbing sound that just wouldn't go away was her first clue that she had TMJ problems. The temporomandibular joints, or TMJs, connect the lower jaw to the skull, and when they act up, the symptoms can be disconcerting, not to mention painful.

After the cracking continued for a while, the 29-year-old Pennsylvania graphic artist recalls having difficulty opening her mouth wide. That was her second sign of trouble.

Finally, something happened to make it all too obvious that her joints were not behaving as good joints should: She yawned, and—to her astonishment—her mouth locked open. Only by shoving her jaw with her hand could she get it to close. After this happened, Lynn decided it was time to seek medical attention.

She did, and now her TMJ problems are gone.

What Troubles the TMJs

What caused Lynn's TMJ disorder in the first place? No one can say for sure, but it might have been related to the car accident she was in several years earlier.

Auto injuries or blows to the face and head are among the most common causes of TMJ problems, says Joseph L. Konzelman, D.D.S., clinical director of oral health research at the Walter Reed Army Medical Center in Washington, D.C., and past president of the American Academy of Oral Medicine.

Other causes of TMJ problems may include excessive teeth clenching or an irregular bite that doesn't allow the jaw to open and close evenly.

It's often hard to pinpoint the exact cause. "There is a large number of disorders that affect the TMJs, just as there are a lot of disorders that affect all joints in the body," says Dr. Konzelman. The problems can be related to muscles, ligaments, bones, cartilage, or a combination of these, he says.

Furthermore, the symptoms vary considerably. A locked jaw, such as Lynn experienced, is rare. More commonly, the prime giveaways of TMJ problems are facial pain and restricted jaw movement.

If you have either of these signs, check with an expert. "Professional diagnosis is the key to determining what is wrong and what to do about it. Call your family dentist and ask if he can help you or refer you to someone who can," says Dr. Konzelman. TMJ disorders tend to fall more under the practice of dentistry than general medicine, he explains.

After you get a professional evaluation, what next? That depends on the nature of your specific problem, but there are a number of things that experts have found often give relief.

Dealing with the pain and discomfort often starts with changing behavior that may be causing, or at least contributing to, your condition.

TMJ PROBLEMS

Extending the neck while working at a desk or a computer is a fairly common cause of TMJ woes, says Dr. Konzelman. A chair with elbow supports should help you to keep your back straight, which will prevent you from leaning over the desk and holding your neck out. You may also find that a support pillow behind your lower back can make a difference.

As a rule of thumb, your cheekbone shouldn't extend past your collarbone, and your ears shouldn't be too far out in front of your shoulders.

Sitting for long periods in a seat where you can't cross your legs, such as on an airplane or bus, may also put your body into the kind of awkward position that spells trouble for your TMJs. What's the answer? "If you can't cross your legs, at least elevate one buttock with a small magazine," says Dr. Konzelman. This can relieve some of the pressure.

The Anti-TMJ Lifestyle

It is possible for you to have perfect posture and still be bothered by pains in the jaw. Some TMJ problems, for instance, are brought on by constant teeth clenching.

You should develop the habit of keeping your teeth slightly apart with the lips lightly touching, says Dr. Konzelman. Unfortunately, clenching sometimes occurs during sleep, when it's hard to control. (If you suspect that you're a night-clencher, turn to the chapter on bruxism on page 107.)

In some cases, TMJ problems may be related to your emotions, says Joseph Marbach, D.D.S., a clinical professor of public health and director of the Pain Research Unit at Columbia University. People with negative attitudes are more likely to suffer more TMJ problems and pain than those who have better self-esteem, he says. So he tells his TMJ patients to get lots of exercise and to work on maintaining good friendships and family relations.

Simple Preventive Measures

You also need to be aware of some common little habits that can contribute to a case of sore jaws. In *The TMJ Book*, author Andrew S. Kaplan, D.M.D., recommends that you avoid the following:

- Lying on your stomach with your head twisted to one side.
- Lying on your back with your head propped up at a sharp angle for reading or watching television.
- Cradling the telephone between your shoulder and chin.
- Propping your chin on one or both hands for extended periods.
- Reaching high overhead to do work, like painting or hammering on walls or ceilings.
- Carrying a heavy shoulder bag with a strap on the same shoulder for a long time.
- Wearing high-heeled shoes.

If, despite all precautions, you do fall victim to the pain of TMJ, you can always reach for the aspirin. Aspirin helps with both aches and inflammation.

Pain in the TMJ area can also be relieved by applying moist heat (such as a wet washcloth) to the jaws, says Dr. Konzelman. Some people find that ice works as well as or better than heat. You should experiment to see which works best for you.

Both heat and cold bring relief by increasing blood flow to the area. You can achieve the same effect by gently stretching your facial muscles and massaging the sides of your face.

Above all, remember that facial pain warrants professional attention, says Dr. Marbach. He recommends that you *always* seek a second opinion and *never* rush into irreversible forms of treatment such as braces or surgery.

Russell Wild

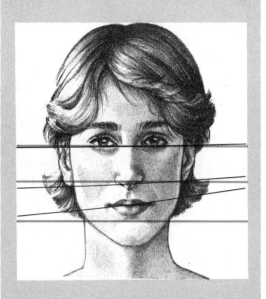

The Joint That's Behind It All

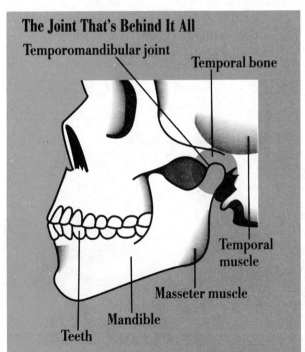

Temporomandibular joint

Temporal bone

Temporal muscle

Masseter muscle

Mandible

Teeth

TMJ is short for temporomandibular joint. TMJ problems occur when these joints and the muscles and ligaments around them are not working together correctly.

Is Your Face On Straight?

You may sometimes feel like your life is out of balance. It's when your *face* is out of balance that you have one of the primary symptoms of a TMJ problem.

We're not talking about anything as chaotic as your nose being where your right ear should be. We're talking about a subtle misalignment. That is, a good hard look in the mirror reveals a certain lopsided look.

As illustrated above, one eye may seem to be slightly higher, maybe even slightly larger than the other. The ears may not be entirely level. And the jawline may be somewhat off center.

With some work in correcting your TMJ problem, you may find that your face and other body parts will follow your jaw back into better alignment.

TMJ PROBLEMS

A Self-Test for TMJ Trouble

Can you give yourself a simple self-examination to tell if you have TMJ problems? Unfortunately, an exact diagnosis of this complicated disorder is sometimes difficult even for medical professionals. You can, however, get an idea of whether you *may* have TMJ by testing yourself in the ways illustrated on these two pages.

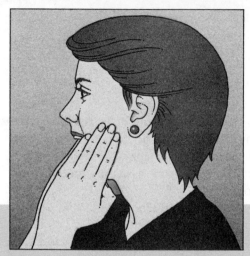

(2) Place your hands on your cheeks with your fingertips pointing toward your ears. All four fingers should rest against the lower jaw on each side, and the index finger should line up with the angle of the jaw. Now open and close your mouth. You should be able to feel the thick muscles that attach to the cheekbone. Notice whether pressing gently is painful.

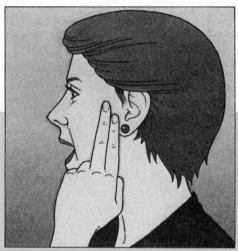

(1) If you put your fingertips directly in front of each ear, you'll be able to feel your TMJs. Open and close your mouth while pressing gently. If you feel pain on one or both sides, your joints could be inflamed. If inflammation exists, even the slightest pressure could prove painful.

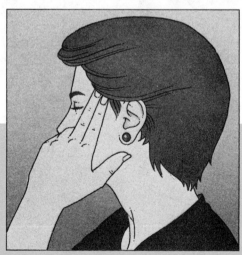

(3) Now place your fingertips on your temples. Do you feel any pain while you open and close your mouth? Pain could be a sign of fatigue or soreness in your temporalis muscles.

392

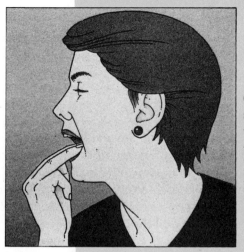

(4) It's not always easy to spot fatigue and soreness in all of the jaws' muscles. Here's a test that gets at less accessible areas. Place three fingers on the biting surfaces of your lower front teeth. Press firmly and try to close your mouth. If this slight resistance is uncomfortable, see your dentist for a professional diagnosis.

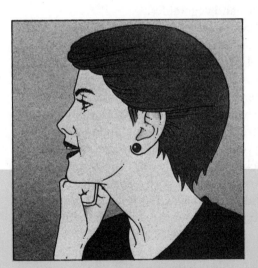

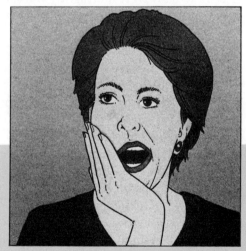

(5) Now close your mouth and place your fist under your chin. Exert a firm but gentle pressure and try to open your mouth. Here again, any discomfort is a sign of trouble and should be checked out.

(6) For your last test, place your palm on your right cheek and press against your lower jaw. Try pushing your jaw against your hand. Does it hurt? Try this on the left side now. If you experience any discomfort, you should seek an expert's advice.

393

VARICOSE VEINS

You're so veined, you probably think this chapter's about you . . . don't you? We're singing the blues, here—those blue-black, knobby veins that tattoo your legs and signal an end to miniskirts. Why do women get them four to ten times more often than men?

Pregnancy, female hormones, and hair play a part. (Well, the hair on men's legs doesn't actually *prevent* unsightly veins, but it does stop most men from ever noticing they have them.)

Pregnancy and childbirth are at fault because they can stretch the veins, damaging valves inside them.

The role of female hormones in causing varicosities isn't clearly understood. But the severity and discomfort of veins and the arrival of spider veins—those purplish threads that bloom mysteriously atop your thighs—seem directly related to menstruation, pregnancy, and taking birth control pills.

"It seems that estrogen opens tiny little channels called shunts between the arteries and the veins. This increases the flow of blood into the capillaries and veins, which puts an extra stress on them," says Luis Navarro, M.D., founder and director of The Vein Treatment Center, New York City, and author of *No More Varicose Veins.*

Another "stress" is our upright posture, which challenges the circulatory system in our legs. Aging might also contribute to the problem.

Heredity, though, is the main cause. "If your father or your mother or both had varicose veins, you are highly predisposed. Usually you will be ten times more likely to get them than someone who has no family history of varicose veins," states Dr. Navarro.

Prolonged standing, obesity, and lack of exercise worsen the condition or increase your chances of getting it. Starting an exercise program is probably one of the most important preventive measures you can take.

Avoiding constipation is also important. To promote regularity, increase your consumption of fiber-rich foods—whole grains, fruits, and vegetables.

If you have varicose veins, elevate your feet as often as possible. Prescription support stockings can help. Your doctor can tell you the weight and length of stocking you need. The pressure of support stockings varies—the heavier pressures control swelling by restricting the amount of blood entering the leg veins. Understand, though, that the stockings do not cure or "fix" anything. They can only relieve discomfort. The condition remains, but it doesn't get worse.

If possible, put the stockings on in bed, before you get up. If you can't put them on until after you shower, elevate your feet before putting them on.

To prevent the condition from worsening, it helps to maintain a trim figure and walk, walk, walk. If you are considering treatment beyond support stockings, seeing a vascular surgeon or a varicose vein specialist is a good idea. Make sure you get a second opinion before any kind of surgery.

Bejou Merry

A Pump a Day Keeps Veins at Bay

To water plants in hanging baskets, someone invented a plastic squeeze bottle with a tall, curving tube at its top. You squeeze the bottle, creating pressure that forces the water up the tube and out the spout. Likewise, your circulatory system, particularly below the knee, has to work against gravity to move blood through your veins back to your heart.

The exercises here and on page 396 are designed to strengthen the muscles of the calves, thighs, and buttocks, the main components of the lower-body muscle pump. Do them daily, in the order indicated, for the suggested number of repetitions, and you may prevent the development of more varicose veins.

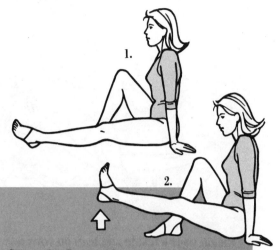

Sit on the floor and extend your legs in front of you. Support yourself with your arms. *(1)* Bend your right knee and place your right foot flat on the floor next to your left knee. Flex your left foot so that the toe points to the ceiling. *(2)* Now raise your left leg without bending the knee. Slowly lower it almost to the floor. Repeat 10 to 15 times. Do this with the right leg. Then repeat with the left leg and the right again.

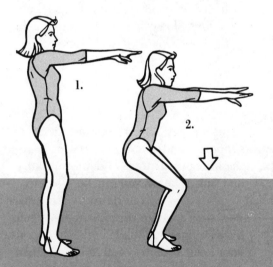

The half squat, not to be done by people with bum knees, will really get those leg veins pumping. *(1)* Stand with your feet about a foot apart, toes pointing slightly outward. Hold your arms out straight.

Throughout the exercise, keep your eyes focused on your fingertips. Bend your knees slowly, keeping your head and back straight. *(2)* Lower your body and hold for a second. Do not let your buttocks sink lower than your knees. Now slowly return to an upright position. Repeat 15 to 20 times. When this becomes easy, add more repetitions.

VARICOSE VEINS

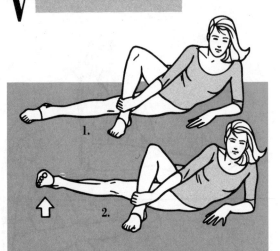

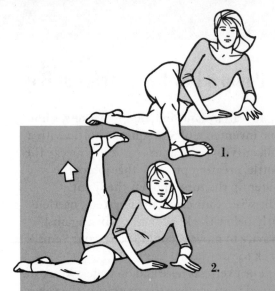

Lie on your left side and lean on your left elbow. Extend your legs and keep them straight. *(1)* Now place your right foot on the floor in front of your left knee and grasp your ankle with your right hand. *(2)* With your left foot flexed, lift your left leg toward the ceiling. You won't be able to raise it far. Lower it slightly, then raise it again. Do this 10 to 15 times.

Prop yourself on your left elbow as you lie on your left side. Both palms should be flat on the floor. *(1)* Bend your left leg for support and straighten your right leg out in front of you at a 90-degree angle from your body. *(2)* With the right foot flexed, lift your right leg toward the ceiling. Slowly lower it without touching the floor. Do this 10 to 15 times.

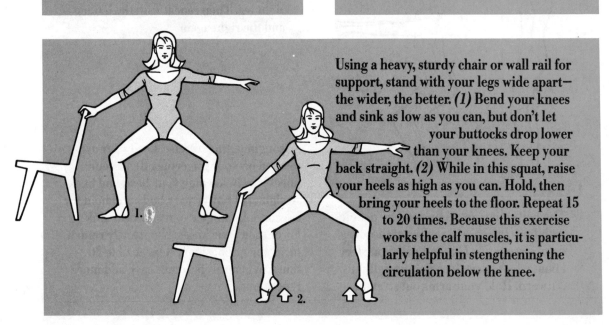

Using a heavy, sturdy chair or wall rail for support, stand with your legs wide apart— the wider, the better. *(1)* Bend your knees and sink as low as you can, but don't let your buttocks drop lower than your knees. Keep your back straight. *(2)* While in this squat, raise your heels as high as you can. Hold, then bring your heels to the floor. Repeat 15 to 20 times. Because this exercise works the calf muscles, it is particularly helpful in stengthening the circulation below the knee.

WRINKLES

Wrinkles are our souvenirs of living. Our smiles and frowns, even our so-called beauty naps, leave us with mementos in the form of fine lines, furrows, and creases on our faces.

Add natural aging, the downward pull of gravity, and sun damage, which robs the skin of the natural support tissues elastin and collagen, and it's a wonder we don't all look like Shar-Pei puppies by the time we're 40.

You are not fated to face the world with these crinkly, age-advertising banners if you are careful to take the proper precautions. And even if you do have wrinkles, there are quite a few things you can do to minimize their appearance.

Prescription for Smooth Skin

A person needs to do four things in life to stay wrinkle-free:

- Avoid the sun
- Use the best sunscreen you can get your hands on
- Use Dove soap
- Get a prescription for Retin-A

This advice comes from Joseph P. Bark, M.D., a Lexington, Kentucky, dermatologist and author of *Retin-A and Other Youth Miracles* and *Skin Secrets*. Staying out of the sun is the most important thing anyone can do to prevent wrinkles, Dr. Bark says.

The sun causes the top, dead layer of skin to thicken and become rough, scaly, dry, and less flexible. The radiation of the sun thins the first living layer of skin and destroys elastin and collagen, the delicate fibers that allow our skin to stretch and snap back.

Begin your daily routine by washing with Dove soap. Dr. Bark recommends this particular brand because "it's the mildest soap in history. It causes few irritations, even in winter."

After you wash, dab on a sunscreen in the place of your usual moisturizer or after-shave lotion.

"I recommend the highest SPF [sun protection factor] number you can get," Dr. Bark says. "A lot of people say you don't get much protection past 15, but I think the higher you go, the better. That way, if you have even a little sunscreen left after you wash or you rub your face, you are still protected. If you decide at the last minute to play golf in the afternoon, you're protected."

You can forget facials, mud packs, masks, gels, glazes, and moisturizers for correction of wrinkles, Dr. Bark says. They make the skin appear plumper and erase lines by softening the dead layer of skin, but their effect is only temporary. They don't erase wrinkles.

Save the Day with Retin-A

Only one ointment—Retin-A—really fills in wrinkles, Dr. Bark says.

Retin-A has a powerful effect on the skin, but it can cause adverse reactions. Ask your doctor whether a prescription is appropriate for you.

WRINKLES

Retin-A speeds up the natural skin repair process, thereby erasing minor sun-caused damage, and also signals the cells to produce more collagen.

The desired effects of using Retin-A may take from six to nine months, says Norman A. Brooks, M.D., a Los Angeles dermatologist. Not only that, Retin-A is not capable of erasing deep wrinkles, facial sags or laugh lines. People who use Retin-A should use it in conjunction with a moisturizer and a sunscreen with an SPF of at least 15, says Dr. Brooks.

There's no way to stop the march of time, but you can arrest the footprints it leaves on your face. Here are some other ways.

Eat Right and Get the Right Kind of Sleep

Maintain overall good nutrition, being especially sure to get the right amounts of the "skin" vitamins—vitamin A, vitamin C, and vitamin E—to help delay premature wrinkling.

Also, wake up to the fact that your beauty sleep may be adding years to your face.

"Try sleeping with the weight of your head centered over the ear area, instead of burying your face deeply into the pillow. Or, sleep on your back if you can," advises Dr. Bark.

Or get the softest goose down pillow you can, he says. A hard pillow will hold skin folds against your face, while a soft pillow may let the folds relax.

Claudia Allen

Give Yourself An Acupressure Face-lift

Can acupressure remove your wrinkles?

Acupressure, based on the ancient art of acupuncture, "calms you down, relaxes you," says David Molony, a certified acupuncturist at the Lehigh Valley Acupuncture Center in Emmaus, Pennsylvania.

"Some 60 percent of all tension shows up in your jaw. People knit their brows and the old blood can't get out, the new blood can't get in," he says. Relaxing those muscles and sending new blood to the area can slow and erase wrinkles.

One reason your skin gets wrinkly, says Harry A. Lusk, M.D., executive director of the Acupuncture Research Institute in Van Nuys, California, is because smiles, frowns, scowls, and laughs exercise the muscles under the skin and force the skin to fold and refold. Muscles become so strong, they pull the face into creases, Dr. Lusk says.

"When you have a tightening of the muscle, you have to relax it." Acupressure is the relaxation method that smoothes the creases.

"The important thing is, your skin must be squeaky clean before you start," says Dr. Lusk. "And when you are finished, let your face relax a bit more. Don't smile and spoil it."

You can use your fingertips or knuckles to follow these acupressure techniques. Massage once a day for the first 30 days and then two or three times a week after that. Spend a minute on each point and use firm pressure, but not enough to hurt. When you are finished, sit quietly for a few minutes.

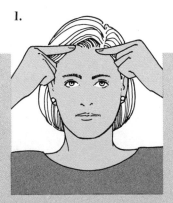

1.

Locate points at your hairline, directly above your eyes. Using steady pressure, massage these points for about 60 seconds. Try making little circles with your fingertips. Keep your forehead relaxed.

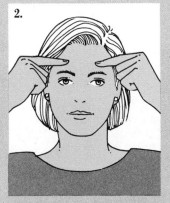

2.

Midway between the hairline and top of the eyebrow are the *Yang Bai* points. Massage them, too, for one minute, keeping your brow unfurrowed. If your fingers get tired, use your knuckles.

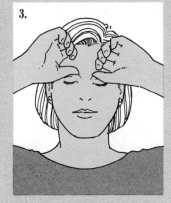

3.

Use your thumbs against the inside of your eye sockets next to your nose. Press gently but firmly against the bone, using the pads of your thumbs. Be wary of long fingernails and do not apply pressure against the eyes.

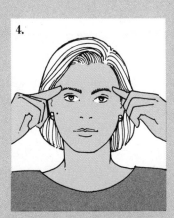

4.

Now, let's erase those unattractive crow's feet. Again, using your fingertips, press and massage the two points found at the outside ends of your eyebrows.

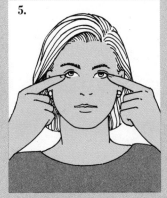

5.

To further smooth the skin around the eyes, lightly massage the acupressure points at the outer edge of the eyes. Massage gently, using firm fingertip pressure. Do not press against the eyes themselves.

(continued)

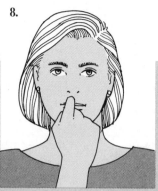

8.

If your fingers are getting tired, use your knuckles. Massage the depression found on your upper lip, just below your nose. Make tiny, soft circles.

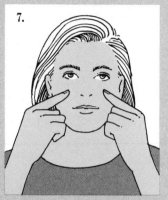

7.

To plump up any tissue that may have succumbed to gravity, find the points located immediately below your eyes and on a plane with your nostrils. Massage for one minute.

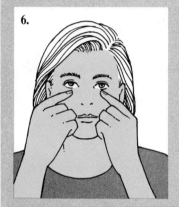

6.

Still firming the area around the eyes, feel for the dip in the cheekbone immediately below each eye. Massaging these points is said to shrink the bags under your eyes.

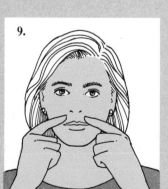

9.

To smooth out the wrinkles at the outside corners of your mouth, slide your fingers about ½ inch from the corners and massage the sensitive points in tiny circles.

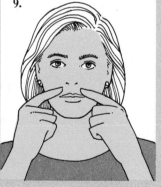

10.

If your chin is developing tiny wrinkles, take special care to massage this point properly. You'll find it halfway between your bottom lip and the tip of your chin. Make tiny circles, using pressure.

11.

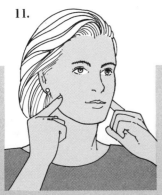

To restore the overall glow of youth, massage the large facial muscle just in front of your ears. (You can find it more easily if you open your mouth a little.)

12.

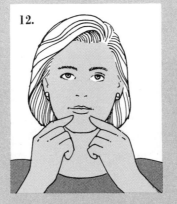

To further smooth the skin and underlying tissue of the skin, massage the spots that are found just below each corner of the mouth. Use firm pressure applied in a clockwise direction.

13.

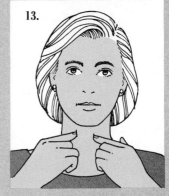

Now, go bobbing for apples. Find your own Adam's apple, that is, and massage the points on either side of the windpipe. Use gentle pressure on these points. You should feel no discomfort.

14.

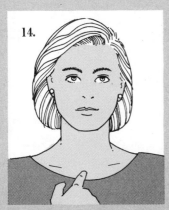

To ease the pathway of energy to your face and neck, find the acupressure point at the center of the collarbone. Using fingertip or knuckle, massage in small circles.

15.

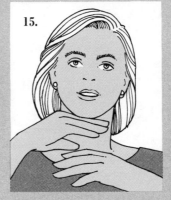

Finish your facelift with an old-fashioned, but effective, exercise that stimulates blood flow. Thrust your chin forward and, using the back of each hand, slap the underside of your chin. Repeat about 40 times, alternating hands.

INDEX

Page references in *italic* indicate illustrations.

A

Abdominal muscles, 91
Acetaminophen, carpal tunnel syndrome and, 130
Achilles tendinitis, 208, 386, 387
Achilles tendon, stretching exercise for, *182*
Acne, 102–3
Acupressure
    for arthritis, 50, *51–53*
    for bruxism, *109*
    for eyestrain, 191, *191*
    foot massage and, 197
    for headaches, *224–25*
    for sinusitis, 371, *371*
    for wrinkles, 399, *399–401*
Acupuncture, 50
Adductor muscles, stretching exercise for, *179*
Adrenaline, 286
Aerobic exercise, 173
    footwear for, 363
    high blood pressure and, 273
Aging
    exercise and, 170, 172
    fainting and, 193
    varicose veins and, 394
Air
    dry, 159
    indoor, sinusitis and, 368–69
Airplanes, ear popping on, 164
Air pollution
    cancer and, 124
    emphysema and, 168
    sinusitis and, 368
Alcohol
    cancer and, 122

    high blood pressure and, 272–73
    hops and, 257
    motion sickness and, 294
    osteoporosis and, 324
    pregnancy and, 353
    rubbing, swimmer's ear and, 163
Allergies, 2–11
    asthma and, 59
    avoidance of, 2, 4, 5–6
    cause of, 2
    in children, 2, *6*
    colic and, 146
    diet and, *6*, 6–7
    from dust and mold, *8–11*
    food, 55
    inhalant, 7
    medications for, 4–5
    shots for, 5
    sinusitis and, 368, 369
Allicin, 254
Almonds, *312*
Aloe, 246
    burns treated by, 112
Altitude changes, headaches from, 222
Amino acids, immune system and, 308
Anal cancer, 240
Anemia, iron deficiency, 196
Anger, acne from, 103
Angina, 12–15, 234
    exercise and, 15
    hardened arteries and, 13, *13*
    nighttime, *12*
    smoking and, 15
    symptoms of, *14*
Animals. *See also* Pets
    bites from, 97–98, 99, *99*

403

Atherosclerosis, 13, *13*, 14, *236*
    cholesterol and, 137, *236*
    exercise and, 15
    heart attack and, 235
    vitamin E and, 308
Athlete's foot, 62, *63*, 299
Attitude
    fatigue and, 196
    stress and, 378–79
Automobiles, back pain and, 78, *79, 81*
Avocados, *312*

B

Babesiosis, 101
Bacitracin, 151
Back
    anatomy of, 64
    functions of, 68
    preventive care of, 67
    range-of-motion exercises for, *35–36*
Back pain, 64–97
    automobiles and, 78, *79, 81*
    body movements and, 78, *79–83*
    causes of, 65
    exercise(s) and, 65, 67–68
        strength and flexibility, 91, *92–94*
        stretching, 72, *72–74*
    incidence of, 64–65
    lifting and, 75, *76–77, 79*
    massage for, 84, *85–90*
    posture and, *66–67*, 68, 70, *70–71*
    in pregnancy, 355
    sex and, 95
    sleep and, 95, *96*
    from stress, 65–67
    treatment of, 68–69
    urgent symptoms of, 69
Back tension, exercise for, *385*
Bacon, cancer and, 121–22
Bacteria
    acne from, 102–3

boils from, 105, *105*
burns and, 110, 111
in dental plaque, 216, 217
food poisoning from, 203–5, *206–7*
wound healing and, 151
Bananas, 311, *313*
Bandaging, 152, *153–54*
    of pets, *348–51*
Barley, *313*
Basis, 160
Bath
    sitz, *214*
    warm, sleepiness from, 279
Beans, flatulence from, 201, 202, *202*
Beards, 278, *278*
Bee stings, 97, *98*
Behavior, heart disease and, 232–33
Benzoyl peroxide, 103
Beta-carotene
    arthritis and, 55
    in diet, 309
Betadine, 112
Biceps, exercise for muscle cramp in, *298*
Bicycling, stationary, 176, *177*
Biofeedback
    for stress relief, 375–76
    for tension headaches, 220
Birth control pills
    headaches from, 222
    high blood pressure from, 274
Bites
    animal
        dog bite prevention, 99, *99*
        from jellyfish, 98
        from snakes, 98
        treatment of, 97–98
    insect
        from bees, wasps, and hornets, 98,
        98
        from spiders, 97
        from ticks, 100–101, *100–101*
Blackheads, *102*

411

INDEX

S

Sacrum, *325*
Safflower oil, *318*
Sage, 264
Salicyclic acid, calluses and, 119
Salmon, *318*
Salmonella, 203, 205
Salt
    dehydration and, 296–97
    high blood pressure and, 271–72
    osteoporosis and, 324
Sardines, *319*
Scalp brushing, headaches and, *223*
Sciatica, 65
Scopolamine, 294
Scrapes and cuts. *See* Cuts and scrapes
Sebum, *102*
Selenium
    cancer and, 121
    immune system and, 308, 309
Septum, deviated, 307
Serotonin, 220
Sex, back pain and, 95
Shinsplints, 362–66
    causes of, 362–63, *363*
    exercise(s) to avoid, 364, *364–65*
Shock, from burns, 112
Shoes
    calluses from, 119
    corns and, 148, *148,* 149, *149, 150*
    footaches and, 208
    proper fit of, *149*
    for running and aerobic exercise, 363
Shoulder blades, stretching exercise for, *183*
Shoulder pain, 301–5
    causes of, 301
    exercises for, 301, 302, *302–3*
    massage for, 304, *304–5*
    treatment of, 301
Shoulders
    range-of-motion exercises for, *31–32*
    stretching exercise for, *178*

tendinitis of, 386, *387*
    tension-relieving exercises for, *198–99*
Shoulder tension
    in bruxism, exercise for, *109*
    exercise for, *385*
Side stitches, 367, *367*
Sinuses, *370*
Sinusitis, 368–71
    acupressure for, 371, *371*
    gravity and, *369*
    prevention of, 368–69
    treatment of, 369
Sitting, back pain and, 72
Sitz bath, *241*
Skeleton, 322, *325, 326*
Skim milk, *319*
Skin, aloe and, 246
Skin cancer, 122–23
Skin moisturizers, 160
Skin problems
    allergy, 5–6, 7
    blemishes, 102–3
    blisters, 104
    boils, 105
    bruises, 106
    burns, 110–17
    calluses, 119
    corns, 148–50
    cuts and scrapes, 151–56
    dry skin, 159–60, *160–61*
    frostbite, 213–15
    rashes, from tick bites, 100, 101, *101*
    witch hazel and, 267
    wrinkles, 159, 397–401
Sleep
    arthritis and, 48, *48–49*
    back pain and, 95, *96*
    hops and, 257
    insomnia, 195, 197, 228, 279–80, *281*
    requirement for, 279
    valerian and, 266
    wrinkles and, 398